A.M. MEDICAL DIAGNOSTICS
10 SWISS HEIGHT DRIVE
OSHAWA, ONTARIO L1H 7K5
723-8477

NONINVASIVE
DIAGNOSIS OF
VASCULAR DISEASE

NONINVASIVE
DIAGNOSIS OF
VASCULAR DISEASE

Falls B. Hershey, MD
Associate Professor of Surgery, Washington University School of
Medicine; Director of Vascular Surgery and Director, Blood Flow
Laboratory, St. John's Mercy Medical Center, St. Louis, Missouri

Robert W. Barnes, MD
Professor and Chairman, Department of Surgery, University of
Arkansas for Medical Sciences, Little Rock, Arkansas

David S. Sumner, MD
Professor of Surgery and Chief, Section of Peripheral Vascular
Surgery, Southern Illinois University School of Medicine, Springfield,
Illinois

Editors

Appleton Davies, Inc.
Publishers in Medicine and Surgery
Pasadena, California

Copyright © 1984 Appleton Davies, Inc.

Publishers in Medicine and Surgery
32 South Raymond Avenue
Pasadena, CA 91105

Design and Production by Graphics Two, Los Angeles, CA
Printed and bound in the United States of America by Kingsport Press, Kingsport, TN

Library of Congress Cataloging in Publication Data

Main entry under title:

Noninvasive diagnosis of vascular disease.

Includes bibliographical references and index.
1. Diagnosis, Noninvasive. 2. Blood-vessels—Diseases—Diagnosis. I. Hershey, Falls B.
II. Barnes, Robert W., 1936-   . III.Sumner, David S. [DNLM:
1. Vascular diseases—Diagnosis. 2. Plethysmography. 3. Ultrasonics—Diagnostic use.
4. Angiography. WG 500
N8125]
RC691.6.N65N65 1984   616.1'30754   83-22310
ISBN 0-941022-01-3

CONTENTS

Contents

Contents

viii

Contents

Contents

BOARD OF ADVISORY EDITORS

LIST OF
CONTRIBUTORS

Arthur I. Auer, MD
Attending Surgeon, Vascular Surgery, St. John's Mercy Medical
Center, St. Louis, Missouri

Robert W. Barnes, MD
Professor and Chairman, Department of Surgery, University of
Arkansas for Medical Sciences, Little Rock, Arkansas

John J. Bergan, MD
Magerstadt Professor of Surgery, Northwestern University Medical
School; Chief, Division of Vascular Surgery, Northwestern Memorial
Hospital, Chicago, Illinois

H. Bradley Binnington, MD
Attending Surgeon, Vascular Surgery, St. John's Mercy Medical
Center, St. Louis, Missouri

Donna R. Blackburn, RN
Assistant Director, Blood Flow Laboratory, Northwestern Memorial
Hospital, Chicago, Illinois

Dennistoun K. Brown, MD
Research Technologist, Blood Flow Laboratory, St. John's Mercy
Medical Center, St. Louis, Missouri

John T. Collins, MS
Clinical Engineer, Northwestern Memorial Hospital, Chicago, Illinois

Donna G. Cox, RN
Clinical Education Coordinator, MedaSonics, Inc. Mountain View,
California

Valerie Crain, RN
Assistant Director, Ocular Pulse and Vascular Laboratory, Tucson
Medical Center, Tucson, Arizona

John J. Cranley, MD
Associate Clinical Professor of Surgery, University of Cincinnati
College of Medicine; Director of Surgery and Director of the Kachel-
macher Memorial Laboratory for Venous Diseases, Good Samaritan
Hospital, Cincinnati, Ohio

William K. Ehrenfeld, MD
Professor of Surgery and Co-Chief, Vascular Division, University of
California, San Francisco, School of Medicine, San Francisco,
California

Falls B. Hershey, MD
Associate Professor of Surgery, Washington University School of
Medicine; Director of Vascular Surgery and Director, Blood Flow
Laboratory, St. John's Mercy Medical Center, St. Louis, Missouri

Joseph J. Hurley, MD
Attending Surgeon, Vascular Surgery, St. John's Mercy Medical
Center, St. Louis, Missouri

Mark M. Kartchner, MD
Medical Director, Ocular Pulse and Vascular Laboratory, Tucson
Medical Center, Tucson, Arizona

Yves E. Langlois, MD
Senior Research Fellow, Department of Surgery, University of
Washington School of Medicine, Seattle, Washington

Robert J. Lusby, MD
Professor of Surgery, University of Sydney, Sydney, Australia; Research Fellow, Concord Hospital, Concord, Australia

Lorin P. McRae, PhD
Technical Director, Ocular Pulse and Vascular Laboratory, Tucson
Medical Center, Tucson, Arizona

Phyllis B. Marszalek, RN
Clinical Research Center, Department of Surgery, Medical College of
Virginia, Virginia Commonwealth University, Richmond, Virginia

John Middleton, MD
Research Assistant, Peripheral Vascular Laboratory, Department of
Surgery, Medical College of Virginia, Virginia Commonwealth Uni-
versity, Richmond, Virginia

Richard D. Miles, PhD
Assistant Professor of Bioengineering, Southern Illinois University School of Medicine, St. John's Hospital, Springfield, Illinois

Terry N. Needham, SRMLSO, MIST
Supervisor, Vascular Laboratory, Saint Anthony Hospital,Columbus, Ohio

M. Lee Nix, RN
Chief Nurse Technologist, Peripheral Vascular Laboratory, Department of Surgery, Medical College of Virginia, Virginia Commonwealth University, Richmond, Virginia

Richard A. J. O'Connor, MD
Associate Professor of Surgery, McGill University Faculty of Medicine; Director, Noninvasive Vascular Laboratory, The Sir Mortimer B. Davis–Jewish General Hospital, Montreal, Quebec, Canada

Linda K. Peterson, RN
Nurse Clinician, Blood Flow Laboratory, Northwestern Memorial Hospital, Chicago, Illinois

William W. Putney, PhD
Bioengineer, Noninvasive Peripheral Vascular Laboratory, McGuire Veterans Administration Medical Center, Richmond, Virginia

Stanley E. Rittgers, PhD
Research Bioengineer, Surgical Service, McGuire Veterans Administration Medical Center, Richmond, Virginia

Ghislaine O. Roederer, MD
Senior Research Fellow, Department of Surgery, University of Washington School of Medicine, Seattle, Washington

James B. Russell, BS
Technologist, Peripheral Vascular Research Laboratory, St. John's Hospital, Springfield, Illinois

Earlene Slaymaker, RN
Vascular Specialist, Peripheral Vascular Laboratory, Veterans Adminstration Medical Center, Iowa City, Iowa

Ronald J. Stoney, MD
Professor of Surgery and Co-Chief, Vascular Division, University of California, San Francisco, School of Medicine, San Francisco, California

D. Eugene Strandness, Jr., MD
Professor of Surgery, University of Washington School of Medicine, Seattle, Washington

David S. Sumner, MD
Professor of Surgery and Chief, Section of Peripheral Vascular Surgery, Southern Illinois University School of Medicine, Springfield, Illinois

D. Glenn Turley, BS
Laboratory Technologist, Peripheral Vascular Laboratory, Department of Surgery, Medical College of Virginia, Virginia Commonwealth University, Richmond, Virginia

James S.T. Yao, MD, PhD
Professor of Surgery, Northwestern University Medical School; Director, Blood Flow Laboratory, Northwestern Memorial Hospital, Chicago, Illinois

PREFACE

This is a practical book written by leaders working in busy laboratories with modern, proven methods. It has been written for those surgeons, physicians, technologists, and nurses who are either new to this growing field or actively involved in running a vascular laboratory. Now that ARDMS certification of vascular technologists and board certification of vascular surgeons are realities, we hope this book will be especially valuable.

Each of the three main parts of the book (i.e., those focusing on the arterial, venous, and cerebrovascular systems) opens with a lucid, practical explanation of anatomy, hemodynamics, pathophysiology, and pathology—the basic background information essential to an understanding of noninvasive diagnostic methodology. Clinically pertinent explanations of the Doppler principle provide the additional information necessary to understand ultrasonic diagnostic technology. Chapter 16 contains a brief outline of Doppler physics, for instance, Chapter 21 offers a detailed account of Doppler physics, and Chapter 23 defines the physical phenomena (e.g., propagation velocity, axial resolution, lateral resolution, etc.) associated with the clinical application of Doppler technology.

Each section proceeds from these essentials to the extremely important matters of selecting, applying, and interpreting the results of particular diagnostic modalities. These chapters form the heart of every section, and it is here that the reader finds invaluable information about clinical techniques, diagnostic pitfalls, special problems of interpretation, diagnostic criteria, relative accuracy, and the importance of the clinical situation.

Finally, discussions of clinically relevant research have been included in each of these sections. The book ends with Part IV, *Associated Technological Considerations,* which provides a practical look into the future of Doppler instrumentation and the present applications of microcomputer technology in the laboratory. Pulsed Dopplers, focused-beam transducers, volume flowmeters, duplex scanners, and the administrative and scientific applications of mini- and microcomputers are some of the subjects of this concluding section.

The Appendix offers the reader the opportunity to test his or her knowledge of the topics covered in this book. Each question is keyed to a particular chapter so that the reader can review specific issues and subjects as conveniently as possible. Although we designed this feature as a posttest, one might benefit just as well by using it as a pretest.

Falls B. Hershey, MD
Robert W. Barnes, MD
David S. Sumner, MD

ACKNOWLEDGMENTS

We are grateful to many people: to the authors for their timely manuscripts and their careful attention to detail, which made the editors' job an easier one; to Mrs. Linda Mostow, who gave us all many gracious reminders while preparing the manuscripts for the publisher; to four people who contributed toward the expense of developing this book for publication, D.E. "Gene" Hokanson of D.E. Hokanson, Inc., Chester A. Smith of Electro-Diagnostic Instruments, John Wells of Zira International, and Clair Smith of Cardiovascular Electronics; and to Appleton Davies, Inc., whose editorial staff and managerial talents produced this attractive book.

Part I

Noninvasive Diagnosis of Arterial Occlusive Disease

CHAPTER 1

PATHOPHYSIOLOGY OF ARTERIAL OCCLUSIVE DISEASE

David S. Sumner

The sole function of the peripheral arterial system is to transport oxygen, nutrients, hormones, enzymes, antibodies, platelets, leukocytes, medications, and other chemical substances to the various tissues of the body. Although arterial disease may look severe on the angiogram, symptoms and signs of arterial insufficiency never appear until this essential function is impaired. Because stress (such as exercise, infection, surgical wounds, and trauma) imposes additional demands on the circulation, a level of perfusion that is sufficient under ordinary resting conditions may not be adequate to permit normal muscular function or normal healing to occur.

BASIC HEMODYNAMICS

To move blood from one point to another in the arterial system requires an energy gradient (Figure 1-1). Left ventricular contraction supplies the energy in the form of blood pressure (potential energy) and blood flow (kinetic energy). As blood moves toward the periphery, energy is dissipated, largely in the form of heat. These energy losses are caused by the viscosity of blood and by its inertia.

Viscosity is a manifestation of intermolecular friction and the friction between the formed elements of the blood. Poiseuille's law summarizes

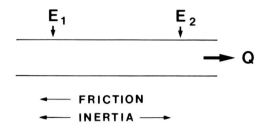

Figure 1-1. An energy gradient (E_1 − E_2) is required to cause flow between any two points in the arterial tree. Flow is impeded by friction and inertia. Inertia also tends to maintain flow.

the relationship among the pressure gradient across an arterial segment (ΔP), its length (L), its radius (r), the quantity of flow (Q), and the viscosity of blood (η):

$$P = Q \ \frac{8 \, L\eta}{\pi r^4}$$

Inertial losses occur when flow accelerates or decelerates—as in pulsatile flow—and when it changes direction. In other words, additional energy must be supplied when the artery bends, branches, narrows, or expands. Inertial losses are proportional to the velocity of blood (v) and to its density (ϱ):

$$P = k \ \tfrac{1}{2} \varrho \ v^2$$

Because the velocity of blood flow is inversely proportional to the cross-sectional area of the vessel and the square of its radius, a 50% reduction in arterial diameter would increase the inertial losses not by a factor of 2, but by a factor of 16! Similarly, from Poiseuille's law (Formula 1-1), we find that a 50% reduction in arterial diameter would also increase energy losses by a factor of 16.

Figure 1-2 illustrates the relationship between pressure and flow in a segment of a normal canine femoral artery. The experimental values show that the amount of energy (pressure drop) required to move a given amount of blood is actually much greater than that predicted by Poiseuille's law (dashed line). The solid line that best fits the observed data has a squared term for flow, indicating that inertial losses and viscosity are of equal importance in determining energy requirements. In fact, as the velocity increases, the values deviate more and more from Poiseuille's law. These intertial losses are related to the pulsatility of the blood.

3

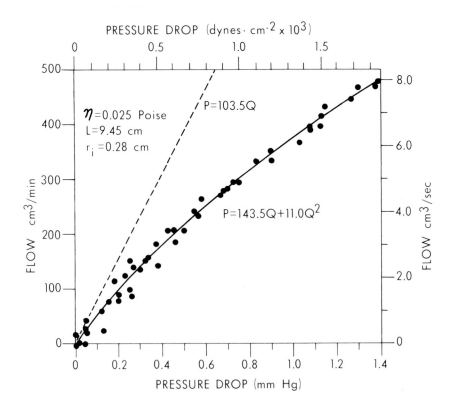

Figure 1-2. Relationship between pressure and flow in a canine femoral artery. Reprinted by permission from Sumner DS: The hemodynamics and pathophysiology of arterial disease. In *Vascular Surgery.* Edited by RB Rutherford. Philadelphia, WB Saunders, 1977.

EFFECT OF ARTERIAL STENOSIS

The common arterial diseases cause stenoses and occlusions. When blood is pushed through a stenosis, several significant hemodynamic effects occur. As the blood goes from a larger tube into a smaller tube (stenosis), it accelerates, causing increased viscous losses (Figure 1-3). But more important, when the blood enters the stenosis, it must change directions as the flow stream narrows; when it leaves the stenosis, it must change directions again as the flow stream expands. Moreover, eddy currents, turbulence, and other disturbances occur at the entrance and exit, all of which create additional inertial losses. When we look at the total energy loss produced by the stenosis—that is, the sum of the potential and ki-

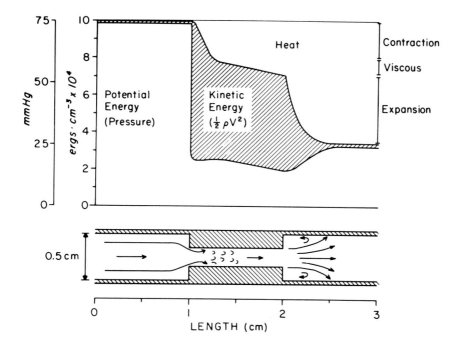

Figure 1-3. Energy losses experienced by blood passing through a stenosis. Reprinted with permission from Sumner DS: The hemodynamics and pathophysiology of arterial disease. In *Vascular Surgery.* Edited by RB Rutherford. Philadelphia, WB Saunders, 1977.

netic energy losses—we see that most of the loss can be attributed to contraction and expansion and relatively little to viscous effects. Thus, the pressure drop across a stenosis is always much greater than Poiseuille's law would predict.

How do these losses affect blood flow across an isolated stenosis? Because both viscous and inertial energy losses are inversely proportional to the fourth power of the radius, there is little change in the pressure gradient across or in the flow through a stenosis until the cross-sectional area of the artery is reduced by about 75% (Figure 1-4). This corresponds to a 50% reduction in arterial diameter when the stenosis is symmetrical. Although increasing the velocity of flow by decreasing the peripheral resistance shifts the curves in Figure 1-4 to the left, the break point continues to occur at about the same degree of narrowing. These observations help us to evaluate the physiologic significance of lesions seen on an arteriogram. A stenosis is likely to be "critical" or "hemodynamically significant" when it appears to narrow the arterial diameter by 50%.

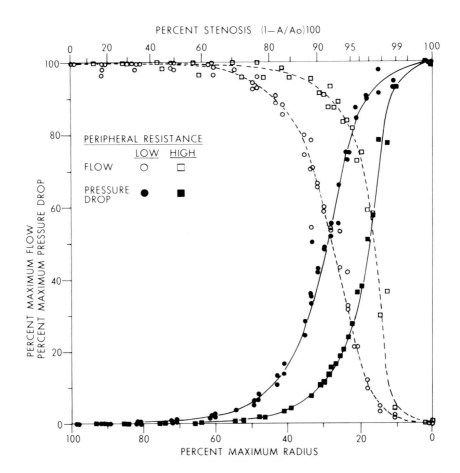

Figure 1-4. Effect of increasing stenosis on pressure and flow through a canine femoral artery. Reprinted with permission from Sumner DS: The hemodynamics and pathophysiology of arterial disease. In *Vascular Surgery*. Edited by RB Rutherford. Philadelphia, WB Saunders, 1977.

Nevertheless, arterial stenoses rarely, if ever, exist in isolation. As the arterial lumen becomes more restricted, the body compensates by developing collateral circulation around the stenosis (Figure 1-5). As in an electrical circuit, resistances in series are additive, while the total resistance offered by two or more vessels in parallel is always less than that of the vessel with the least resistance. Thus, the "segmental" resistance (R_{seg}) offered by the collaterals (R_c) and the stenotic or occluded vessel (R_s) is less than one would expect if all the flow destined for the periphery (Q_t) were forced to traverse the affected artery. Nevertheless, even when the

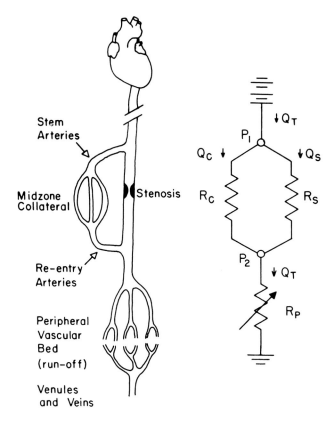

Figure 1-5. Arterial circuit containing a stenosis in a major artery and an electrical analogue of this circuit. Collateral resistance (R_c) and resistance imposed by the stenosis (R_s) are in parallel and constitute a "fixed" segmental resistance (R_{seg}). Segmental resistance is in series with the peripheral arteriolar resistance (R_p), which is "variable." Reprinted with permission from Sumner DS: The hemodynamics and pathophysiology of arterial disease. In *Vascular Surgery*. Edited by RB Rutherford. Philadelphia, WB Saunders, 1977.

collaterals are well developed, the segmental resistance is usually much higher than that of the artery in its undiseased state. For example, it would take 246 collaterals with diameters of 2.5 mm or 10,000 collaterals with diameters of 1.0 mm to reduce the segmental resistance to that of a major vessel with a diameter of 10 mm.

Because segmental resistance is always increased in cases of arterial obstruction, adequate flow to the tissues depends mainly on the ability of the peripheral arterioles to dilate. The peripheral resistance (R_p) imposed by these microvascular components of the circulation is "in series" with the segmental resistance (R_{seg}); therefore, the total resistance of the arterial circuit is the sum of the two resistances (Figure 1-5). As long as the peripheral arterioles retain the ability to dilate, the tissues will be adequately supplied with blood.

Resistance is merely a convenient term for describing the ratio of the pressure gradient across an arterial segment to the flow through the segment. It is not a fixed value. Even when the arterial stenosis itself remains unchanged, resistance increases as the flow through the stenosis increases (Figure 1-2). If the proximal pressure is labeled P_1 and the distal P_2, the following formulas can be developed:

$$R_{seg} = \frac{P_1 - P_2}{Q}$$

$$P_2 = P_1 - (Q \times R_{seg})$$

The latter formula (1-4) is very important in the noninvasive evaluation of arterial function. It reveals that the pressure distal to a stenosis falls as segmental resistance rises, provided that the flow through the segment remains constant. This fact is the basis for our use of resting ankle pressures to diagnose the presence of hemodynamically significant disease and for our use of segmental pressures to localize the site or sites of obstruction. It also explains why increasing the flow through a stenotic segment causes the ankle pressure to fall. Again, this is the basis for our use of pressures following either exercise or reactive hyperemia to evaluate the functional impairment caused by an arterial stenosis.

EFFECT OF EXERCISE

Hydraulic models can be used to illustrate the effect of arterial stenosis on pressure-flow patterns in the human leg at rest and during exercise (Figure 1-6). Under normal circumstances, the resistance of the main supplying artery (i.e., the segmental resistance) is quite low. In the diagram, this is indicated by the fact that the screw clamp is wide open. The resistance of the arterioles is high at rest, as indicated by the faucet which is almost shut off. The normal flow to the leg is 300 cm³/min. During exercise, the arterioles dilate in response to the production of metabolic products, and blood flow increases five times to 1500 cm³/min. Despite the marked increase in flow through the low-resistance arterial segment, the distal pressure falls only 4 mmHg.

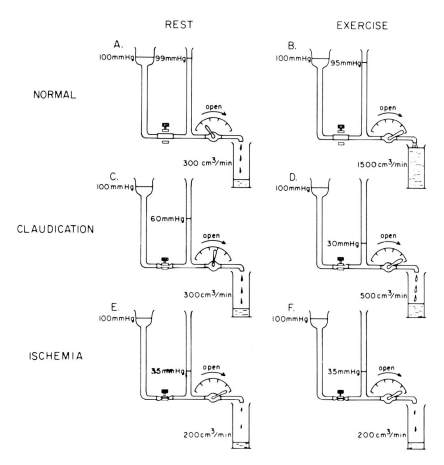

REST   EXERCISE

A.   B.

NORMAL

CLAUDICATION

ISCHEMIA

Figure 1-6. Hydraulic models of an arterial circuit with varying degrees of stenosis in the main supplying artery (screw clamp). Faucet represents the resistance imposed by the peripheral arteriolar bed. Reprinted with permission from Sumner DS: The hemodynamics and pathophysiology of arterial disease. In *Vascular Surgery*. Edited by RB Rutherford. Philadelphia, WB Saunders, 1977.

When the patient has no symptoms at rest but suffers from claudication, the segmental resistance is increased, as indicated by the partially closed screw clamp. Because the arterioles have partially dilated to compensate for the increased proximal resistance, resting flow remains unchanged at 300 cm³/min. But because the same amount of flow is now passing through increased segmental resistance, the resting peripheral pressure is only 60 mmHg and a gradient of 40 mmHg exists across the stenotic segment.

With exercise, the arterioles dilate completely (faucet completely open) in an effort to achieve maximal flow. Since the total resistance of the circuit is increased, the flow rate rises only to 500 cm³/min, which is inadequate to supply the nutritional needs of the exercising muscle. As a result, the patient experiences claudication. Because of the increased blood flow across the stenosis, the distal pressure falls 30 mmHg.

In patients with ischemia at rest, the segmental resistance is quite high (screw clamp almost closed) and the peripheral arterioles are maximally dilated (faucet completely open); yet the total blood flow is reduced to 200 cm³/min, and the patient experiences pain at rest. Despite the decreased flow, the segmental resistance is so high that the peripheral pressure is reduced to 35 mmHg. Because the peripheral arterioles are already maximally dilated at rest, a further increase in flow is not possible with exercise.

Table 1-1 lists the blood flow in human gastrocnemius muscles measured by the xenon clearance method. At rest, the blood flow in normal extremities and in limbs with arterial obstruction does not differ appreciably, but during exercise the blood flow in normal limbs is three to five times higher than that in limbs with arterial obstruction. Under resting conditions, the ankle/arm pressure index exceeds 1.0 in normal individuals (Table 1-1). In limbs with arterial obstruction, however, the resting ankle/arm pressure index is decreased even though blood flow is normal, and with exercise the index drops even further in response to the increased flow through the stenotic segment or segments. Limbs with multiple levels of obstruction (e.g., iliac and superficial femoral)

Table 1-1. Blood Flow and Blood Pressure in Normal Legs and in Legs with Arterial Obstruction, at Rest and during Exercise[a]

Location of Obstruction	Ankle Pressure Index		Muscle Blood Flow (ml/100 g min)	
	Resting	Postexercise	Resting	During Exercise
No obstruction	1.09 ± 0.09[b]	1.10 ± 0.09	4.1 ± 2.0	36.6 ± 11.4
Superficial femoral	0.70 ± 0.13	0.33 ± 0.21	2.0 ± 1.3	11.6 ± 7.6
Aortoiliac	0.66 ± 0.19	0.24 ± 0.19	1.5 ± 1.3	9.7 ± 5.7
Multilevel	0.54 ± 0.18	0.20 ± 0.23	2.3 ± 2.3	7.1 ± 12.8

[a] Data from Wolf EA Jr, Sumner DS, Strandness DE Jr: Correlation between nutritive blood flow and pressure in limbs of patients with intermittent claudication. Surg Forum 23: 238–239, 1972.
[b] ± One standard deviation.

have the lowest resting and postexercise ankle/arm pressure index and show the least increase in gastrocnemius blood flow. These observations are all well explained by both Formula 1-4 and the hydraulic models.

During exercise a flow debt develops, which is repaid after exercise by a period of increased flow, the so-called postexercise hyperemia. Normally, hyperemia decreases rapidly and flow returns to preexercise levels within a few minutes (Figure 1-7). In limbs with arterial obstruction, however, the peak blood flow is less and the hyperemic period is pro-

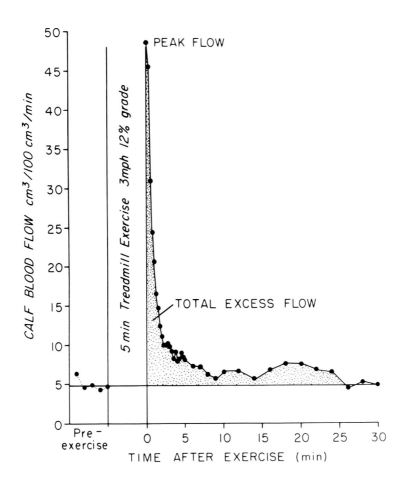

Figure 1-7. Postexercise hyperemia in a normal human calf. Reprinted with permission from Strandness DE Jr and Sumner DS: *Hemodynamics for Surgeons*. New York, Grune & Stratton, 1975.

longed, often for more than 20 minutes (Figure 1-8). This occurs because the claudicating muscles build up a greater flow debt during exercise and because the inflow following exercise is restricted by the stenotic or occlusive disease. Again, Formula 1-4 explains why the ankle pressure is depressed following exercise and why it requires several minutes to return to preexercise levels (Figure 1-8). As the flow rate decreases, the pressure drop across the stenotic or obstructed segment decreases and the ankle pressure rises.

A more complex situation exists when there are multiple levels of arterial obstruction. Figure 1-9 shows the pre- and postexercise pressure-flow data in a patient with stenosis of the iliac artery and occlusion of the superficial femoral artery. During exercise, the arterioles in both the thigh and calf muscles dilate. Because of their more proximal posi-

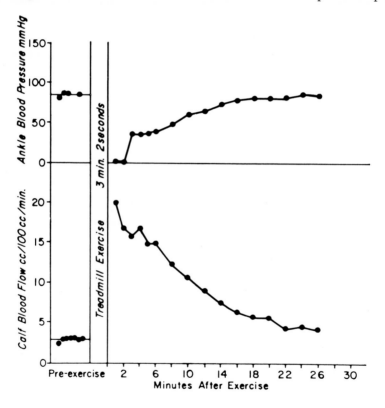

Figure 1-8. Ankle blood pressure and calf blood flow before and after exercise in a limb with superficial femoral arterial stenosis. Reprinted with permission from Sumner DS and Strandness DE Jr: The relationship between calf blood flow and ankle blood pressure in patients with intermittent claudication. Surgery 65: 763–771, 1969.

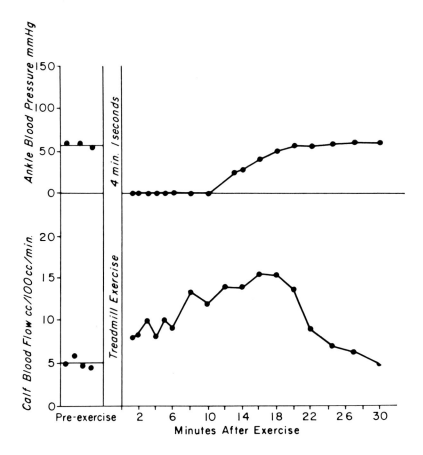

Figure 1-9. Ankle blood pressure and calf blood flow before and after exercise in a limb with stenosis of the iliac artery and occlusion of the superficial femoral artery. Reprinted with permission from Sumner DS and Strandness DE Jr: The relationship between calf blood flow and ankle blood pressure in patients with intermittent claudication. Surgery 65: 763–771, 1969.

tion, blood is diverted into the thigh muscles at the expense of the calf muscles. The increased flow through the iliac stenosis reduces the femoral artery pressure to such an extent that there is little pressure left to perfuse the calf muscles. After exercise, calf blood flow is initially low but begins to rise as the postexercise hyperemia in the thigh muscles subsides. The ankle pressure is unrecordable for many minutes and rises only after blood begins to return to the calf; the hyperemia in the calf finally decreases when the flow debt incurred by the calf has been repaid.

The physiologic significance of multilevel disease is therefore much greater than that of single-level disease, not only because of the increased resistance imposed by two or more stenoses in series, but also because the proximal muscles steal blood from those more peripherally located.

THERAPY

The treatment of arterial obstructive disease should be directed toward correcting the physiologic defects discussed above. Segmental resistance must be reduced by removing or by bypassing the obstruction. Therapeutic measures designed to increase arteriolar dilation, on the other hand, have no theoretically valid rationale (Figure 1-10). Although sympathectomy or vasodilating drugs will decrease the resting peripheral

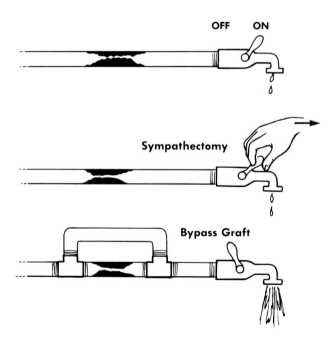

Figure 1-10. Diagram contrasting the effects of sympathectomy and arterial bypass on blood flow through an arterial circuit containing a hemodynamically significant stenosis.

resistance in claudicants and increase resting blood flow (which is unnecessary), they cannot increase blood flow during exercise because the arteriolar bed is already maximally dilated by the metabolic products of the exercising muscle. Similarly, in limbs with ischemia at rest, the arterioles are already maximally dilated and further vasodilation is rarely possible.

BIBLIOGRAPHY

1. Shepherd JT: *Physiology of the Circulation in Human Limbs in Health and Disease.* Phildephia, WB Saunders, 1963.
2. Strandness DE Jr, Sumner DS: *Hemodynamics for Surgeons.* New York, Grune & Stratton, 1975.
3. Sumner DS: The hemodynamics and pathophysiology of arterial disease. In *Vascular Surgery.* Edited by RB Rutherford. Philadelphia, WB Saunders, 1977, chapter 4.
4. Sumner DS, Strandness DE Jr: The relationship between calf blood flow and ankle blood pressure in patients with intermittent claudication. Surgery 65: 763–771, 1969.
5. Wolf EA Jr, Sumner DS, Strandness DE Jr: Correlation between nutritive blood flow and pressure in limbs of patients with intermittent claudication. Surg Forum 23: 238–239, 1972.

CHAPTER 2

SEGMENTAL LIMB PRESSURES, DOPPLER WAVEFORMS, AND STRESS TESTING

H. Bradley Binnington

The measurement of segmental limb blood pressures both at rest and after exercise or reactive hyperemia, together with the evaluation of Doppler arterial waveforms, are well-established functions of the vascular laboratory. The primary function of the laboratory is to gather—noninvasively—objective physiologic data on individuals with symptoms of peripheral arteriosclerosis. It is also possible to detect arterial stenosis and occlusion with reasonable accuracy in the vascular laboratory, and it is here that patients can be objectively evaluated following reconstructive surgery (see Chapter 5).

Several studies have demonstrated that there is a critical level of arterial stenosis that reduces flow at rest. This level ranges from 70% to 90% of the cross-sectional area of the vessel lumen, depending on the diameter of the artery; the larger the vessel, the greater the stenosis must be to decrease flow. When narrowing increases beyond the critical level, pressure drops rapidly and markedly. Because several investigators have shown that pressure changes across stenotic lesions correlate well with decreased blood flow through that stenosis, and because pressure measurements are easier to measure than flow, these measurements are used in the clinical vascular laboratory to determine flow.

Measurements taken at rest may not, on the other hand, be sufficient to detect significant stenosis, and this fact explains the practical importance of stress testing. The stenosis required to decrease pressure and flow is less at higher rates of flow. Because exercise or reactive hyperemia normally increases the flow of blood to a limb, stress testing offers a solution to the problem of diagnosing stenosis that has not reached the critical level. A mild arterial stenosis, insufficient to lower pressure at rest, may well be detected with exercise or reactive hyperemia.

THE DOPPLER WAVEFORM

The Doppler waveform is a graphic representation of the way blood is flowing through an artery. In the peripheral artery of a normal limb, there is a rapid forward flow of blood at the onset of systole, followed by slowing and then a small amount of reverse flow during early diastole. The picture created by the Doppler waveform tracing reflects this. There is a rapid upstroke, a sharp peak, a rapid downstroke (which may be slightly bowed toward the baseline), and a short peak below the baseline representing reverse flow (Figure 2-1).

R Arm 144

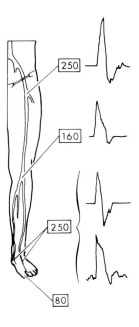

Figure 2-1. Normal waveforms in open arteries; pressures elevated falsely because of calcification of the arterial wall.

Distal to a critical arterial stenosis or occlusion, systolic flow cannot increase rapidly with systole, nor can it decrease as rapidly; rather, flow is more continuous than normal. Diastolic reversal is eliminated, and the Doppler waveform reveals this alteration. The upstroke is slower, the peak is rounded, and the slower downstroke often is bowed away from the baseline. There is no tracing below the baseline (Figure 2-2). The more severe the disease proximal to the vessel being examined and the less adequate the collateral circulation, the more dramatic the waveform changes. A flat Doppler tracing indicates a lack of flow in the vessel.

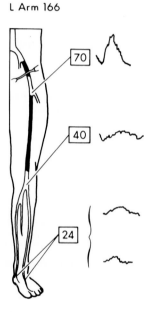

L Arm 166

Figure 2-2. Tandem occlusions with progressively abnormal waveforms. Severe pressure drops.

TECHNIQUES

Our laboratory uses standard 12-cm-wide blood pressure cuffs to measure pressure at high and low thigh levels and at the proximal calf and ankle. Two-centimeter cuffs can be used on digits. Our experience indicates that oversized or tapered cuffs for thigh measurements are troublesome to use and, contrary to the reports of others, no more accurate than those of conventional size.

Measurements are taken in the supine position, using a bidirectional Doppler (capable of showing diastolic reversal), with an 8-MHz probe over the loudest signal. In the event that foot or ankle flow is difficult to detect, the examiner listens over the popliteal artery for thigh pressure measurements. Bernstein et al. have presented data showing that the sensing site affects high-thigh pressure measurements.[2] Measurements of low pressures in the upper thigh sensed by toe or ankle signals should be repeated by placing the probe over the popliteal artery, as suggested; otherwise, the low high-thigh pressure may wrongly imply inflow stenosis. It also is important to measure both arm pressures, as one subclavian artery may be stenotic.

Results are expressed as absolute pressures and as the ankle brachial index (highest ankle pressure/highest systolic brachial pressure). The pressure measured is that of the artery underlying the cuff, not that of the vessel over which the Doppler probe is placed. Waveforms, on the other hand, are from the artery directly under the probe.

For stress testing we use a small treadmill set at a 10% grade and at a speed of 1.5 miles per hour. After the segmental blood pressures have been measured at rest, the patient, with ankle cuffs in place, walks for five minutes or until symptoms occur. Exercise is stopped and a note made if dyspnea, chest pain, or tachycardia occur. (With these precautions we find it unnecessary to monitor ECGs.) The patient lies down and ankle and arm pressures are measured immediately. Repeat pressures are obtained 1, 2.5, and 5 minutes later. It is important to obtain the brachial systolic pressure immediately after exercising since it may increase significantly. When the resting ankle pressure is less than 40 mmHg, stress testing may be omitted because it adds no new information.

Occasionally, in debilitated patients or amputees, the only feasible stress test is reactive hyperemia, the results of which closely parallel those of treadmill exercise. The thigh cuff is inflated 40–50 mmHg above systolic pressure for 4 minutes and then released. Pressures are measured at the ankle immediately and at 30-second intervals for up to 2.5 minutes thereafter.

INTERPRETATION

Interpreting the data is usually simple. The normal high-thigh pressures as we measure it usually exceeds the brachial pressure by a factor of 1.2. Pressure differences of less than 20 mmHg between limbs at the same level are considered normal variation. The normal ankle brachial index (ABI) is greater than 1.0, with smaller ratios indicating arterial narrowing or obstruction. An ABI of 0.5–0.9 usually indicates single-level disease, while a ratio of less than 0.5 suggests multilevel obstruction to flow.

Pressure differences that exceed 30 mmHg between segmental levels are considered abnormal, and those over 40 mmHg usually signify occlusion. Frequently, differences between limbs at the same level that exceed 20 mmHg are also significant. These criteria are not without qualification, however.

VARIABILITY OF ANKLE PRESSURE

Baker and Dix have found that the variation in mean ABI measured daily in 35 men with stable claudication was 0.18, with a range of 0.40 and a standard deviation of 0.03.[3] Therefore, any single pressure reading must be interpreted with care.

CORRELATION OF PRESSURE READINGS AND ARTERIOGRAPHIC FINDINGS

Pressure readings taken at rest provide physiologic data, while arteriography supplies a map of the arteries of the extremity. In a personal communication, Sumner reports that segmental pressures correlate poorly with arteriographic findings. According to Sumner, the usual criteria cited above were not very predictive, particularly in the presence of multiple segmental lesions. Segmental pressures did correlate with the anatomic extent of disease, but they did not accurately predict arteriographic findings. Localized 50% stenosis of aortofemoral and superficial femoral segments were frequently missed, and disease of the tibial artery was consistently recognized only when severe and involving all three vessels. Nevertheless, Sumner suggests (and we agree) that pressures may reveal the physiologic severity of the disease more accurately than arteriography. Further stress testing and waveform analysis might have improved the accuracy of these correlations.

TOE VERSUS ANKLE PRESSURES

Toe pressures appear more useful than ankle pressures, according to new data from Ramsey et al.[4] Using a digital pneumatic cuff and photoplethysmography, they found that the severity of ischemia and the prediction of healing correlated better when based on toe pressures. The ABI and the toe/brachial index (TBI) were correlated; TBIs usually were lower, with a regression coefficient of 0.76, $P < 0.0001$. For asymptomatic limbs they report a TBI of 0.70 ± 0.19; in claudicants, 0.37 ± 0.17;

and in 51 limbs with severe ischemia, 0.11 $\pm$ 0.09. Ninety percent of the patients with ischemic limbs had toe pressures of 35 mmHg, and ischemic lesions did not heal when toe pressures fell to 30 mmHg. According to these results, toe pressures appear more reliable than ankle pressures, especially for diabetics and persons with incompressible arteries.

MISLEADING ESTIMATIONS OF THIGH PRESSURE

We have had difficulty with decreased thigh pressures that suggest iliac stenosis or occlusion where none exists radiologically. Occasionally, the decreased pressure results from occlusion of the superficial femoral artery at its origin, with accompanying stenosis of the profunda femoris artery. There are occasions, however, when this is not the case. An experimental study by Bernstein et al. may explain this phenomenon.[2] They found that stenosis of the superficial femoral artery distal to the thigh cuff, particularly when there is more than one area of stenosis, gives a false estimation of the actual high-thigh pressure. The presence of a normal femoral arterial pulse, as well as the absence of bruit over the lower abdomen and femoral area, ought to alert one to this possibility.

ANALYZING DOPPLER WAVEFORMS AND SEGMENTAL PRESSURES IN THEIR CLINICAL CONTEXT

We evaluate Doppler waveforms qualitatively, by pattern recognition, rather than quantitatively. Vessels are judged to be either normal or diseased on the basis of the waveform, and the extent of an abnormality reflects the degree to which blood flow is altered. There are, however, a number of clinical situations in which the diagnosis is problematic.

Diabetes and Renal Failure

In the presence of diabetes mellitus or renal failure, arteries may calcify and become difficult to compress. Pressures exceeding 250–300 mmHg may be required to stop flow during cuff inflation. In these cases, an analysis of the Doppler waveform falsely indicates occlusive disease (Figure 2-1). Toe pressures are less likely to be misleading in such cases (see above).

Effect of Ambient Temperature

Ambient temperature may also affect the waveform. When a patient is examined too soon after arriving in cold weather, or when the examining room is cold, the Doppler waveform may be abnormal. In particular, the normal diastolic reversal may be lost.

Differentiating Occlusive Disease from Congestive Heart Failure

In a healthy person, the stress test either fails to change or, more usually, elevates the ankle pressure. Decreased ankle pressure with exercise, on the other hand, usually indicates stenosis or obstruction; the decrease is proportional to the severity of the disease. When the femoral/popliteal or several of the outflow vessels are abnormal, the fall is usually precipitous. The time it takes to recover pressure is proportional to the adequacy of collateral circulation. With exercise, however, uncompensated congestive heart failure may also produce a fall in ankle pressure because the heart cannot increase its output acutely.

Differentiating True Claudication from Pseudoclaudication

"Pseudoclaudication"—pain on walking due to musculoskeletal or neurologic problems—must be distinguished from true claudication. Segmental pressure measurement, plus stress testing, can distinguish patients with true claudication from those whose lower extremity symptoms are not caused by arterial disease. In the diabetic, however, neurogenic pain may coexist with arterial insufficiency. Occasionally, diabetics are treated for vascular insufficiency with good objective results, but continue to experience pain at rest because of their diabetic neuropathy. Pure ischemic neuropathy, on the other hand, may resolve over a year's time. If there is doubt concerning neuropathy, nerve conduction studies may be helpful.

Stress testing should confirm the arterial basis of symptomatic calf pain with exercise; the ABI should fall from baseline values. Because recovery may be rapid when the blockage is at one level only and when collateral circulation is well established, postexercise measurements must be taken quickly once exercise ceases.

Determining Amputation Level and Prognosis

Attempts to determine amputation level on the basis of segmental blood pressures are unsuccessful. Only the probabilities of healing can be suggested. Some investigators report good predictability, others poor. Barnes has published data that reveal poor correlation between postsurgical healing and toe pressures in diabetic patients.[5] Clinical judgment based on all available data, including the results of arteriography and noninvasive studies, seems the best guide. Measurements of skin blood flow by radioactive ^{133}Xe clearance at the level of proposed amputation appears promising, too,[6] and toe pressures may be more helpful predictors than ankle pressures. Meanwhile, a patient should not be denied distal amputation solely on the basis of a low segmental arterial pressure.

Monitoring ECGs

Several investigators report the value of recording a V-5 ECG lead during treadmill tests, citing a good correlation between ischemic events during the test and postoperative myocardial ischemia.[7,8]

Monitoring Ankle/Brachial Indices

ABIs may change during the course of a patient's disease, and changes greater than 0.15–0.18 have been shown to be significant. Other chapters discuss further applications of segmental pressure measurements in the detection and diagnosis of postoperative complications, including that of vein-graft stenosis (Chapter 5).

REFERENCES

1. Moore WS, Malone LM: Effect of flow rate and vessel calibre on critical arterial stenosis. J Surg Res 26:1–9, 1979.
2. Bernstein EF, Witzel TH, Scotts JS, et al: Thigh pressure artifacts with noninvasive techniques in an experimental model. Surgery 89:319–323, 1981.
3. Baker TD, Dix DE: Variability of Doppler ankle pressures with arterial occlusive disease: an evaluation of ankle index and brachial-ankle pressure gradient. Surgery 89:134–137, 1981.
4. Ramsey DE, Lambeth A, Manke DA, et al: Toe pressure measurements in peripheral arterial disease. International Vascular Symposium, London, 1981.
5. Barnes RW, Thornhill B, Nix L, et al: Prediction of amputation wound healing. Roles of Doppler ultrasound and digit photoplethysmography. Arch Surg 116:80–83, 1981.
6. Moore WS, Henry RE, Malone JM, et al: Prospective use of xenon Xe 133 clearance for amputation selection level. Arch Surg 116:86–88, 1981.
7. Carroll RM, Rose HB, Vyden J, et al: Cardiac arrhythmias associated with treadmill claudication testing. Surgery 83:284–287, 1978.
8. McCabe CJ, Reidy NC, Abbott WM, et al: The value of electrocardiogram monitoring during treadmill testing for peripheral vascular disease. Surgery 89:183–186, 1981.

CHAPTER 3

DIGITAL
PLETHYSMOGRAPHY AND
PRESSURE MEASUREMENTS

David S. Sumner

Plethysmographs record changes in the volume of toes, fingers, or entire limbs.[1] Transient changes in volume occur with each pulse beat as blood flows in or out of the digit or extremity. Over the years, several types of plethysmographs have been devised. The earliest, and perhaps the most accurate, enclose the part being examined in a container of water. Although water-filled plethysmographs are useful for physiologic experiments, they are much too cumbersome to be used routinely for clinical diagnostic purposes. Commonly used varieties include air-filled cuffs, mercury in Silastic rubber strain gauges, photophethysmographs, and impedance plethysmographs. For studying pulses in the fingers and toes, we prefer the photoplethysmograph for routine work and the mercury strain gauge when quantitation is necessary.[2,3]

EFFECT OF TEMPERATURE AND SYMPATHETIC
ACTIVITY ON DIGITAL PULSE AND VOLUME

Plethysmographic pulse contours are similar in various areas of the body (Figure 3-1). The normal waveform has a rapid systolic upslope and a downslope that bows toward the baseline. Usually, a dicrotic notch or wave is evident on the downslope. The volume of the plethysmographic

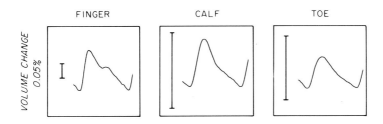

Figure 3-1. Plethysmographic pulse recordings from normal finger, calf, and toe. Reprinted with permission from Strandness DE Jr, and Sumner DS: *Hemodynamics for Surgeons.* New York, Grune & Stratton, 1975.

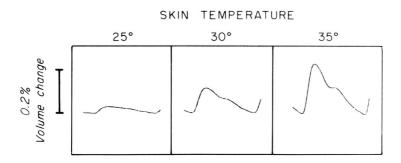

Figure 3-2. Effect of different finger temperatures on digit pulse volume. Reprinted with permission from Strandness DE Jr, Sumner DS: *Hemodynamics for Surgeons.* New York, Grune & Stratton, 1975.

pulse is very sensitive to changes in temperature (Figure 3-2), and when the part being examined is cold, the pulse volume diminishes and may assume an "obstructive" contour or disappear entirely. Because of this behavior, all plethysmographic studies should be performed in a warm room (about 25°C). Supplementary warming of the digits may be necessary in some cases.

Sympathetic nerve activity regulates the volume of blood in the digit by controlling the arteriolar sphincter mechanism and venous diameter. When the sympathetic nerves are intact, the volume of the digit decreases with inspiration and increases with expiration (Figure 3-3). When the breath is held, the plethysmographic tracing becomes level. More gradual, less frequent changes in digital volume (the so-called alpha waves) are also attributable to sympathetic activity.[4] Often, these sympathetically induced changes in volume far exceed those that occur with

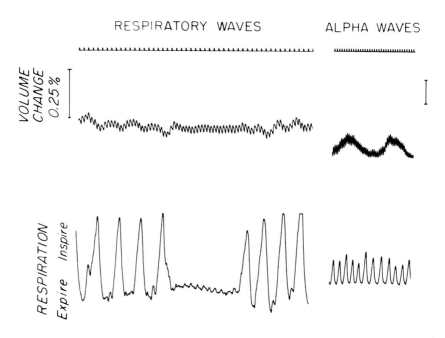

Figure 3-3. Respiratory waves and alpha waves from a normal fingertip. Reprinted with permission from Strandness DE Jr, Sumner DS: *Hemodynamics for Surgeons.* New York, Grune & Stratton, 1975.

each pulse beat, making it difficult for the examiner to keep the plethysmographic tracing on the recording paper, especially when the amplifier is in the dc mode. By using an ac amplifier, one can suppress the respiratory and alpha waves and obtain a more stable tracing for observing pulse contours.

Sympathectomy abolishes these respiratory responses. A simple test for detecting and for assessing the degree of sympathetic activity is illustrated in Figure 3-4. With a plethysmographic sensor placed on the finger (or toe), the patient is asked to take a deep breath, to hold it for a moment, and then to release it rapidly. Often there is a transient rise in digital volume because the venous outflow backs up in response to a temporary rise in intrathoracic pressure. In a sympathectomized extremity, there is no change in pulse volume or in the total volume of the digit; but in a normally innervated limb, there is a marked decrease in both the pulse volume and the finger volume. This test must be performed with a dc amplifier, since it is necessary to follow prolonged changes in volume as well as those that occur with each pulse beat.

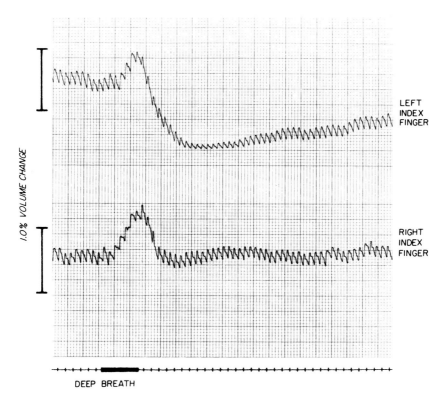

1.0% VOLUME CHANGE

LEFT
INDEX
FINGER

RIGHT
INDEX
FINGER

DEEP BREATH

Figure 3-4. Effect of a deep breath on digit pulse volume and the volume of the finger-tip in a patient who had undergone a right cervicothoracic sympathectomy. Response on the left side (intact sympathetic innervation) is normal. Tracings were made simultaneously. Reprinted with permission from Strandness DE Jr, Sumner DS: *Hemodynamics for Surgeons.* New York, Grune & Stratton, 1975.

ISCHEMIC SYNDROMES OF THE UPPER EXTREMITY

Ischemia of the upper extremity may be intermittent or constant.[4,5] When symptoms of intermittent digital ischemia occur in response to cold exposure or emotional stimuli, they are called *Raynaud's phenomenon.* Claudication, another form of intermittent ischemia, is less common in the arm or hand than it is in the leg, but the etiology is similar. The presence of claudication always implies a "fixed" arterial obstruction involving the subclavian, brachial, or (rarely) distal arteries. Raynaud's phenomenon, on the other hand, may occur in extremities with anatomically intact vessels or in extremities with fixed arterial obstruction, usually in the digital, palmar, or forearm arteries.

When the ischemia is due only to digital arterial spasm, the condition is called *Raynaud's disease,* but when the intermittent ischemia is due to the normal vasoconstrictive responses of the arterioles or digital arteries superimposed on a fixed arterial obstruction, the condition is called *secondary Raynaud's phenomenon.* Although true Raynaud's disease is a rather benign condition with an excellent prognosis, secondary Raynaud's phenomenon may be the first manifestation of a collagen vascular disease, Buerger's disease, heavy metal intoxication, or traumatic vascular occlusive disease.

When the ischemia is constantly present, there is always a fixed arterial obstruction. The extent of the ischemia depends on the location of the obstructive process. The process may be confined to a single finger when the obstruction is limited to the digital arteries, or it may involve the entire hand when the brachial and forearm arteries are occluded.

ANALYZING PULSE CONTOURS

The major diagnostic challenge is to differentiate fixed arterial obstruction from vasospasm.[6] Plethysmographic tests may be very helpful in this regard. Figure 3-5 illustrates pulse contours typical of patients complaining of cold sensitivity. The normal pulse contour (Figure 3-5C) is seen in patients with Raynaud's disease when vasospasm has been aborted by warming the hand. Arterial occlusion anywhere proximal to the end of the finger—in the digital, hand, or arm arteries—causes the pulses to assume an "obstructive" form that is characterized by a slow upslope, a rounded peak, and a downslope that bows away from the baseline (Figure 3-5B). An intermediate form has been identified, which we call the "peaked" pulse (Figure 3-5A). This pulse shares some of the characteristics of both the normal and abnormal forms. The upslope is somewhat slower than normal, a rather sharp anacrotic notch is present, and the dicrotic notch is located high on the downslope. We have found that the peaked pulse is commonly seen in the early stages of collagen vascular disease.[7]

As Table 3-1 indicates, these pulses constitute a fairly good method of distinguishing among the various causes of digital ischemia. Those patients whose symptoms suggest Raynaud's disease and whose pulses are peaked or obstructive may eventually turn out to have Raynaud's phenomenon secondary to an underlying cause, such as scleroderma or another collagen vascular disease.

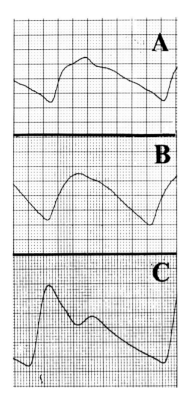

Figure 3-5. Plethysmographic pulses from fingers of patients with cold sensitivity. **A** Peaked, **B** obstructive, **C** normal. Reprinted with permission from Sumner DS, Strandness DE Jr: An abnormal finger pulse associated with cold sensitivity. Ann Surg 175:294–298, 1972.

Table 3-1. Digit Pulse Contours in Patients with Cold Sensitivity[a]

Clinical Classification	Pulse Classification		
	Normal	Peaked	Obstructive
Raynaud's disease[b]	7 (44%)	4 (25%)	5 (31%)
Etiology unknown[c]	4 (8%)	39 (81%)	5 (10%)
Etiology known[d]	0 (0%)	11 (69%)	5 (31%)
Collagen vascular disease[e]	2 (8%)	11 (44%)	12 (48%)

[a] Data from Sumner and Strandness.[7]

[b] Based on criteria of Allen, Barker, and Hines.[5]

[c] No diagnosis 26; suspected collagen disease, Buerger's disease, causalgia, traumatic arteritis, 22.

[d] Buerger's disease 5, vibratory arteritis 3, thoracic outlet (emboli) 2, causalgia 2, frostbite 2, cryoglobulinemia 2.

[e] Scleroderma 11, rheumatoid arthritis 6, SLE 4, dermatomyositis 3, polyarteritis 1.

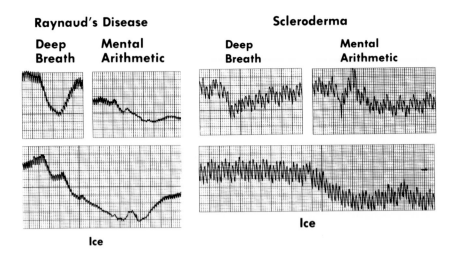

Figure 3-6. Responses to sympathetic stimuli in a patient with primary Raynaud's disease (*left panels*) and in a patient with scleroderma (*right panels*). Pulse volumes are larger in the right-hand panels because the amplification of the recorder was greater. Reprinted with permission from Sumner DS, Lambeth A, Russell JB: Diagnosis of upper extremity obstructive and vasospastic syndromes by Doppler ultrasound, plethysmography, and temperature profiles. In *Hemodynamics of the Limbs—1*. Edited by P Puel, H Boccalon, A Enjalbert. Toulouse, France, GEPESC, 1979, pp 365–373.

ASSESSING THE POTENTIAL BENEFITS OF SYMPATHECTOMY

A question that often arises in cases of cold sensitivity is whether a sympathectomy would be beneficial. Figure 3-6 contrasts the plethysmographic tracings observed in a finger of a patient with primary Raynaud's disease with those in a finger of a patient with scleroderma. Responses to sympathetic stimuli were normal in the patient with Raynaud's disease: both the digital volume and the pulse volume were markedly decreased following a deep breath, mental arithmetic, and the application of ice to the forehead. These changes were not seen in the patient with scleroderma, indicating that the stiffened peripheral arteries and arterioles were not affected by the increased sympathetic outflow. When the plethysmographic tracing fails to demonstrate an active response to sympathetic stimuli, it is doubtful that sympathetic ablation would afford much symptomatic relief.

The increased blood flow that follows restoration of the circulation after a period of ischemia is known as reactive hyperemia. Although reactive hyperemia may occur in a sympathectomized extremity, sympathectomy is unlikely to produce increased flow in an extremity that fails to show reactive hyperemia. Normally, in response to a 3- to 5-minute period of ischemia of the hand produced by the inflation of a pneumatic cuff, the finger pulse reappears immediately after the cuff is released and rapidly increases in volume until its maximum volume is at least double that present under control conditions (Figure 3-7). In contrast, the digital pulse in a patient with scleroderma (or other arterial disease that results in a fixed microvasculature) may not show an increase in volume (Figure 3-7). Such an extremity is unlikely to benefit from vasodilators or surgical sympathectomy.

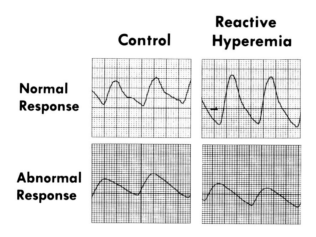

Figure 3-7. Reactive hyperemic response in a patient with primary Raynaud's disease (*upper panels*) and in a patient with scleroderma (*lower panels*). Reprinted with permission from Sumner DS, Lambeth A, Russell JB; Diagnosis of upper extremity obstructive and vasospastic syndromes by Doppler ultrasound, plethysmography, and temperature profiles. In *Hemodynamics of the Limbs—1*. Edited by P Puel, H Boccalon, A Enjalbert. Toulouse, France, GEPESC, 1979, pp 365–373.

TAKING AND ANALYZING FINGER PRESSURES

Digital pressure measurements are among the most helpful of the methods employed in diagnosing and evaluating arterial disease of the upper extremity.[8,9,10] A pneumatic cuff, which should have a width at least 1.2 times that of the finger, is wrapped around the proximal or middle phalanx. A photoplethysmograph or a mercury strain gauge is placed on the distal phalanx (Figure 3-8). The cuff is inflated above the systolic pressure well beyond the point at which the digital pulses disappear. While

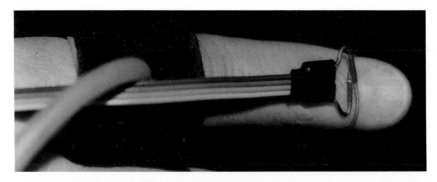

Figure 3-8. Method for measuring digital arterial pressure with a mercury strain gauge and a pneumatic cuff. Reprinted with permission from Sumner DS: Noninvasive measurement of segmental arterial pressure. In *Vascular Surgery*. Edited by RB Rutherford. Philadelphia, WB Saunders, 1977, pp 115–131.

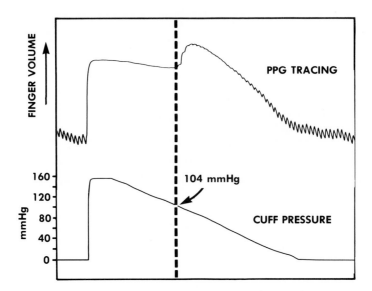

Figure 3-9. Simultaneous pneumatic cuff pressure and PPG tracing in a normal finger. Note the sharp increase in finger volume and the reappearance of digital pulses when the cuff pressure reaches the systolic pressure in the finger.

the cuff is inflated, the volume of the digit usually falls at a slow, steady rate. As the cuff is gradually deflated, digital pulses reappear and the digital volume begins to rise when the systolic pressure is reached (Figure 3-9).

Although these measurements can be made with a hand-held bulb pump and sphygmomanometer, it is often difficult to maintain a steady pressure or to deflate the cuff gradually because of the small volume of the bladder and the inevitable leakage of air. Consequently, it is easier to use an automatic cuff inflator (D.E. Hokanson, Inc., Issaquah, Washington). This device automatically maintains the pressure in the cuff at any prescribed level. As the pressure is gradually decreased, the point at which the pulse reappears is easily noted on the gauge and can be read even after the cuff is fully deflated.

An index can be calculated by dividing the systolic pressure in the finger by the ipsilateral brachial systolic pressure. The normal finger/brachial indices cluster around 1.0, similar to normal ankle pressure indices (Figure 3-10). About 90% of the normal values lie above an index of

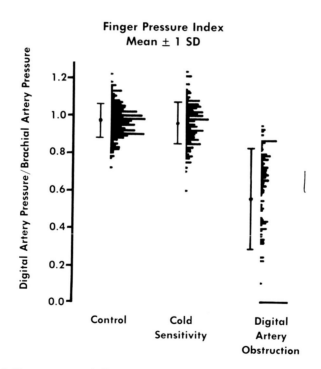

Figure 3-10. Finger-pressure indices in normal (control) subjects, patients with primary Raynaud's disease, and patients with obstructive disease of the palmar or digital arteries. Reprinted with permission from Sumner DS, Lambeth A, Russell JB: Diagnosis of upper extremity obstructive and vasospastic syndromes by Doppler ultrasound, plethysmography, and temperature profiles. In *Hemodynamics of the Limbs—1*. Edited by P Puel, H Boccalon, A Enjalbert. Toulouse, France, GEPESC, 1979, pp 365–373.

0.79.[6] Patients who have cold sensitivity associated with primary Raynaud's disease tend to have normal finger/brachial indices, indicating the absence of any proximal digital, palmar, forearm, or brachial arterial obstruction. Digital and palmar arterial occlusive disease, on the other hand, cause a decrease in the finger/brachial index. As Figure 3-10 indicates, the indices vary with the degree of ischemia, and an appreciable number of fingers have indices of zero. A low finger/brachial index in a patient with cold sensitivity immediately places the disease in the category of secondary Raynaud's phenomenon.

ISCHEMIC SYNDROMES OF THE LOWER EXTREMITY

Plethysmography can assist in the diagnostic evaluation of suspected arterial disease of the lower extremity by (1) demonstrating the presence or absence of arterial obstruction, (2) assessing its severity, (3) predicting a patient's response to sympathectomy, and (4) evaluating the likelihood that ulcers, localized gangrene, or distal amputations will heal. The studies are similar to those used in the examination of the upper extremity.

ANALYZING PULSE CONTOURS

The plethysmographic pulse in the normal toe closely resembles that in the finger.[11] When there is obstruction at any point proximal to the tip of the toe, the pulse becomes rounded and the downslope bows away from the baseline (Figure 3-11). As the disease becomes more severe, the volume of the pulse diminishes, and in the most severe cases it becomes undetectable. An obstructive toe pulse in a limb with a normal ankle pressure localizes the disease to the pedal or digital arteries. In certain cases when arterial calcification makes it impossible to obtain accurate pressure data at the ankle, an abnormal toe pulse may provide the only objective physiologic confirmation of clinically suspected arterial disease.

TESTING RESPONSE TO REACTIVE HYPEREMIA

As shown in Figure 3-11A, the volume of the toe pulse will more than double in a normal limb following a reactive hyperemia test. This test is performed by inflating a pneumatic cuff placed around the ankle to pressures exceeding systolic for five minutes. In the absence of arterial ob-

Digit Pulse — Second Toe

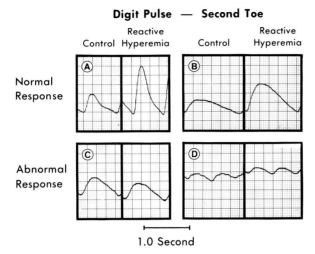

Figure 3-11. Toe pulse contours and reactive hyperemic response. **A** Normal, **B** superficial femoral arterial obstruction, **C** diabetic with pedal arterial disease and normal ankle pressure, and **D** combined iliac and superficial femoral obstruction. Reprinted with permission from Sumner DS: Digital plethysmography. In *Vascular Surgery*. Edited by RB Rutherford. Philadelphia, WB Saunders, 1977, pp 73–78.

struction, the maximum response to reactive hyperemia occurs within a few seconds after the cuff is deflated, but the maximum pulse volume may not be attained for several minutes in limbs with arterial disease. Nevertheless, the pulse volume may double even in the presence of proximal arterial obstruction, implying that the peripheral arterioles still retain the ability to dilate (Figure 3-11B). This response is characteristic of a limb which experiences intermittent claudication but which does not suffer from ischemia at rest (see Chapter 1). When the peripheral arteriolar bed is already maximally dilated either because of peripheral neuropathy or to compensate for a high proximal resistance, there will be little or no increase in pulse volume (Figure 3-11C and D). A sympathectomy would not be expected to increase blood flow in a limb that shows no response to a reactive hyperemia test, but it might afford some relief from neuropathic pain.

Taking and Analyzing Toe Pressures

Toe Pressures and Healing Potential

Predicting the likelihood that a foot lesion will heal or that a toe or transmetatarsal amputation will be successful is difficult when one must rely solely on the clinical examination. Reports in the literature indicate that such predictions are erroneous in from 18% to 46% of cases.[12-15] Ankle pressures have not fared much better.[13] Recent studies, however, suggest that toe pressures are reasonably reliable.[16-18] For example, Holstein and associates found that only 34% of foot lesions healed spontaneously when the toe pressure was less than 30 mmHg; when the toe pressure was greater than 30 mmHg, 91% healed.[17]

Our results are similar (Table 3-2).[18] When the toe pressure was less than 30 mmHg, 95% (35/37) of foot and toe ulcers failed to heal, but when toe pressure exceeded 30 mmHg, 86% (18/21) eventually healed with con-

Table 3-2. Relationship of Toe Pressure to Healing of Foot Ulcers[a]

Clinical Classification	Toe Pressure (mmHg)	Number of Limbs		Total
		Nonhealing	Healed	
Diabetic	0–29	19	2	21
	> 30	1	10	11
Total		20	12	32
Nondiabetic	0–29	16	0	16
	> 30	2	8	10
Total		18	8	26
Both groups	0–29	35	2	37
	> 30	3	18	21
Total		38	20	58

[a] Data derived from Ramsey et al.[18]

servative therapy. The figures were similar for both diabetics and nondiabetics. That ankle pressures were far less reliable in our experience is documented in Table 3-3. The criteria chosen were those published by Raines and colleagues,[19] who found that foot lesions were unlikely to heal in diabetics when ankle pressure was less than 80 mmHg; in nondiabetics they were not likely to heal when the ankle pressure was less than 55 mmHg. Although a low ankle pressure carried a poor prognosis, a high ankle pressure could not be relied upon to predict healing. In fact, only 55% (18/33) of those limbs with an ankle pressure exceeding 80 mmHg healed spontaneously.[18]

Table 3-3. Relationship of Ankle Pressure to Healing of Foot Ulcers[a]

Clinical Classification	Ankle Pressure (mmHg)	Number of Limbs		Total
		Nonhealing	Healed	
Both groups	0–54	11	1	12
	> 55	27	19	46
Total		38	20	58
Both groups	0–79	23	2	25
	> 80	15	18	33
Total		38	20	58
Nondiabetic	0–54	7	0	7
	> 55	11	8	19
Total		18	8	26
Diabetic	0–79	12	1	13
	> 80	8	11	19
Total		20	12	32

[a] Data derived from Ramsey et al.[18]

This discrepancy between the results obtained with the ankle and toe pressures has two possible explanations: (1) the ankle pressure was distortedly high as a result of medial calcification, or (2) the ankle pressure was reliable indicating satisfactory perfusion at the ankle level, but pedal arterial disease was so severe that perfusion of the distal foot was limited. Both of these factors are often operative in the diabetic patient with peripheral arterial disease.

Toe Pressures and Symptoms

Toe pressures correlate well with the patient's symptoms (Table 3-4). In a study of 200 patients with arterial disease, those with no symptoms had toe pressures that hovered around 90 to 100 mmHg. When the only complaint was intermittent claudication, the pressures were in an intermediate range, but they averaged about 20 mmHg when the feet were ischemic. There was little difference between the toe pressures of diabetics and nondiabetics—a point of some significance, since ankle pressures are often quite different in the two groups.

Table 3-4. Toe Pressures and Toe Indices in Patients with Arterial Disease

Symptoms	Nondiabetic		Diabetic	
	Pressure (mmHg)	Index[a]	Pressure (mmHg)	Index
None	99 ± 24	0.71 ± 0.18	94 ± 26	0.66 ± 0.24
Claudication	55 ± 25	0.37 ± 0.18	63 ± 25	0.38 ± 0.15
Ischemia	17 ± 16	0.10 ± 0.09	22 ± 17	0.12 ± 0.09

[a] Index: toe systolic pressure/brachial systolic pressure.

Toe Pressures and Digital Plethysmography

Toe pressures and digital plethysmographic tracings often complement one another.[20] An example indicating good perfusion and good healing potential is shown in the upper panel of Figure 3-12. The digital plethysmogram is relatively normal, except for a little bowing away from the baseline, and the toe pressure is well above ischemic levels (< 30 mmHg). The lower panel in this figure illustrates a case with poor healing potential despite a high ankle pressure: the toe pressure is in the ischemic

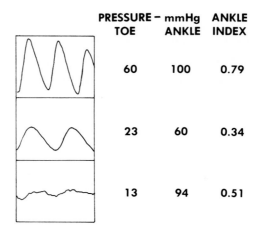

	PRESSURE – mmHg		ANKLE
	TOE	ANKLE	INDEX
	60	100	0.79
	23	60	0.34
	13	94	0.51

Figure 3-12. Pressure data and toe pulse contours in three patients with arterial disease. *Upper panel:* good perfusion. *Middle panel:* borderline perfusion, *Lower panel:* ischemia. Reprinted with permission from Sumner DS: Rational use of noninvasive tests in designing a therapeutic approach to severe arterial disease of the legs. In *Hemodynamics of the Limbs—2.* Edited by P Puel, H Boccalon, A Enjalbert. Toulouse France, GEPESC, 1981, pp 369–376.

range (< 30 mmHg), and the digital waveform is attenuated and irregular. The middle panel presents a more difficult problem. Here the toe pressure is ischemic, but the plethysmographic pulse, although abnormal, has reasonably good volume. In these cases, the reactive hyperemic response may afford some insight.

Toe Pressures and Reactive Hyperemia

When a reactive hyperemia test was performed on the patient whose tracing was illustrated in Figure 3-12 (middle panel), the pulse volume actually decreased at 30 seconds after release of cuff compression, and even at 4 minutes there was no evident hyperemia (Figure 3-13, upper panel). This response suggests that the proximal portions of the foot were actually stealing blood from the toes, implying that the adequacy of the circulation and healing potential were at best borderline.

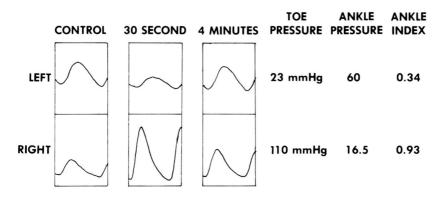

	CONTROL	30 SECOND	4 MINUTES	TOE PRESSURE	ANKLE PRESSURE	ANKLE INDEX
LEFT				23 mmHg	60	0.34
RIGHT				110 mmHg	16.5	0.93

Figure 3-13. Toe pulses showing abnormal (*upper tracings*) and normal (*lower tracings*) reactive hyperemic responses. Upper tracings are from the same patient illustrated in the middle panel of Figure 3-12. Reprinted with permission from Sumner DS: Rational use of noninvasive tests in designing a therapeutic approach to severe arterial disease of the legs. In *Hemodynamics of the Limbs—2*. Edited by P Puel, H Boccalon, A Enjalbert. Toulouse, France, GEPESC, 1981, pp 369–376.

Toe Pressure Technique and Instrumentation

The technique for measuring toe pressures is entirely analogous to that used for measuring finger pressures, but because many toes tend to be short and broad, it is difficult to apply a pneumatic cuff of sufficient width while still leaving room for a flow sensor. All too often, the cuff overlaps a mercury strain gauge that is wrapped around the terminal phalanx, thereby distorting the tracing. For this reason, we have found the photo-plethysmograph, which can be attached to the very tip of the toe, more useful than the mercury strain gauge.

Clinical Application of Toe Pressures

Toe pressures and the toe plethysmogram may be used to document the presence or absence of arterial obstructive disease in diabetics or other patients whose arteries are incompressible at the ankle. No matter what the level of the ankle pressure might be, distal foot or toe lesions seldom heal and digital or transmetatarsal amputations are likely to fail if the toe pressure is ischemic. On the other hand, a patient may have an ankle pressure that is below the level ordinarily considered conducive to healing (diabetic < 80 mmHg, nondiabetic < 55 mmHg) and yet have a toe pressure exceeding 30 mmHg. In this event, there is an excellent chance that a foot lesion will respond to local therapy.

When a patient presents with ischemic pain at rest, a distal foot or toe ulcer, or localized gangrene, my approach has been to rely heavily on the toe pressure and plethysmogram in formulating a therapeutic plan.[20-22]

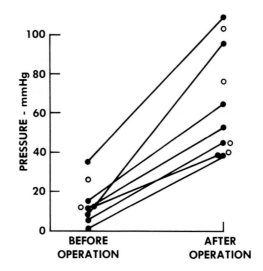

Figure 3-14. Improvement in toe pressures following femorotibial bypass grafting. *Closed circles and interconnecting lines:* preoperative and postoperative values for the same limbs. *Open circles:* isolated values. Reprinted with permission from Sumner DS: Defining the need for and assessing the results of tibial-peroneal-dorsalis pedis bypass grafts by noninvasive tests. In *Hemodynamics of the Limbs—2.* Edited by P Puel, H Boccalon, A Enjalbert. Toulouse, France, GEPESC, 1981, pp 425–433.

If (1) the toe pressure is in the ischemic range, (2) the plethysmographic tracing is flat or very obstructive, and (3) there is no reactive hyperemic response, no local procedures are attempted. Rather, an arteriogram is obtained, and if an obstruction amenable to surgical therapy is seen, revascularization is performed. Successful reconstructions elevate the toe pressure above ischemic levels (Figure 3-14). Benefitted by the increased perfusion, over 90% of the lesions heal spontaneously or respond successfully to local amputation or skin grafting.[20] On the other hand, if no reconstructable lesion is discovered, a below-the-knee or more proximal amputation must be considered.

When the toe pressure is above the ischemic range and the plethysmogram reveals a pulse of good volume, it is safe to proceed with local therapy. Reconstruction is not necessary. In a carefully selected, good-risk patient whose arteriogram demonstrates an optimum anatomic situation, however, one might elect to perform a revascularization with the expectation that the additional perfusion pressure would accelerate the healing process.

CONCLUSION

Digital plethysmography and pressure measurements provide valuable information about the arterial supply to the most distal parts of the extremities. These tests, which should be a part of the diagnostic investigation of ischemic syndromes of the arms and hands, permit vasospasm to be distinguished from arterial obstruction, help locate the site or sites of arterial obstruction, evaluate its severity, suggest etiologies, and predict the response to sympathectomy. In the lower extremity, they are the most objective methods for evaluating arterial disease of the foot and toes and for predicting the likelihood that lesions in these areas will heal. Consequently, they should be an integral part of all peripheral vascular investigations for ischemic syndromes of the foot.

REFERENCES

1. Sumner DS: Volume plethysmography in vascular disease: an overview. In *Noninvasive Diagnostic Techniques in Vascular Disease.* Edited by EF Bernstein. St Louis, CV Mosby, 1978, pp 68–92.

2. Sumner DS: Digital plethysmography. In *Vascular Surgery.* Edited by RB Rutherford. Philadelphia, WB Saunders, 1977, pp 73–78.

3. Sumner DS: Mercury strain-gauge plethysmography. In *Noninvasive Diagnostic Techniques in Vascular Disease.* Edited by EF Bernstein. St Louis, CV Mosby, 1978, pp 126–147.

4. Strandness DE Jr, Sumner DS: *Hemodynamics for Surgeons.* New York, Grune & Stratton, 1975.

5. Allen EV, Barker NW, Hines EA Jr: Raynaud's phenomenon and allied vasospastic conditions. In *Peripheral Vascular Diseases.* Philadelphia, WB Saunders, 1962, pp 124–171.

6. Sumner DS, Lambeth A, Russell JB: Diagnosis of upper extremity obstructive and vasospastic syndromes by Doppler ultrasound, plethysmography, and temperature profiles. In *Hemodynamics of the Limbs—1.* Edited by P Puel, H Boccalon, A Enjalbert. Toulouse, France, GEPESC, 1979, pp 365–373.

7. Sumner DS, Strandness DE Jr: An abnormal finger pulse associated with cold sensitivity. Ann Surg 175: 294, 1972.

8. Gunderson J: Segmental measurements of systolic blood pressures in the extremities including the thumb and the great toe. Acta Chir Scand [Suppl] 426: 1–90, 1972.

9. Hirai M: Arterial insufficiency of the hand evaluated by digital blood pressure and arteriographic findings. Circulation 58: 902–908, 1978.

10. Nielsen PE, Bell G, Lassen NA: The measurement of digital systolic blood pressure by strain gauge technique. Scand J Clin Lab Invest 29: 343–379, 1972.

11. Strandness DE Jr: *Peripheral Arterial Disease: A Physiologic Approach.* Boston, Little, Brown, 1969.

12. Baker WH, Barnes RW: Minor forefoot amputation in patients with low ankle pressure. Am J Surg 133: 331, 1977.

13. Gibbons GW, Wheelock FC Jr, Siembieda C, et al: Noninvasive prediction of amputation level in diabetic patients. Arch Surg 114: 1253, 1979.

14. Johnson WC, Patten DH: Predictability of healing of ischemic leg ulcers by radioisotopic and Doppler ultrasonic examination. Am J Surg 133: 485, 1977.

15. Verta MJ Jr, Gross WS, van Bellen B, et al: Forefoot perfusion pressure and minor amputation for gangrene. Surgery 80: 729, 1976.

16. Bone GE, Pomajzl MJ: Toe blood pressure by photoplethysmography: an index of healing in forefoot amputation. Surgery 89: 569–574, 1981.

17. Holstein P, Noer I, Tønnesen KH, et al: Distal blood pressure in severe arterial insufficiency. In *Gangrene and Severe Ischemia of the Lower Extremities.* Edited by JJ Bergan, JST Yao. New York, Grune & Stratton, 1978, pp 95–114.

18. Ramsey DE, Manke DA, Sumner DS: Toe blood pressure: a valuable adjunct to ankle pressure measurement for assessing peripheral arterial disease. J Cardiovasc Surg 22: 449, 1981.

19. Raines JK, Darling RC, Buth J, et al: Vascular laboratory criteria for the management of peripheral vascular disease of the lower extremities. Surgery 79: 212, 1976.

20. Sumner DS: Rational use of noninvasive tests in designing a therapeutic approach to severe arterial disease of the legs. In *Hemodynamics of the Limbs—2.* Edited by P Puel, H Boccalon, A Enjalbert. Toulouse, France, GEPESC, 1981, pp 369–367.

21. Sumner DS: Algorithms using non-invasive data as a guide to therapy of arterial insufficiency. In *Hemodynamics of the Limbs—1.* Edited by P Puel, H Boccalon, A Enjalbert. Toulouse, France, GEPESC, 1979, pp 543–546.

22. Sumner DS: Defining the need for and assessing the results of tibial-peroneal-dorsalis pedis bypass grafts by non-invasive tests. In *Hemodynamics of the Limbs—2.* Edited by P Puel, H Boccalon, A Enjalbert. Toulouse, France, GEPESC, 1981, pp 425–433.

CHAPTER 4

POSTOPERATIVE NONINVASIVE EVALUATION OF FEMOROTIBIAL BYPASS GRAFTS

Joseph J. Hurley

Pathologic changes in vein grafts are a significant cause of graft thrombosis.[1-4] Regrettably, the first sign or symptom of graft failure may be catastrophic, complete thrombosis, and successful restoration of flow usually requires replacement of the entire vein graft. Early detection of grafts in jeopardy is possible in the noninvasive laboratory, however, where signs of stenoses can be detected before they cause symptoms. If they are detected before thrombosis occurs, the pathologic changes may be localized and easily correctable. Arteriography is indicated in those patients whose laboratory or clinical signs suggest arterial insufficiency after apparently successful bypass vein grafts.

This chapter illustrates the value of conducting frequent postoperative examinations that include recordings of the Doppler velocity tracings and measurements of the ankle brachial index (ABI) of systolic pressure. In a study conducted in our laboratory, these measurements revealed significant decreases in the ABIs of 11 patients, signaling the need for arteriograms and corrective surgery. Obstructive changes in the Doppler velocity tracings, which may occur before significant decreases in ankle pressure, were also noted. Because the laboratory criteria are more sensitive than the history or physical examination, we recommend systematic postoperative examination of patients in the vascular laboratory.[5]

METHODS AND RESULTS

Figure 4-1 presents a life table analysis of the patency of 148 distal tibial bypass vein grafts performed from 1963 to 1981. Since 1977, all 83 patients with bypass vein grafts have been followed with both routine postoperative visits and noninvasive laboratory examinations. During

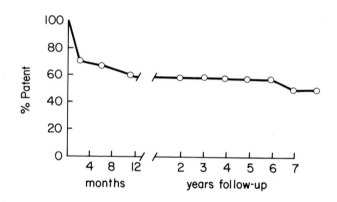

Figure 4-1. Life table analysis of graft patency of 134 distal tibial bypass vein grafts performed from 1963 to 1981.

these years, stenoses of the vein grafts were detected in 11 cases. The follow-up examinations included a history of walking distances, claudication, and pain at rest, and a physical examination—healing or non-healing lesions or recurrences of ischemic lesions were noted, pulses in the graft and foot were palpated, and so forth. Table 4-1 shows the clinical status of the patient when stenosis was suspected and proven.

Vascular laboratory examinations included ankle and brachial pressures and calculation of the mean ankle brachial index (ABI) of systolic pressure.[6] The ABIs of the 11 patients who developed stenosis of their vein grafts are shown in Figure 4-2 and Table 4-2. Toe pressures instead of ankle pressures were measured when the graft extended onto the foot (see *Toe versus Ankle Pressures*, Chapter 2). Toe pressures, now part of our routine examination, are normally 10–20 mmHg lower than ankle

Table 4-1. Signs or Symptoms
When Proven Vein-Graft Stenosis
was First Detected

Preoperative Clinical Signs	N
Asymptomatic	7
Claudication	2
Nonhealing ulcers[a]	2

[a] Pain at rest eliminated in both.

pressures when determined with photoplethysmographic sensor on the toe. Doppler velocity tracings over the graft and over the pedal pulses were also recorded (Figure 4-2). Experimentally and clinically, the change to a monophasic waveform was and is the earliest sign of obstruction; we noted such a waveform in one case of vein-graft stenosis in which

Table 4-2. Summary of Ankle/Brachial Indices of Systolic Pressure before and after Vein Grafting, at the Time of Vein-Graft Stenosis, and after its Correction by Reoperation

Case	Before Vein Graft	After Vein Graft[a]	After Graft Stenosis[b]	After Reoperation
1	0.38	1.0 (0.62)	0.72 (0.28)	0.91
2		1.0	0.67 (0.33)	1.05
3	0.45	0.65 (0.20)	0.57 (0.08)	0.87
4	0.18	0.83 (0.65)	0.40 (0.43)	0.75
5		0.9	0.43 (0.47)	1.0
6	0.42	1.10 (0.68)	0.53 (0.57)	0.95
7	0.10	0.34 (0.24)	0.34 (—)	0.93
8	0.37	0.85 (0.48)	0.85 (—)	1.0
9		1.0	1.0 (—)	1.0
10	0.75	1.0 (0.25)	0.51 (0.49)	0.95
11	0.46		0.64	1.06

[a] Numbers in parentheses denote improvements in the ABI.
[b] Numbers in parentheses denote decreases in the ABI.

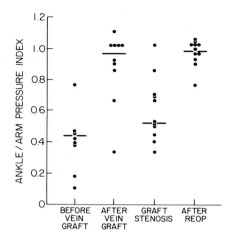

Figure 4-2. Mean ankle/brachial indices of systolic pressure in 11 cases of vein-graft stenosis.

the resting ABI remained normal. (The term "vein-graft stenosis" as used in this chapter means narrowing of the graft at or between the anastomoses.)

Table 4-3 shows the sites of the anastomoses in the 11 cases. Note that seven were distal to the tibioperoneal trunk and that one graft extended onto the foot. No multiple stenoses were seen, although one graft (Case I) had multiple mural thrombi in the distal third. Stenoses in these 11 cases involved only the vein, and those cases with new or progressive arterial plaques or arterial stenosis are not reported in this chapter.

Table 4-3. Sites of the
Distal Anastomoses in 11 Vein Grafts
that Developed Stenosis

Initial Vein-Graft Procedures	N
Femoropopliteal	4
Femoral–posterior tibial	2
Femoral–anterior tibial	2
Femoroperoneal	2
Femoral–dorsalis pedis	1

TREATMENT

All cases were treated by resecting and replacing the segments involved. In two cases this involved revision of the arterial graft anastomosis. All grafts originated from the common femoral artery, which is the customary site for the proximal anastomosis of vein grafts in the leg.

No cases were treated by percutaneous transluminal angioplasty (PTA) as suggested by Berkowitz et al.[7] In Berkowitz's series, 27 of 30 grafts harboring vein-graft stenosis were initially treated by PTA. Four of these vein grafts became occluded, and five additional grafts developed restenosis after having been successfully dilated. This experience represents a 33% failure rate for PTA. We prefer to replace the diseased segment with a new healthy living sleeve of vein inserted end-to-end with interrupted sutures.

The stenoses we treated were easily accessible because of the subcutaneous graft bed utilized in our series. Results of this treatment have been excellent, with one occlusion and one recurrent stenosis in 11 cases (the result of a mismatched sleeve graft of PTFE). Figure 4-2 shows the improvement in the ABI following surgery. After reoperation, the Doppler waveforms indicated improvement in one patient whose vein-graft stenosis was detected solely by changes in the Doppler velocity tracings. Systematic follow-up and reexamination are essential following surgery.

ARTERIOGRAPHY

Arteriography is essential to confirm the diagnosis and to plan the treatment. In our series, arteriograms revealed two stenoses in the vein at the anastomosis. All others were randomly distributed at the sites of valves or near tributaries. As in Sladen and Gilmour's series,[1] fibrosis identifiable at valve sites was detected in 10 of our 11 patients. Valve stenosis is felt to be related to fusion of valves, fibrotic thickening caused by the movement of arterial pulsation, and platelet fibrin precipitation and/or trauma induced by application of "atraumatic clamps." One graft (Case I) contained many mural thrombi in its distal third two weeks after placement. Figure 4-3 shows stenoses of vein grafts demonstrated by arteriograms in three cases. None of these stenoses were present when the vein graft was inserted, because it is our practice to fill the graft with one-quarter strength radiopaque media and to take films so as to detect and correct any lesions before the grafts are inserted.

A **B** **C**

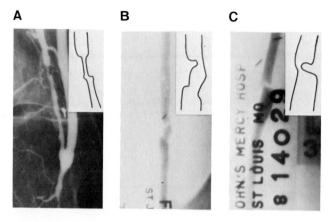

Figure 4-3. Arteriograms of three cases showing vein-graft stenoses. *Insets:* diagrams of the stenotic segment.

Poor outflow due to progression of the atherosclerosis in the inflow or outflow is another cause of recurrent ischemia and graft failure. These cases are not reported here.

Noninvasive Laboratory Findings

The mean ABIs of the 11 patients who developed stenosis of their vein grafts are shown in Figure 4-2. Mean ABI decreased less than 0.28 in 6 cases. Claudication was noted in other cases in which the ABI did not decrease. In two cases, even though pain at rest was relieved by the functioning vein graft, the postoperative ABI remained low, and ischemic ulcers did not heal. Toe pressures might have been more revealing in some patients whose arteries at the ankle were inelastic and poorly compressible. (Toe pressures correlate better with clinical findings than the ABI, particularly in diabetics,[8] and toe pressures are now part of our routine peripheral arterial examination.) Treadmill stress tests can cause decreases of pressure and reveal stenoses too mild to reduce the resting ABI, but such tests were not always feasible.

The Doppler velocity tracings showed loss of the reversed phase in all cases. The Doppler waveform generated over the pedal arteries became monophasic in all patients with vein-graft stenosis, whose waveforms were previously triphasic (i.e., normal). Changes in amplitude were sometimes noted, but these changes are not reliable indicators of stenosis.

Vein-graft stenoses were detected in two patients during the first post-operative month. The intervals between graft and stenosis ranged from 2 weeks to 3½ years, with 8 of the 11 stenoses appearing during the first year (Table 4-4).[9] Atherosclerotic plaques have been reported in vein grafts and occur early in hyperlipidemic patients. In all of our resected specimens, however, the stenosis was the result of fibrosis and hypertrophy. Doubtless atherosclerotic plaques will appear later in some patients.

Table 4-4. Interval between Initial and Reconstructive Surgery

Case	Vein Graft (Date)	Reoperation for Stenosis (Date)	Elapsed Time (Months)
1	6/78	6/78	0.5
2	5/78	11/78	6.0
3	12/78	6/79	6.0
4	1/81	4/81	3.0
5	7/75	12/78	41.0
6	3/77	1/79	22.0
7	10/78	4/79	6.0
8	6/76	11/79	41.0
9	10/79	11/79	1.0
10	6/80	12/80	6.0

CASE REPORTS

The following narrative case reports illustrate interesting points.

CASE I

A 64-year-old man had ischemic pain at rest in his left foot. He also had coronary artery disease, hypertension, and diabetes mellitus, and he smoked heavily. PTFE (polytetrafluoroethylene) was inserted during two previous operations because the donor vein was unsuitable. These grafts failed, and an umbilical vein biograft was inserted. It also thrombosed. Our arteriograms revealed an open posterior tibial artery with sufficient outflow. On June 14, 1978, we performed a left common femoral-to-distal-posterior-tibial reversed autogenous vein graft with four segments of brachial vein spliced together end to end. The ABI was 1.0 on June 16, 0.86 on June 18, and 0.72 on June 26 (Figure 4-4). A new left femoral angiogram revealed numerous intraluminal filling defects in the distal third of the venous bypass. This abnormal segment was resected and replaced with additional vein on June 27. Six months postoperatively, the patient's ABI was 0.92, and he continued to do well until February 1981, when claudication, new pain at rest, and gangrene of the toes developed. This time arteriograms showed inadequate distal outflow. The left leg was amputated above the knee on April 9, 1981.

This case illustrates the value of serial noninvasive examinations during the early postoperative course. Fewer than one of every five distal tibial bypass vein grafts fail in the first month. Early noninvasive detection of grafts in jeopardy may permit salvage of some of these, however.

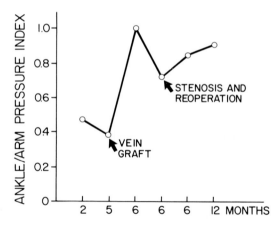

Figure 4-4. Case I. Ankle/brachial indices of systolic pressure before and after insertion of vein graft, before and after development of vein-graft stenosis, and after its correction by reoperation.

CASE II

A 72-year-old woman was admitted to the hospital in May 1978 with multiple ischemic ulcers of the left foot. She did not smoke. Her medications were oral hypoglycemics and antihypertensives. Arteriograms revealed occlusions of her superficial femoral, popliteal, posterior tibial, and anterior tibial arteries. Because the peroneal artery had satisfactory outflow, we performed a common femoral-to-distal-peroneal vein graft bypass on May 31, 1978. The ulcers were debrided and gradually healed except for a small ulceration of the great toe, which became indolent. The ABI fell 0.33 to 0.67, so she was readmitted in November 1978, six months after her initial vein graft (Figure 4-5). New arteriograms revealed 50%–60% stenosis at the take-off of the vein graft on the common femoral artery. After repair with a short vein interposition, the ABI was restored to 1.05 and the toe lesions healed rapidly.

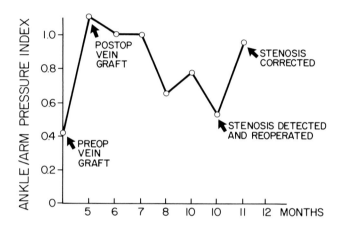

Figure 4-5. Case II. Ankle/brachial indices of systolic pressure before and after insertion of vein graft, before and after development of vein-graft stenosis, and after its correction by reoperation.

CASE III

A 60-year-old miner with severe claudication of the left leg was hospitalized, and on December 28, 1978, a left femoropopliteal bypass vein graft was performed. His postoperative ABI improved somewhat to 0.57, but remained a matter of concern. Five months after surgery, walking caused numbness of the forefoot, and a minor drop in the ABI was noted. Arteriograms revealed severe stenosis. On June 7, 1979, the stenosis was resected and a new vein segment interposed. The ABI improved markedly and the numbness with walking disappeared, but angina became more frequent and prevented him from returning to work.

Poor improvement of the ABI after the first operation was interpreted to be the result of poor outflow. The slight drop in the ABI five months postoperatively was associated with return of mild claudication and signaled the need for arteriograms. The return of ischemic symptoms in individuals with salvageable limbs requires angiographic evaluation regardless of the change in ABI. Toe pressures might have been more revealing.

CASE IV

An 80-year-old woman with ischemic pain at rest and discoloration of the right forefoot had no history of diabetes, smoking, or heart disease, only hypertension. Arteriograms suggested that a long graft was feasible, but at operation on January 26, 1981, suitable veins were sufficient only for the distal portion. She underwent a right common femoral-to-popliteal PTFE bypass, and the vein graft was inserted from the distal PTFE to the distal anterior tibial artery. Postoperatively, she did well until April 22, 1981, when her ABI decreased from 0.83 to 0.40. She was admitted to the hospital, where arteriograms revealed a high-grade stenosis at the take-off of the vein graft from the PTFE graft. Utilizing cephalic vein from the right arm, the stenosis was replaced, flow was restored, and the ABI increased to 0.75.

In this case, routine measurements of the ABI revealed a high-grade stenosis in an asymptomatic patient three months after surgery. Because vein grafts seem to tolerate low flow better than PTFE, a high-grade stenosis apparently can exist for some time without producing complete occlusion. It is doubtful that attempts to detect high-grade stenosis in PTFE grafts would be as successful.

DISCUSSION

All vein grafts are susceptible to pathologic changes, but the most troublesome are the long bypasses to the lower leg.[10] The cumulative patency curve for femoral-to-distal-tibial or -peroneal bypass grafting procedures reveals three relatively different slopes or phases (Figure 4-1). The initial, steepest slope occurs during the first month and represents a combination of technical misadventure, poor patient selection as regards outflow capabilities, and other morbid events related to hypoperfusion or coagulopathies. Thirteen grafts occluded during the first month of this study. Two correctable stenoses were found in the first month. Case I developed mural thrombi in the distal part of the vein graft. Other correctable lesions may be found during this phase if careful noninvasive testing is employed.

The second phase may be arbitrarily designated as the period from one month to one and one-half years. Here the rate of thrombosis is greater than that in the last phase, but considerably less than the first. Five of the 10 stenoses occurred during the first year and were corrected. Six other grafts thrombosed irretrievably and without warning during this interval, most commonly because of fibrous hyperplasia at the sites of anastomoses or venous valves.

Graft failure during the final phase, from 18 months on, is usually attributable to progression of atherosclerosis. The short life expectancy of patients with widespread atherosclerosis is reflected in the calculations of cumulative patency,[11] because one-half of the patients who die are assumed to have occluded grafts. The 11 vein grafts salvaged by reoperation, therefore, affect cumulative patency very little, unless they survive a considerable period.

Failure of the operation is most common during the first month; vein-graft stenosis and poor runoff appear to be the main causes of early failure. Can noninvasive testing predict success and improve our ability to select patients for operation? Corson et al. presented a group of patients undergoing femoropopliteal bypass grafting, noting that 21 of 22 early failures occurred in limbs whose preoperative ABI was 0.5 or less.[12] Femoral-to-distal-tibial or -peroneal bypass grafting is rarely considered in patients who are not threatened with the loss of a limb, however, and those who are threatened all have ABIs of less than 0.5. Corson's work revealed no predictive value in subsets of patients with ABIs below 0.5; neither early nor late success could be predicted. Although the lowest preoperative ABI did indicate the greatest danger to the leg, it did not predict surgical success or failure.

Noninvasive testing in the early postoperative period does, however, help to assess the chances of graft success.[4,12,13] (A significant drop in ankle pressure is considered to be 0.15 mmHg; measured repeatedly in the same patients, ankle pressures may vary two standard variations.) Corson's study demonstrates the value of postoperative noninvasive testing. When the ABI improved only 0.1 or less, the rate of early failure was exceptionally high. With each progressive rise in postoperative ABI, though, early failure became less likely. If the ABI is to suggest a hopeful prognosis, it must, evidently, increase at least 0.1 within four hours after surgery,[12] and when it is twice the preoperative pressure within four hours of surgery, a successful graft is likely.[13]

Arterial stenoses proximal or distal to the vein graft or faulty anastomoses, emboli, and the like also decrease the ABI, and low postoperative ABIs signify the need for arteriograms.

The rate of vein-graft failure during the first year is variously reported to be from 8% to 37% for femoropopliteal grafts and from 36% to 46% for longer grafts to the tibial arteries.[13] Frequent noninvasive testing can detect correctable lesions in some of these patients. Indeed, clinical evaluation is not sufficient in cases of early lesions. Thrombosis sometimes occurs without any previous claudication, particularly in patients whose activity is limited by disease of the other leg or by cardiopulmonary disease. Such limitations restrict exercise and, of course, claudication. Even when claudication suggests the need for an arteriogram, the vascular laboratory's confirmation is reassuring.

Reoperation rarely succeeds after thrombosis of vein grafts.[1] The simplicity and success of early reoperation is far superior. Transluminal balloon dilation also can correct vein-graft stenoses that do not involve the anastomoses[7,14] and might have been suitable for some of our cases. Nevertheless, it remains to be seen whether stenosis recurs after dilation.

CONCLUSIONS

During the early postoperative period, ankle pressures should be measured every 2–3 hours with vital signs, then daily while the patient is hospitalized. Also, during early office visits two and four weeks following surgery and for the first one and one-half years, measurements of ankle and/or toe pressures, Doppler velocity tracings, and, when feasible, treadmill tests are recommended every two to three months. Arteriograms are indicated when the ABI decreases more than 0.15. Further, patients with recurrent or persistent ischemic symptoms should be considered for arteriograms even when there are no changes in noninvasive tests, for these patients may have significant lesions. Because diabetic arterial calcification may prevent decreases in Doppler ankle pressures, pressures in the great toes should also be determined. Detection and early operation for correctable lesions, such as vein-graft stenosis, may prevent catastrophic thrombosis and thereby salvage legs. It also may improve cumulative patency.

REFERENCES

1. Sladen JG, Gilmour JL: Vein graft stenosis. Characteristics and effect of treatment. Am J Surg 141:549–553, 1981.
2. Szilagy ED, Elliott JP, Hageman JH, et al: Biologic fate of autogenous vein implants as arterial substitutes. Ann Surg 178:232–246, 1973.
3. Whitney DG, Kahn EM, Estes JW: Valvular occlusion of the arterialized saphenous vein. Am J Surg 42:879–887, 1976.
4. Whittemore AD, Alexander CW, Couch N, et al: Secondary femoropopliteal reconstruction. Ann Surg 193:35–42, 1971.
5. Sumner DS: Defining the need for and assessing the results of tibial-peroneal-dorsalis pedis bypass grafts by non-invasive tests. In *Hemodynamics of the Limbs—2.* Edited by P. Puel, H. Boccalon, A Enjalbert. Toulouse, France, GEPESC, 1981, pp 425–433.
6. Holstein P, Noer I, Tønneson KH, et al: Distal blood pressure in severe arterial insufficiency. In *Gangrene and Severe Ischemia of the Lower Extremities.* Edited by JJ Bergan, JST Yao. New York, Grune & Stratton, 1978, pp 95–114.
7. Berkowitz HD, Hobbs CL, Roberts B, et al: Value of routine vascular laboratory studies to identify vein graft stenosis. Surgery 90:971–979, 1981.
8. Thulesius O: Principles of pressure measurement. Sixth Annual San Diego Vascular Symposium, 1979.
9. DePalma RG: Atherosclerosis in vascular grafts. Atherosclerosis Rev 6: 157–177, 1979.
10. DePalma RG: A technique for preparation of saphenous vein grafts. Surgery 143:800–801, 1976.
11. Mehta S: A statistical summary of the results of femoropopliteal bypass surgery. Technical Note 175. Newark, WL Gore & Assoc, 1980, pp 14, 21.
12. Corson JD, Johnson WC, LoGerfo FW, et al: Doppler ankle systolic blood pressure. Arch Surg 113:932–935, 1978.
13. Yao JST, Nicolaides AN: Transcutaneous Doppler ultrasound in the management of lower limb ischemia. In *Investigation of Vascular Disorders.* Edited by AN Nicolaides, JST Yao. London, Churchill Livingstone, 1981, pp 249–273.
14. Alpert JR, Ring EJ, Berkowitz HD: Treatment of vein graft stenosis by balloon catheter dilation. JAMA 242:2769–2771, 1979.

CHAPTER 5

NEW TECHNIQUES TO ASSESS AORTOILIAC STENOSIS

Robert W. Barnes and Donna G. Cox

Patients with claudication or is-
chemic pain at rest must be accurately assessed for the anatomic location
of arterial occlusive disease. The history and physical findings often
identify aortoiliac (inflow), femoropopliteal (outflow), or tibioperoneal
(runoff) arterial disease; many patients, however, may present with pal-

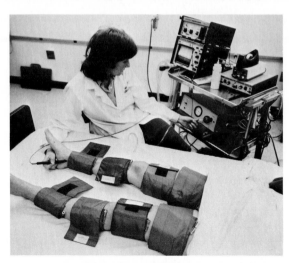

Figure 5-1. Technique of measuring segmental limb blood pressures.

pable femoral pulses and iliac or femoral artery bruits. The clinician must decide whether such aortoiliac disease constitutes significant hemodynamic obstruction to the circulation of the leg. Unfortunately, contrast arteriography usually presents a single-plane view of the aortoiliac morphology and does not show the physiologic significance of the aortoiliac occlusive disease. Intraarterial pressure measurements from the femoral artery provide hemodynamic evidence of aortoiliac obstruction, but this technique has not been routinely used in clinical practice. Recently, however, several noninvasive screening techniques have become available to document objectively the hemodynamic significance of aortoiliac obstruction. In this chapter we describe the techniques, diagnostic criteria, and results of several of these new methods.

PROXIMAL THIGH PRESSURE MEASUREMENT[1,2]

TECHNIQUE

The patient is studied in the supine position. A pneumatic cuff with an inflatable bladder measuring 12.5 cm × 40 cm is placed on the proximal thigh just below the inguinal ligament. Similar cuffs are placed more distally at the above-knee, below-knee, and ankle locations (Figure 5-1). Using a Doppler ultrasonic flow probe, the examiner elicits a distal arterial velocity signal from the posterior tibial or dorsalis pedis artery. Using an aneroid manometer or an automatic cuff inflator, the examiner inflates the proximal thigh cuff until the distal arterial velocity signal disappears, and then deflates the cuff until the arterial signal reappears at the point of systolic pressure in the proximal thigh. The segmental leg pressures are measured at the other locations on the leg.

DIAGNOSTIC CRITERIA

Normally, the systolic proximal thigh pressure is at least 20 mmHg, or greater, above that of the arm, and there should be no more than a 20-mmHg pressure gradient between adjacent levels of measurement. The systolic ankle pressure should equal or slightly exceed that of the arm. If the proximal thigh pressure is less than 20 mmHg above that of the arm, hemodynamically significant obstruction of the arterial inflow to the limb is implied. Arterial occlusive disease of the aorta, common iliac, external iliac, common femoral, or combined superficial femoral and profunda femoris arteries may result in an abnormally low proximal thigh pressure. An abnormal pressure gradient between the proximal thigh and above-knee cuffs suggests obstruction of the superficial femoral artery. An abnormal pressure gradient between the below-knee and ankle cuffs suggests occlusive disease of the tibioperoneal artery.

RESULTS

The accuracy of proximal thigh pressure measurements in the detection or exclusion of hemodynamically significant aortoiliac obstruction ($>50\%$ diameter reduction) was assessed by independent comparison with contrast arteriography in 173 extremities (Table 5-1). The sensi-

Table 5-1. Comparison of Proximal Thigh Pressures with Arteriogram

Aortoiliac Arteriogram	Number of Arteries	Thigh Pressure	
		Normal	Abnormal
Normal	62	43	19
< 50%	33	21	12
≥ 50%	56	10	46
Occluded	22	0	22

tivity of an abnormal proximal thigh pressure was 87% (68 of 78 extremities). The specificity of a normal thigh pressure measurement was 67% (64 of 95 limbs). The positive predictive value of an abnormal proximal thigh pressure measurement was 69% (68 of 99 extremities). The negative predictive value of a normal proximal thigh pressure measurement was 86% (64 of 74 limbs). The sensitivity and specificity of proximal thigh-leg pressure gradients in evaluating femoropopliteal occlusive disease were 93% and 72%, respectively.

DISCUSSION

Segmental leg pressure measurements may be artifactually elevated because of calcification (rigidity) of the arterial wall or obesity of the limb.

Nevertheless, segmental pressure measurements provide simple, rapid, and inexpensive quantification of the presence and location of arterial occlusive disease in the lower extremity.

FEMORAL ARTERIAL DOPPLER WAVEFORM

TECHNIQUE

The patient is studied in the supine position. At an angle of about 45 degrees, a bidirectional Doppler probe (Model D9, MedaSonics, Inc., Mountain View, California) is coupled with acoustic gel to the skin overlying the common femoral artery (Figure 5-2). The Doppler probe is moved about until the maximal femoral artery velocity signal is ob-

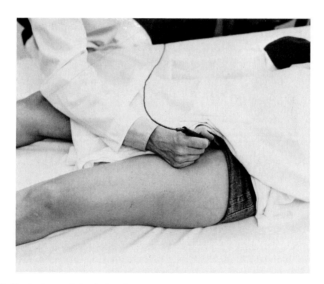

Figure 5-2. Technique of obtaining femoral arterial blood velocity waveform by Doppler ultrasound.

tained. With the Doppler instrument connected to a strip-chart recorder, the blood flow velocity of the femoral artery is recorded at a paper speed of 25 mm/sec.

DIAGNOSTIC CRITERIA

The normal femoral arterial velocity waveform is multiphasic with a prominent systolic component and one or more diastolic sounds, the first of which represents transient reverse flow (Figure 5-3). Distal to hemodynamically significant aortoiliac stenosis, the waveform is attenuated, with a monophasic signal including a prominent systolic component and absence of the diastolic waveforms. Distal to aortoiliac occlusion, the femoral velocity signal is attenuated even further with a low-pitched, monophasic waveform.

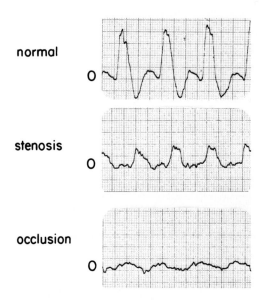

Figure 5-3. Doppler velocity waveforms from the femoral artery in the presence of normal circulation (*top*), aortoiliac stenosis (*middle*), and iliac artery occlusion (*bottom*).

RESULTS

The accuracy of femoral arterial Doppler velocity waveforms in detecting or excluding aortoiliac occlusive disease was determined by independent comparison with contrast arteriography of 185 extremities (Table 5-2). The sensitivity of an abnormal femoral Doppler velocity waveform was 85% (73 of 78 extremities). The specificity of a normal Doppler ve-

Table 5-2. Comparison of Femoral Velocity with Arteriogram

Aortoiliac Arteriogram	Number of Arteries	Doppler Waveform	
		Normal	Abnormal
Normal	72	61	11
< 50%	35	30	5
≥ 50%	58	5	53
Occluded	20	0	20

locity waveform was 85% (91 of 107 limbs). The positive predictive value of an abnormal Doppler waveform was 82% (73 of 89 extremities). The negative predictive value of a normal Doppler velocity waveform was 95% (91 of 96 limbs). Doppler velocity recordings may also be obtained from more distal arteries in the leg, including the popliteal, posterior tibial, dorsalis pedis, and peroneal arteries. The same diagnostic criteria apply for the presence or absence of significant arterial occlusive disease in these more distal arteries of the extremity, except that a diastolic reverse-flow velocity may not be present, particularly when the limb is vasodilated.

VOLUME PULSE RECORDINGS[4,5]

TECHNIQUE

The recording of pressure changes in pneumatic cuffs applied at the proximal thigh, above-knee, below-knee, and ankle levels permits the assessment of volume pulse waveforms from the extremity (Figure 5-4). A dual-channel instrument (Volume Pulse Recorder, Medical Sales Specialty, Concord, California) allows the simultaneous recording of volume pulses from both limbs.

DIAGNOSTIC CRITERIA

The normal volume pulse waveform of the leg is similar to that of a pressure waveform with a steep upslope, a relatively sharp peak, and a dicrotic wave on a downslope that is concave toward the baseline (Figure 5-5). In the presence of aortoiliac obstruction, the proximal thigh recording

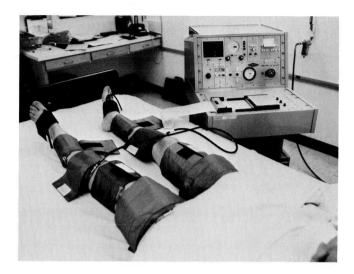

Figure 5-4. Technique of measuring segmental limb volume pulses.

normal

stenosis

occlusion

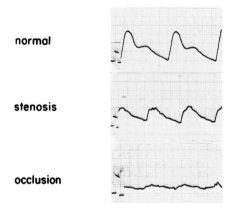

Figure 5-5. Segmental volume pulse recordings from the proximal thigh in the presence of normal circulation (*top*), aortoiliac stenosis (*middle*), and iliac artery occlusion (*bottom*).

is abnormal. When the femoropopliteal artery is obstructed, the volume pulse recording from the proximal thigh is normal, but the waveform at the above-knee or below-knee level is abnormal. In the presence of tibio-peroneal arterial occlusive disease, the volume pulse recordings are normal except for an abnormal waveform at the ankle.

RESULTS

The accuracy of the proximal thigh volume pulse recording in detecting hemodynamically significant aortoiliac occlusive disease was independently compared with contrast arteriography in 28 extremities (Table 5-3). The sensitivity of an abnormal proximal thigh volume pulse recording was 91% (10 of 11 extremities). The specificity of a normal pulse waveform in the proximal thigh was 94% (16 of 17 extremities). The positive predictive value of an abnormal proximal thigh volume pulse recording was 91% (10 of 11 extremities). The negative predictive value of a normal pulse waveform was 94% (16 of 17 limbs).

Table 5-3. Comparison of Volume Pulse Recordings with Arteriogram

Aortoiliac Arteriogram	Number of Arteries	Pulse Waveform	
		Normal	Abnormal
Normal	15	14	1
< 50%	2	2	0
≥ 50%	10	1	9
Occluded	1	0	1

FEMORAL ARTERIAL PRESSURE MEASUREMENT[6,7]

TECHNIQUE

Intraarterial pressure measurements may be obtained at the time of contrast arteriography, in the vascular laboratory, or during surgery. At the time of arteriography, measurements of femoral arterial pressure may be obtained and compared to aortic pressures using the intraarterial catheter; the femoral arterial pressure may also be compared to arm pressure measured either invasively or noninvasively. In the vascular laboratory, femoral arterial pressures may be measured by direct needle puncture and compared to pressures in the arm measured noninvasively. In the operating room, the femoral arterial pressure may be measured by needle puncture and compared to intraarterial pressure in the upper extremity, which may be measured either invasively, with an indwelling monitoring catheter, or noninvasively, by the anesthesiologist. Pressures may be measured both at rest and following hyperemia induced by intra-arterial injection of a vasodilator (such as papaverine, 15–30 mg).

DIAGNOSTIC CRITERIA

The normal systolic blood pressure of the femoral artery should be equal to that of the aorta or the arm. Hemodynamically significant obstruction of the aortoiliac segment is suggested by a resting systolic pressure gradient of 10 mmHg or greater. During hyperemia, a pressure gradient of 15–20 mmHg or greater between the arm and the femoral artery suggests significant obstruction of the aortoiliac segment.

CONCLUSIONS

The clinical assessment of aortoiliac occlusive disease begins with the history and physical examination. Patients with significant hip or thigh claudication should be considered to have hemodynamically significant aortoiliac occlusive disease until proven otherwise.

The absence of a femoral pulse should not present a diagnostic dilemma; in the presence of a normal femoral pulse and a bruit over the iliac or common femoral artery, however, the clinician must determine whether or not hemodynamically significant aortoiliac stenosis exists. Unfortunately, a single-plane contrast arteriogram does not document the physiologic significance of aortoiliac occlusive disease. Some patients may have minimal angiographic abnormalities but nevertheless suffer from severe inflow obstruction to the extremity. On the other hand, many patients with significant arterial lesions on arteriogram have no significant obstruction to blood flow to the extremities.

Objective physiologic methods of documenting aortoiliac occlusive disease are now available to the clinician. The most simple noninvasive technique to assess aortoiliac stenosis is the recording of femoral arterial velocity waveforms using Doppler ultrasound. Absence of a reverse flow signal in early diastole is the single best sign of significant aortoiliac stenosis. This occlusive disease may be quantified by measuring systolic blood pressures at the proximal thigh. Unfortunately, segmental leg pressure measurements may be in error because of calcification of the arterial wall or obesity of the limb. An alternative to femoral-velocity waveform recordings is the recording of volume pulse waveforms at the level of the proximal thigh. A normal proximal-thigh waveform or a normal femoral velocity recording is the best index of the adequacy of the inflow to the arterial circulation of the limb.

Physiologic confirmation of aortoiliac occlusive disease may be obtained by intraarterial pressure measurements, either at the time of contrast arteriography or intraoperatively. A systolic pressure gradient of 10 mmHg or greater or a hyperemic femoral artery pressure gradient of 20 mmHg or greater, relative to that of the arm, signifies aortoiliac occlusive disease.

REFERENCES

1. Winsor T: Influence of arterial disease on the systolic blood pressure gradients of the extremity. Am J Med Sci 220:117–126, 1950.
2. Heintz SE, Bone GE, Slaymaker EE, et al: Value of arterial pressure measurements in the proximal and distal part of the thigh in arterial occlusive disease. Surg Gynecol Obstet 146:337–343, 1978.
3. Barnes RW, Wilson MR: *Doppler Ultrasonic Evaluation of Peripheral Arterial Disease*. Iowa City, University of Iowa Press, 1976, p 296.
4. Winsor T: The segmental plethysmograph: a description of the instrument. Angiology 8:87–101, 1957.
5. Darling RC, Raines JK, Brener BV, et al: Quantitative segmental pulse volume recorder: a clinical tool. Surgery 72:873–887, 1972.
6. Moore WS, Hall AD: Unrecognized aortoiliac stenosis. Arch Surg 103:633–638, 1971.
7. Brener BJ, Raines JK, Darling RC, et al: Measurement of systolic femoral arterial pressure during reactive hyperemia. An estimate of aortoiliac disease. Circulation 50 [suppl]: 259–267, 1974.

CHAPTER **6**

SEGMENTAL VOLUME PULSE RECORDER: IMPROVED ANATOMIC DISCRIMINATION BY REFINEMENT IN TECHNIQUE

Donna G. Cox and Robert W. Barnes

Anatomic localization of arterial occlusive lesions is important for the diagnosis and management of patients with peripheral arterial disease. There are several noninvasive diagnostic techniques that can provide objective physiologic information about the locations and extent of arterial occlusive lesions. Both segmental systolic pressure measurements and segmental volume pulse plethysmography are widely accepted means of obtaining functional data to complement the history and physical examination. These studies also help to confirm the diagnosis, to predict therapeutic results, and to monitor medical and surgical therapy.

In the past, segmental pulse volume recordings have been obtained by using a single wide cuff on the thigh and narrow cuffs below the knee and at the ankle. Segmental pressure measurements have been obtained by using either a single wide thigh cuff or narrow proximal and distal thigh cuffs along with narrow cuffs below the knee and at the ankle. It has been found, however, that the narrow proximal and distal thigh cuff technique localizes arterial occlusive lesions more accurately, especially those of the aortoiliac and femoropopliteal segments.[1] In light of this finding, we conducted a prospective study to determine if the level of accuracy for detecting aortoiliac and femoropopliteal lesions could be improved by using segmental volume pulse plethysmography with the four-cuff technique, using segmental systolic pressure measurements and contrast arteriography as standards for comparison. In addition, we obtained Doppler velocity recordings of the common femoral artery in an attempt to differentiate aortoiliac from common femoral or combined superficial femoral and profunda femoris disease.

PATIENTS AND METHODS

One hundred thirty-one patients with suspected atherosclerotic occlusive disease were studied. There were 68 men and 63 women, ranging in age from 14 to 82 years (mean age, 61). Forty-eight patients (36%) were diabetic. A total ot 251 limbs were studied. One hundred ten limbs (43%) were evaluated for claudication, 26 limbs (10%) for pain at rest, and 30 limbs (12%) for necrotic lesions.

Seventy-one limbs (27.5%) underwent standard single-plane arteriography. The distal aorta, iliac system, common femoral, superficial femoral, popliteal, anterior tibial, posterior tibial, and peroneal arteries were read blindly by an arteriographer who was unaware of both the clinical status of the patients and the results of their noninvasive tests.

A complete history and limb examination were obtained from each patient prior to the noninvasive testing. The history included past and present conditions as well as family history. Examination of the limbs included notation of hair loss, nail changes, trophic skin changes, and palpation of peripheral pulses.

Femoral arterial velocity waveforms were obtained over the femoral artery bilaterally at the level of the inguinal crease with the use of an 8-MHz bidirectional Doppler probe and a chart recorder (MedaSonics P-92A bidirectional Doppler and R12A chart recorder). The normal velocity patterns of peripheral vessels reflect both positive and negative flow, which are manifested by a multiphasic arterial Doppler signal. A sharp upstroke is noted during early systole with a rapid decline back to the baseline. In early diastole there is a reversal of flow directly proportional to arterial resistance. With vasoconstriction a prominent negative deflection is noted, whereas with vasodilation little or no flow reversal occurs. In patients with lesions of the aortoiliac segment, the femoral arterial velocity waveform is dampened and there is loss of the negative deflection. When there are lesions just distal to the common femoral artery, the velocity waveform is abnormal as well. The popliteal, posterior tibial, dorsalis pedis, and peroneal arteries were assessed audibly for their multiphasic characteristics.[1,2]

Segmental systolic pressure measurements were taken as described by Barnes and Wilson[3] using the four-cuff technique. Pneumatic cuffs measuring 12.5 cm × 40 cm were placed high on the thigh, above the knee, below the knee, and at the ankle. Care was taken to make sure that the cuffs were placed on the limb snugly, but not tight enough to occlude venous return, and that the bladders were over the arterial pathways. The pressure measurements were obtained by using either the posterior tibial or dorsalis pedis arteries. In a normal patient tested with the narrow cuff, the high-thigh pressure is approximately 30 mmHg higher than the brachial systolic pressure. Other values indicate the presence of arterial occlusive disease of the aorta, iliac, common femoral, or both the superficial femoral and profunda femoris arteries. A pressure gradient of 20–30 mmHg between two consecutive cuffs on the leg indicates arterial occlusive disease at the level between the cuffs.

Segmental volume pulse recordings were obtained with the same pneumatic cuffs used to take the pressure measurements. The cuffs were snugly placed on the high thigh, above the knee, below the knee, and at the ankle. Using a Cardioline Pulsorette (Cardio-Vascular Electronics, Concord, California), also known as a volume pulse recorder, the examiner inflated the cuffs to 60 mmHg at each position, but evaluated both legs simultaneously. All measurements were recorded on a three-channel chart recorder at a paper speed of 25 mm/sec while the patient was resting in a supine position. The volume pulse recordings were assessed for pulse amplitudes and pulse volume contours as previously described (Figure 6-1).[4-6]

normal

stenosis

occlusion

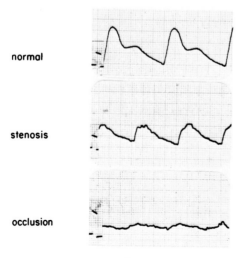

Figure 6-1. Segmental pulse volume recordings taken at the proximal thigh.

RESULTS

The results of the femoral arterial velocity waveforms, segmental limb blood pressures, segmental volume pulse recordings, and contrast arteriograms are presented in Table 6-1.

The sensitivity of the femoral arterial velocity waveforms was 100%, their specificity 70%, and their overall accuracy 80% in the detection or exclusion of significant ($>50\%$) stenosis or occlusion of the aortoiliac segment. Their negative predictive value was 100% and their positive predictive value 63%.

The sensitivity of the proximal thigh pressure was 100%, its specificity 72%, and its overall accuracy in detecting or excluding significant aortoiliac disease 82%. Its negative predictive value was 100% and its positive predictive value 65%. Segmental limb blood pressures were less sensitive to femoropopliteal and tibioperoneal arterial occlusive disease (73% and 53%, respectively) and somewhat nonspecific (59% and 89%, respectively). Their negative and positive predictive values were 88% and 66% respectively.

The sensitivity of the proximal thigh pulse recordings was 79% and their specificity 79%, giving an overall accuracy of 79% in the detection or exclusion of significant aortoiliac disease. The pulse volume recordings were relatively insensitive to femoropopliteal and tibioperoneal arterial disease, 67% and 60% respectively. The recordings were, however, somewhat more specific: 91% and 78%, respectively. The negative predictive values were poor—56% and 55%, respectively—but the positive predictive values were better, 94% and 81%, respectively.

Table 6-1. Results of Noninvasive and Arteriographic Studies

Contrast Arteriogram		Femoral Arterial Velocity		Segmental Pressure		Volume Pulse Recording	
Level	Stenosis	Normal	Abnormal	Normal	Abnormal	Normal	Abnormal
Aortoiliac	$<50\%$	33	14	34	13	37	10
	$\geq 50\%$	0	24	0	24	5	19
Femoropopliteal	$<50\%$	—	—	13	9	20	2
	$\geq 50\%$	—	—	13	35	16	32
Tibioperoneal	$<50\%$	—	—	24	3	21	6
	$\geq 50\%$	—	—	20	23	17	26

DISCUSSION

Segmental limb pressures were first described by Winsor[7] and later by Strandness and Bell,[5] using a four-level pressure measurement system. Pressures were obtained on the proximal thigh, above the knee, below the knee, and at the ankle. It was noted that a narrow cuff (10 × 40 cm) would result in an artificially elevated high-thigh pressure measurement because of the discrepancy between the width of the cuff and the girth of the limb. Thus, some investigators (Gundersen,[8] Yao and Bergan,[9] and Raines et al.[10] among them) have recommended the use of a single wide thigh cuff to minimize the artifact in the thigh pressure measurement. The wider cuff results in a thigh pressure measurement that normally approaches that of the brachial systolic pressure.

Heintz and colleagues questioned whether arterial occlusive lesions of the aortoiliac and femoropopliteal segments could be accurately localized using either the narrow proximal and distal thigh cuffs or the single wide thigh cuff.[1] They found that the proximal and distal thigh pressures correctly localized aortoiliac, femoropopliteal, or combined disease in 78% of the diseased extremities, whereas the wide cuff correctly localized only 19% of the arterial obstructions.

Darling and colleagues also noted some diagnostic limitations of wide cuffs placed on the thigh for volume pulse recordings taken to localize arterial occlusive disease. They found that volume pulse contours and amplitudes, as well as pressure measurements, were often identical in patients with aortoiliac, femoropopliteal, and combined lesions.[2]

CONCLUSIONS

The use of narrow proximal and distal thigh cuffs in obtaining volume pulse recordings increases the accuracy of diagnosing arterial occlusive lesions of the aortofemoral and femoropopliteal segments. Nevertheless, it is still difficult to determine the level of occlusive lesions involving the aortoiliac segment, the common femoral, the profunda femoris, or a combination of these arteries. Femoral arterial Doppler velocity waveforms can be used in conjunction with segmental pressures or pulse volume recordings to help differentiate aortoiliac disease from lesions of the common femoral artery and its two branches.

REFERENCES

1. Heintz SE, Bone GE, Slaymaker EE, et al: Value of arterial pressure measurements in proximal and distal part of the thigh in arterial occlusive disease. Surg Gynecol Obstet 146:337–343, 1978.

2. Darling CR, Raines JK, Brener JB, et al: Quantitative segmental pulse volume recorder: a clinical tool. Surgery 72:873–877, 1973.

3. Barnes RW, Wilson MR: *Doppler Ultrasonic Evaluation of Peripheral Arterial Disease: A Programmed Audio-Visual Instruction.* Iowa City, Iowa: University of Iowa Press, 1976, pp 71–128.

4. Kappert A, Winsor T: *Diagnosis of Peripheral Vascular Disease.* Philadelphia, FA Davis, 1972, pp 38–39.

5. Strandness DE Jr, Bell JW: Peripheral vascular disease: diagnosis and objective evaluation using a mercury strain gauge. Ann Surg [suppl] 161:3–35, 1965.

6. Winsor J, Sibley AE, Fisher EK, et al: Peripheral pulse contours in arterial occlusive disease. Vasc Dis 5:61–69, 1968.

7. Winsor T: Influence of arterial disease on the systolic blood pressure gradients of the extremity. Am J Med Sci 220:117–126, 1950.

8. Gundersen J: Segmental measurements of systolic blood pressure in the extremities including the thumb and the great toe. Acta Chir Scand [suppl] 426:1–90, 1972.

9. Yao JSR, Bergan JJ: Application of ultrasound to arterial and venous diagnosis. Surg Clin North Am 54:23–38, 1974.

10. Raines JK, Darling RC, Buth J, et al: Vascular laboratory criteria for the management of peripheral vascular disease of the lower extremities. Surgery 79:12–29, 1976.

CHAPTER 7

INTRAVENOUS DIGITAL ANGIOGRAPHY IN THE ASSESSMENT OF ARTERIAL DISEASE

Robert J. Lusby, William K. Ehrenfeld, and Ronald J. Stoney

Digital subtraction imaging of arterial structures following the intravenous injection of contrast media may revolutionize the approach to diagnosis of atherosclerotic vascular disease (hence its inclusion in a book otherwise devoted to noninvasive techniques). It is a radical departure from the conventional use of x-ray film to detect and record shadows. Real-time digital video processing of the fluoroscopically detected signal combined with digital subtraction techniques make it possible to detect small concentrations of iodine moving through the arterial system. The subsequent display of images following a variety of electronic enhancement procedures adds yet another dimension to this new technology.

Sporadic reports of digital subtraction angiography (DSA) followed its early application to cardiovascular imaging,[1-3] but the need for large volumes of toxic contrast media and the poor quality of the images made its application fairly impractical.[3] The introduction of photographic subtraction techniques to suppress the bony and soft-tissue backgrounds still did not result in a satisfactory intravenous image. The introduction of the image intensifier did make it possible to visualize the arterial tree in real time, however, and the arterial catheterization studies commonly

Supported by a grant from the Fogarty International Center, National Institutes of Health, USA; Grant No. 1 FO5 TWO3103-01.

used today were developed. Now the present boom in video techniques and electronic digital processing enables the signal obtained from an image intensifier (coupled to a television camera) to be recorded and processed. The storage of digital images in memories with identical specifications permits the processing of all data through an identical analog channel and the successful implementation of identical channel subtraction imaging.[4] Unlike film subtraction, the digital technique is ideal for enhancing the small iodine signals isolated by the subtraction process, and as a result it has renewed interest in an intravenous route for dye injection.[4-7]

Visualization of accessible vascular lesions is essential in planning surgery and justifies the small morbidity associated with conventional angiography. Because complications increase with age and in the presence of advanced atheromatous disease, however, some physicians have been deterred from proceeding to conventional angiography when the cause of symptoms is in doubt. It is in these patients with atypical or asymptomatic extracranial disease that the apparent safety of DSA is most appealing. This chapter outlines the principles of the intravenous digital subtraction techniques and demonstrates their clinical potentials.

TECHNOLOGY

Existing digital fluoroscopic systems differ greatly in their design, imaging capabilities, and fluoroscopic requirements.[5-7] Two independently developed systems are currently in use at the University of California, San Francisco. Radiographs from a fluoroscopic x-ray tube are detected by an image intensifier that is coupled to a television camera, and the resulting signal is digitized and transferred into a digital memory. With a pulse-mode system, the first image is obtained before the arrival of the contrast media and stored in one of two parallel digital memories to act as a mask for subsequent subtraction. During the passage of the iodine bolus, additional images are digitized into the second memory. For static images, the real-time data is integrated at a rate tailored for each study, usually about one image per second. The most important element in the imaging process is the subsequent subtraction, which isolates the clinically relevant subset of signals present in the unsubtracted image. The signal thus detected can be defined as the difference in the x-ray transmission with time.[7] In the absence of motion, this signal is created by the transient presence of iodine within the artery.

Dynamic studies with continuous-mode systems are also available. These systems use either tandem digital processing or rapid subtraction prior to enhancement, and then reconversion to analog form for display. The dynamics of flow of contrast through the field can thus be studied. The images are stored on video discs and tapes for subsequent display on a television monitor and for hard-copy production of the relevant images (Figures 7-1 and 7-2). Radiation exposure is no less than standard fluoroscopic examinations, ranging from 50–150 mrad/image for extracranial and extremity views to 200–300 mrad/image for abdominal views.[7,8]

The injection technique currently favored is via the femoral vein, which allows the rapid infusion of a bolus of contrast into the central venous system. A power injector is routinely used to obtain a rate of 12–16 ml/second. Usually 40 ml of contrast is sufficient to visualize the aortic arch and the extracranial and intracranial vessels; 60 ml is usually necessary for the abdominal and lower-limb vessels. In order to view the extracranial vessels separately, up to four runs are performed at varying angles.

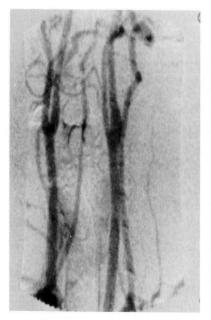

Figure 7-1. Intravenous digital subtraction images of normal extracranial vessels.

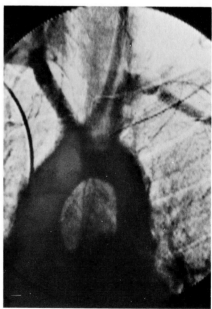

Figure 7-2. Intravenous digital subtraction angiogram of aortic arch and great vessels.

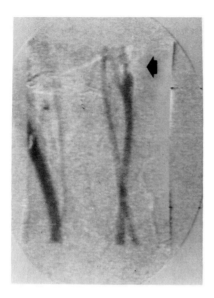 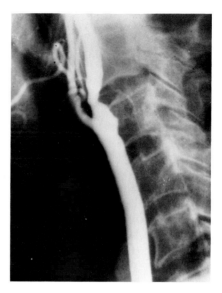

Figure 7-3. Intravenous digital subtraction image and conventional angiogram showing high-grade lesion of left internal carotid artery.

DISCUSSION

It is in the field of extracranial vascular disease that our preliminary experience is greatest. The main contribution of this new technology is its ability to demonstrate the carotid and vertebral arteries with safety. In Figure 7-3, high-grade stenosis of the internal carotid artery is demonstrated and the subsequent conventional angiogram is displayed for comparison. The need for multiple views to separate the origins of the internal and external carotid arteries and to separate the vertebral artery has become apparent. Heavy calcification may add to the difficulty of subtracting at the carotid bifurcation. Blurring of the image due to arterial motion is another limiting factor.[8] Also, the great distensibility[9] of the carotid bulb may limit high-grade resolution unless ECG gating is used.

In a study comparing the morphology outlined by DSA to the operative findings, we found an overall agreement between the two in 29 out of 33 (88%) of vessels. In the detection of lesions greater than 50% diameter reduction, the sensitivity of DSA when compared to the operative findings was 96% and its specificity was 86%, with an overall accuracy of 93.5%. Twenty-seven vessels were operated on without conventional angiography, and in 26 of 27 (96%) the pathological findings confirmed the appearance on DSA.[10]

The study indicated that in the majority of patients DSA provides the morphologic criteria necessary to allow surgical intervention. Occasionally (in approximately 12% of cases), the DSA study proved inadequate, and a conventional angiographic examination was necessary to demonstrate more precisely the pathologic anatomy. We proceeded to operate on 27 vessels with good-quality DSA studies, but were not content to proceed on the basis of a doubtful study. The use of conventional angiographic studies is strongly recommended when any doubt exists. In the presence of an abnormal screening test, such as a positive oculopneumoplethysmographic test, or in the presence of increased frequency and spectral broadening using Doppler detection of carotid blood flow, a normal DSA test should be regarded with suspicion. In these circumstances the quality of the DSA is often inadequate, and we have proceeded to conventional angiography with multiplanar views in order to determine the cause of the abnormal functional tests. Good-quality carotid DSA, in patients with appropriate symptomatology and functional tests, permits operations to proceed without further angiographic investigation, and it may become the imaging modality of choice in carotid artery disease.

Conventional angiography has its own well-defined limitations, such as the underestimation of atherosclerotic disease because of layering of contrast or persistence of an unopacified boundary layer. Vessels such as the internal carotid and profunda femoris arteries, which arise from the posterolateral aspect of their feeding vessels, require oblique and biplanar projections to help identify them. With DSA these limitations must clearly be defined and caution must be exercised until such multiplanar studies are complete. Nonetheless, in carefully selected patients DSA has proved to be of value, particularly when intraarterial catheterization poses the risk of dislodging an embolus. For instance, the patient in Figure 7-4 was referred with an abdominal aortic aneurysm and left-leg claudication. His accompanying digital study showed a short-segment occlusion of the left iliac artery and a patent external iliac and femoral arterial system, providing a thorough preoperative evaluation without the risk of an intraarterial study.

A further benefit of computerized enhancement technology is the ability to use small-dose (< 10 ml) contrast for intraarterial studies in patients with renal failure, iodine allergy, or combined extracranial and aortic atherosclerotic disease. It has the potential for expanding the information gained, using conventional-dose angiograms, in the delineation of

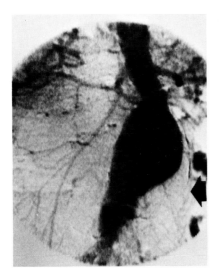 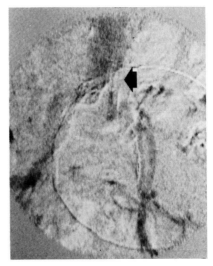

Figure 7-4. Intravenous digital subtraction images of abdominal aortic aneurysm with a short-segment occlusion of the left common iliac artery (*arrows*). Late views show patency of iliac system distal to the stenosis.

popliteal trifurcation disease in severe ischemia and in the runoff of patients with aortic aneurysms, in whom slow flow rates limit the conventional study. In the investigation of renal hypertension, the combination of DSA and urography could become the most helpful routine.

CONCLUSIONS

DSA represents a major advance in vessel imaging. Early experience comparing DSA to noninvasive carotid artery studies reveals its superiority in detecting occlusion of the carotid artery, a major limitation of the noninvasive technologies. It provides the surgeon with an image similar to a conventional angiogram, and provides diagnostic information that appears superior to the present array of complex noninvasive studies. DSA may overtake these modalities in the quest for safe and reliable morphologic information. Certainly the safety, quality, and economy of this modality suggest broad application in many surgical settings.

REFERENCES

1. Bernstein EF, Greenspan RH, Loken MK: Intravenous abdominal aortography. A preliminary report. Surgery 44:529–535, 1958.
2. Steinberg I, Finby N, Evans JR: A safe and practical intravenous method for abdominal aortography, peripheral arteriography and cerebral angiography. AJR 82:758–772, 1959.
3. Robb GP, Steinberg I: Visualization of the chambers fo the heart, the pulmonary circulation and the great blood vessels in man. AJR 41:1–17, 1939.
4. Mistretta CA, Crummy AB: Diagnosis of cardiovascular disease by digital subtraction angiography. Science 214:761–765, 1981.
5. Kruger RA, Mistretta CA, Lancaster J, et al: A digital video image processor for real time x-ray subtraction imaging. Optical Eng 17:652–654, 1978.
6. Ovitt TW, Christenson PC, Fisher HD, et al: Intravenous angiography using digital video subtraction: x-ray imaging system. AJR 135:1114–1144, 1980.
7. Gould RG, Lipton MJ, Mengers P, et al: Digital subtraction fluorscopic system with tandem video processing units. SPIE 274:125–131, 1981.
8. Crummy AB, Strother CM, Sackett JF, et al: Computerized fluoroscopy: digital subtraction for intravenous angiocardiography and arteriography. AJR 135:1131–1140, 1980.
9. Lusby RJ, Machleder HI, Jeans W, et al: Vessel wall and blood flow dynamics in arterial disease. Philos Trans R Soc Lond B294:231–239, 1981.
10. Lusby RJ, Ehrenfeld WK: Carotid artery surgery based on digital subtraction angiography. Am J Surg 144:211–214, 1982.

CHAPTER 8

OBSERVATIONS ON VASCULOGENIC IMPOTENCE

John J. Bergan

In 1940, Rene Leriche described the syndrome caused by thrombotic obliteration of the terminal aorta. Later he said, "if the disease is left to itself, sexual impotency will soon be permanent."[1] He recognized that the condition was not rare, and that the patients were young adults, mostly males. He knew that such patients presented themselves to the physician because of their inability to keep a stable erection and because of extreme fatigue in both lower extremities. He described the findings of global atrophy of the muscles of the limbs and absence of ischemic trophic changes of the skin and nails of the feet. In time, the attention of surgeons was directed toward consideration of restoration of blood flow to the genitalia. As techniques of aortic reconstruction became standardized, surgeons became aware of sexual dysfunction persisting after aortic surgery or occurring de novo after aortoiliac reconstruction. Now there is increasing interest by surgeons in trying to prevent postoperative sexual dysfunction and in attempting preoperatively to plan arterial reconstructions that will increase blood supply to the genitalia.

PHYSIOLOGY

Erotic stimuli initiate a series of changes in the male, of which penile erection is the first response. This is a vascular phenomenon produced by neural mediation. The neural control allows dilation of the arterial supply to the erectile tissues of the penis (corpora cavernosa and corpus spongiosum).[2] These erectile tissues are large venous sinuses which contain little blood when the penis is flaccid. Flow from these sinuses is blocked by valvelike structures (polsters or Ebner pads). The autonomic nerve supply to this arterialized smooth muscle is derived from both the parasympathetic and sympathetic levels of the spinal cord. The implication of this fact is that an intact sympathetic nervous system, parasympathetic nervous system, and arterial inflow are necessary for the production of an erection.

In assessing sexual function in patients who are about to undergo operation, it should be remembered that several forms of drug therapy, common in patients with arterial disease, can cause sexual dysfunction. For example, clonidine, methyldopa, and reserpine decrease libido and impair potency.[3] The ganglionic blocker trimethaphan impairs ejaculation, as does guanethidine, while the receptor antagonists phenoxybenzamine, phentolamine, and prazosin frequently impair ejaculation.[3] Also, diabetes mellitus manifests itself with neural and vascular elements. The neuropathy is frequent and may be an important cause of the impotence which occurs in one-fourth of all diabetic males under age 40.[4]

On the other hand, it has been found that there is no significant difference between diabetic and nondiabetic patients in extent of stenosis of the iliac arteries (both the common and internal).[5] This suggests that the vascular lesions which occur in diabetics are as important to the genesis of impotence in nondiabetics as they are in diabetics.

LABORATORY DIAGNOSIS OF IMPOTENCE

PENILE BLOOD PRESSURE

By far, the easiest laboratory test for the objective assessment of impotence is penile blood pressure. The various arteries of the penis, including the dorsal artery, are derived from the internal pudendal artery, which is a branch of the internal iliac artery (Figure 8-1). To obtain penile blood pressure, an inflatable cuff is placed at the base of the penis, inflated above systolic pressure, and then deflated until arterial flow returns to the penis (Figure 8-2). The return of such arterial flow has been measured by spectroscopy,[6] strain-gauge plethysmography,[7] impedance plethysmography,[8] Doppler ultrasound, and even pulse palpation. In the normal

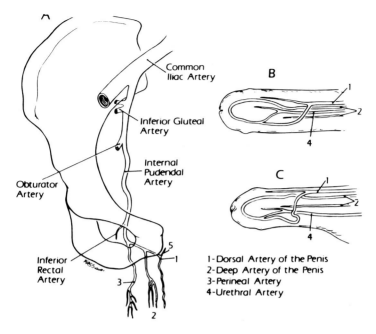

Figure 8-1. Major blood supply to the penis is from the deep and dorsal penile arteries and the urethral artery. All these arteries are branches of the internal pudendal artery, which is a large branch of the internal iliac artery. Reprinted with permission from Queral LA, Flinn WR, Bergan JJ, et al: Sexual function and aortic surgery. In *Surgery of the Aorta and its Body Branches.* Edited by JJ Bergan, JST Yao. New York, Grune & Stratton, 1979.

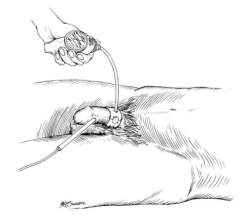

Figure 8-2. Technique of recording penile systolic pressure using the Doppler ultrasound technique. Reprinted with permission from Queral LA, Whitehouse WM Jr, Flinn WR, et al: Pelvic hemodynamics after aortoiliac reconstruction. Surgery 86:799–809, 1979.

81

patient, the penile blood pressure is about the same as the brachial systolic pressure. The penile/brachial index (PBI)[9] is of great value in comparing results between patient populations (Figure 8-3). It is generally felt that a PBI of 0.6 is useful as a guideline for the diagnosis of vascular impotence.[10-12] It is important to recognize that a penile blood pressure greater than 0.6 is reassuring, but that a pressure below this level cannot be taken as the only cause of the patient's sexual dysfunction.

An attempt has been made to analyze arterial pulse waveforms in assessing vasculogenic impotence.[8] A flattening of the pulse curve is the usual pathologic finding, but the significance of waveform signals is difficult to interpret. Such waveforms are a manifestation of vascular tone and may be related to apprehension during testing.

Kempczinski[10] has called attention to the fact that, in young patients who are capable of having an erection, the PBI is always greater than 0.80 and the penile volume waveform is of good or fair quality. Since young impotent patients have such findings, it is reasoned that the majority of such patients are impotent as a result of neurogenic factors or causes other than arterial blood flow. Beyond 40 years of age, Kempczinski says, all measured variables of penile blood flow deteriorate. The penile/brachial systolic gradient increases, the PBI falls, and the penile volume waveforms assume a more abnormal configuration. Other investigators have corroborated these findings.[13, 14]

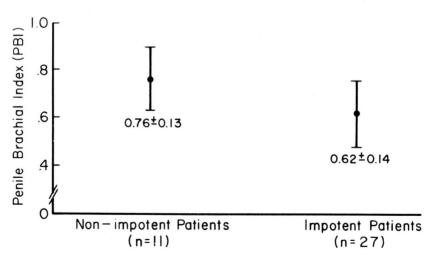

Figure 8-3. Penile/brachial index (PBI) in patients with normal potency and in impotent patients ($P < 0.05$). Reprinted with permission from Queral LA, Whitehouse WM Jr, Flinn WR, et al: Pelvic hemodynamics after aortoiliac reconstruction. Surgery 86:799–809, 1979.

Nocturnal Tumescence

In an attempt to separate organic from nonorganic causes of impotence, nocturnal penile tumescence has been measured.[15, 16] This test is based on the fact that all normal males from three to 79 years of age have nocturnal penile tumescence during normal sleep.[17-20] Therefore, this tumescence is measured in a carefully controlled atmosphere by special teams who are aware of the many implications of the method. The laboratory evaluation of nocturnal penile tumescence is complicated and time-consuming, and it requires a high degree of technical expertise.[16] Nevertheless, the measurement of nocturnal penile tumescence in combination with a thorough exploration of organic and psychogenic factors is helpful in assigning a cause to the symptom of impotence.[15]

Surgery and Impotence

While a number of surgical procedures have been advocated for the correction of impotence, the most applicable surgery relates to aortoiliac reconstruction.[11, 21-23] In such reconstructions, it is necessary to preserve the autonomic nerve fibers.[24, 25] Generally, autonomic nerve fibers crossing the aorta in the region of the inferior mesenteric artery should be avoided. Those of the aortic bifurcation, which contain ramifications of the anterior aortic plexus, and nerves surrounding the common iliac arteries and their superior hypogastric plexi should also be spared.

In the study by Hallbook and Holmquist, it was found that, in nine of ten men who reported absence of ejaculation after aortoiliac reconstruction, a dissection of the aorta and aortic bifurcation had been done. In contrast, those patients who had normal ejaculatory function had less dissection in the region of the aortic bifurcation.[26] Sabri and Cotton have also emphasized that the superior hypogastric sympathetic plexus should be preserved in order to maintain sexual function.[27] Queral has emphasized the hemodynamics of maintaining flow to the internal iliac system during arterial reconstruction.[11, 28] Also, Michal has called attention to the importance of maintaining stable hemodynamics in the pelvic territory.[21-23]

The general conclusions reached by careful study of the cases reported follow:

1. Aortic surgery should be done in such a way that the sympathetic fibers crossing the aorta and comprising the hypogastric plexus at the aortic bifurcation are preserved.

83

2. Pulsatile arterial blood flow should be maintained through the aorta, common iliac arteries, and internal iliac arteries whenever possible.

3. If transection of the aorta is necessitated by the type of aortic surgery to be done, blood flow should be restored to the internal iliac arteries through a nonobstructed arterial pathway, e.g., a noncompromised external iliac artery above the femoral anastomosis in aortofemoral bypass.

Sometimes abnormal pelvic hemodynamics are found—common iliac artery occlusion above a normally patent hypogastric artery, for example, when the contralateral internal iliac artery is occluded. In such cases, blood flow can be restored to the normal internal iliac artery by femorofemoral bypass with expectation of correction of the vasculogenic impotence and avoidance of sympathetic nerve damage (Figure 8-4).

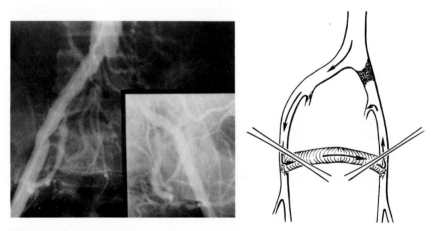

Figure 8-4. In a patient with total obstruction of the left common iliac artery and marked stenosis of the right internal iliac artery, a right-to-left femorofemoral graft augmented pelvic perfusion by retrograde flow through the left external iliac artery. Reprinted with permission from Queral LA, Whitehouse WM Jr, Flinn WR, et al: Pelvic hemodynamics after aortoiliac reconstruction. Surgery 86:799–809, 1979.

CONCLUSIONS

Patients with arterial insufficiency of the aortoiliac system frequently have sexual dysfunction. This dysfunction can be separated into its various components by use of noninvasive monitoring[29] and by careful history-taking, including the documentation of drug usage. When appropriate preoperative data are evaluated in light of arteriography, reconstructive operations frequently can be planned so as to maintain genital blood flow in patients who are capable of having erections preoperatively or to restore pulsatile arterial blood flow in those patients who are impotent.

REFERENCES

1. Leriche R, Morel A: The syndrome of thrombotic obliteration of the aortic bifurcation. Ann Surg 127:193–206, 1948.
2. deGroat WC, Booth AM: Physiology of male sexual function. Ann Intern Med 92: 329–331, 1980.
3. Reichgott MJ: Problems of sexual function in patients with hypertension. Cardiovasc Med 4:149–156, 1979.
4. Queral LA, Flinn WR, Bergan JJ, et al: Sexual function and aortic surgery. In *Surgery of the Aorta and its Body Branches*. Edited by JJ Bergan, JST Yao. New York, Grune & Stratton, 1979, pp 263–276.
5. Herman A, Adar R, Rubinstein Z: Vascular lesions associated with impotence in diabetic and nondiabetic arterial occlusive disease. Diabetes 27:975–981, 1978.
6. Gaskell P: The importance of penile blood pressure in cases of impotence. Can Med Assoc J 105:1047, 1971.
7. Britt DB, Kemmerer WT, Robison JR: Penile blood flow determination by mercury strain-gauge plethysmography. Invest Urol 8:673–678, 1971.
8. Canning JR, Bowers LM, Lloyd FA, et al: Genital vascular insufficiency and impotence. Surg Forum 14:298–299, 1963.
9. Gaylis H: Penile pressure in the evaluation of impotence in aortoiliac disease. Surgery 89:277–278, 1981.
10. Kempczinski RF: Role of the vascular diagnostic laboratory in the evaluation of male impotence. Am J Surg 138:278–282, 1979.
11. Queral LA, Whitehouse WM Jr, Flinn WR, et al: Pelvic hemodynamics after aorto-iliac reconstruction. Surgery 86:799–809. 1979.
12. Engel G, Burnham S, Carter MF: Penile blood pressure in the evaluation of erectile impotence. Fertil Steril 30:687, 1978.
13. Abelson D: Diagnostic value of the penile pulse and blood pressure: a Doppler study of impotence in diabetics. J Urol 113:636–639, 1975.
14. Malvar T, Baron T, Clark SS: Assessment of potency with the Doppler flowmeter. Urology 11:396–400, 1973.
15. Wasserman JD, Pollak CP, Spielman AJ, et al: The differential diagnosis of impotence. The measurement of nocturnal penile tumescence. JAMA 243:2038–2042, 1980.
16. Karacan I, Ware JC, Dervent B, et al: Impotence and blood pressure in the flaccid penis: relationship to nocturnal penile tumescence. Sleep 1:125–132, 1978.
17. Karacan I, Hursch CJ, Williams RL, et al: Some characteristics of nocturnal penile tumescence in young adults. Arch Gen Psychiatry 26:351–356, 1972.
18. Karacan I, Williams RL, Thornby JI, et al: Sleep-related tumescence as a function of age. Am J Psychiatry 132:932–937, 1975.

19. Karacan I, Salis PJ, Thornby JI, et al: The ontogeny of nocturnal penile tumescence. Waking Sleeping 1:27–44, 1976.

20. Hursch CJ, Karacan I, Williams RL: Some characteristics of nocturnal penile tumescence in early middle-aged males. Comp Psychiatry 13:539–548, 1972.

21. Michal V, Kramar R, Pospichal J, et al: Arterial epigastricocavernous anastomosis for the treatment of sexual impotence. World J Surg 1:515–520, 1977.

22. Michal V, Kramar R, Bartak V: Femoro-pudendal bypass in the treatment of sexual impotence. J Cardiovasc Surg 15:356–359, 1974.

23. Michal V, Kramar R, Pospichal J: Femoro-pudendal bypass, internal iliac thrombo-endarterectomy and direct arterial anastomosis to the cavernous body in the treatment of erectile impotence. Bull Soc Internat Chir 4:344–350, 1974.

24. Weinstein MH, Machleder HI: Sexual function after aortoiliac surgery. Ann Surg 181:787–790, 1975.

25. DePalma RG, Levine SB, Feldman S: Preservation of erectile function after aorto-iliac reconstruction. Arch Surg 113:958–962, 1978.

26. Hallbook T, Holmquist B: Sexual disturbances following dissection of the aorta and the common iliac arteries. J Cardiovasc Surg 11:255–260, 1970.

27. Sabri S, Cotton LT: Sexual function following aorto-iliac reconstruction. Lancet 2:1218–1219, 1971.

28. Queral LA, Dagher FJ, Yao JST, et al: Femoral steal syndrome: a report of five cases. Surg Forum 32:344–345, 1981.

29. Nath RL, Menzoian JO, Kaplan KH, et al: The multidisciplinary approach to vasculogenic impotence. Surgery 89:124–133, 1981.

Part II

NONINVASIVE
DIAGNOSIS OF
VENOUS DISEASE

CHAPTER 9

VENOUS
ANATOMY AND
PATHOPHYSIOLOGY

David S. Sumner

The venous system seems to stimulate less interest than the arterial system, perhaps because veins are perceived as rather passive conduits of blood that lack the dynamism of the arteries. Yet venous diseases, particularly in the legs, affect a large portion of the population, cause a tremendous amount of disability, and result in enormous economic losses. Moreover, emboli originating from the leg veins are a major cause of death. Increasing awareness of these problems has encouraged new research directed toward the diagnosis, treatment, and pathophysiology of venous disease.

In this chapter, some of the practical aspects of venous anatomy and physiology are discussed. These subjects are appreciably more complicated than they are in the arterial system.

ANATOMY

Unlike their arterial counterparts, the veins of the leg are divided into two systems: the superficial and the deep. The two principal veins in the superficial system are the greater (or long) saphenous vein and the lesser (or short) saphenous vein. Beginning just anteriorly and laterally to the medial malleolus, the greater saphenous vein courses up the medial aspect of the calf and thigh to enter the common femoral vein at the groin. The lesser saphenous vein, which is found posterior to the lateral malleolus, runs up the posterior aspect of the calf and terminates in the popliteal vein. Both of these veins are rather deeply situated, lying on the surface of the investing fascia. Draining into the saphenous veins are numerous tributaries, which lie more superficially in the subcutaneous areolar tissue. One of these veins, the posterior arch vein, deserves special mention because it represents the superficial connection of the three ankle perforating veins, which are of major importance in the genesis of venous stasis ulcers. The posterior arch vein begins behind the medial malleolus and passes up the medial aspect of the calf to enter the greater saphenous vein at knee level.

The major deep veins are analogues of the corresponding arteries. They lie adjacent to the arteries of the same name. In the calf, these deep veins are usually duplicated into venous comitantes, one lying on each side of the artery. Large spindle-shaped veins called *soleal sinusoids* collect the venous drainage from the soleus muscle and terminate in the posterior tibial and peroneal veins. The veins draining the gastrocnemius muscle are tributaries of the popliteal vein. These large muscular "sinusoids" are important physiologically, because they act as the principal "bellows" of the muscle pump (see below), and pathologically, because they are a favored site for the formation of thrombi.

Connecting the deep and superficial systems are a series of perforating or communicating veins. In the thigh there is a constant perforating vein—the so-called *Hunterian perforator*—that connects the superficial femoral vein to the greater saphenous vein. More numerous and more important are the perforating veins in the calf, three of which have been alluded to above in the discussion of the posterior arch vein.

Perhaps the most significant feature of venous structure is the presence of bicuspid valves. These valves are oriented to permit blood to flow in a cephalad direction only. When functioning properly, they preclude retrograde flow down the leg. Valves in the perforating veins direct blood from the superficial to the deep system. Just cephalad to and surrounding the valve cusps, the vein is dilated to form a small sinus. This aides the function of the valves by facilitating their closure. Without the dilated area, the valves when open would be closely approximated to the venous wall. Because blood flow at the base of the valve cusp is relatively stagnant, venous thrombi tend to form in the valve sinuses.

Valves are much more numerous in the veins below the knee than they are in the more proximal veins. The vena cava and common iliac veins are valveless. Only about one-fourth of the external iliac veins contain a valve, and about three-quarters of the femoral veins have a valve. One to four valves are present in the superficial femoral vein, one to three in the popliteal, about seven in the peroneal, and nine in the anterior tibial and posterior tibial veins. A valve is constantly present in the profunda femoris vein just before it joins the superficial femoral vein to form the common femoral vein. Within the terminal 2 to 3 cm of the saphenous vein, there are one or two valves. The remainder of this vein contains 10 to 20 valves, most of which are below the knee. The lesser sephenous vein has 6 to 12 valves.

At first glance a phlebogram appears quite confusing because there are so many veins. However, if one remembers the distribution of the major arteries of the leg, it is relatively easy to identify all of the deep veins. The greater saphenous vein is best seen in an anterior-posterior view, where it lies medial to the deep veins. A lateral view demonstrates the lesser saphenous vein more clearly. Soleal and gastrocnemial veins are more difficult to fill with contrast and often are not visualized. When they do fill, however, they stand out most clearly in a lateral projection, where they can be identified because of their shape, position, and termination in the posterior tibial or popliteal veins. Because it is not in the mainstream of the drainage from the foot, ascending phlebography seldom demonstrates the profunda femoris vein, although a very short segment distal to its terminal valve is often seen.

PHYSIOLOGY

VENOUS RESISTANCE

When distended, the cross-sectional area of the veins is about 3 to 4 times than of the corresponding arteries. It is not surprising, then, that the extra pulmonary veins contain about two-thirds of the blood in the body. Nevertheless, it is somewhat surprising that—despite their large diameter—veins offer about the same resistance to flow as arteries. One usually thinks of the veins as a low-pressure, low-resistance system; but when one recalls that the pressure drop from the heart to the arterioles is about 15 mmHg, that the pressure drop from the venules to the right atrium is about the same, and that both the arteries and the veins carry the same amount of blood, it becomes obvious that the total peripheral venous and arterial resistances are similar. This paradoxic situation is explained by the collapsible nature of the venous wall. Veins are seldom completely full. In the partially empty state, they assume a flattened or elliptical cross section, which offers a great deal more resistance to blood flow than a circular cross section. This ability to go from an elliptical to a circular cross section is distinctly advantageous. It permits the veins to accommodate a great increase in blood flow without an increase in the pressure gradient from the periphery to the heart. In other words, as the rate of flow increases, the vein becomes more circular, lessening resistance.

HYDROSTATICS

Hydrostatic pressure is equivalent to the weight of the column of blood extending from the heart to the level where the pressure is being measured. Expressed mathematically:

$$P \text{ (hydrostatic)} = \varrho gh \tag{9-1}$$

where ϱ is the density of blood (approximately 1.056 g/cm³), g is the acceleration due to gravity (980 cm/sec²), and h is the distance in centimeters below the heart. This formula gives the pressure in dynes/cm², which can be converted to mmHg by dividing by 1333.

The pressure at any point in an artery or vein is the sum of the dynamic pressure derived from the contraction of the left ventricle and the hydrostatic pressure. Although hydrostatic pressure affects both the arterial and venous pressures equally, its effect is more noticeable on the venous side because of the lower dynamic pressure in the veins. Some of these relationships are illustrated in Figure 9-1, which depicts a six-foot man

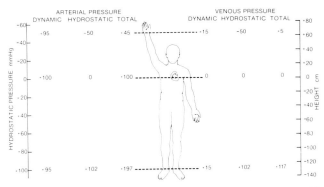

Figure 9-1. Effect of hydrostatic pressure on venous and arterial pressures. The reference point for zero pressure is at the right atrium. If the subject were supine, total intravascular pressure would closely approximate the dynamic pressure. Reprinted with permission from Sumner DS: The hemodynamics and pathophysiology of venous disease. In *Vascular Surgery*. Edited by RB Rutherford. Philadelphia, WB Saunders, 1977, pp 147–163.

whose heart and ankles are separated by a vertical distance of 131 cm in the standing position. When the subject is supine, all of the veins and arteries are roughly at the same level as the heart; consequently, the differences in hydrostatic pressure are negligible, and the pressures at various points in the arterial and venous sytems are almost totally represented by the dynamic pressure derived from the heart. The pressure in the centrally located great veins is close to zero (i.e., atmospheric pressure) and that in the ankle veins is 15 mmHg. When the subject stands, a hydrostatic pressure of 102 mmHg is added to the dynamic pressure, giving a total venous pressure of 117 mmHg at the ankle.

The same phenomenon occurs in the arteries at ankle level, where the mean pressure rises from 95 mmHg to 197 mmHg as the subject shifts from the supine to the vertical position. Since the increase in pressure in both the arteries and veins is identical, the pressure gradient across the capillaries at ankle level is unchanged (80 mmHg in both positions). As will be discussed later, contraction of the leg muscles in the upright position reduces the venous pressure, often to values as low as 5 mmHg. Since exercise has no direct effect on the arterial pressure, the gradient across the capillaries is increased from 80 mmHg to 192 mmHg (197 mmHg − 5 mmHg). This increased gradient greatly facilitates the increased flow required during exercise and, thus, reflects a major contribution of hydrostatic pressure to the functioning of the muscle pump mechanism.

The situation is remarkably different in the uplifted arm. In the example given (Figure 9-1), the hydrostatic pressure is "negative," subtracting 50 mmHg from the dynamic pressure in the arteries at wrist level. The venous pressure, however, cannot fall below the tissue pressure of 5 mmHg; otherwise, the veins would be completely collapsed and no blood would flow. Therefore, the perfusion pressure across the capillaries at wrist level falls from 80 mmHg in the supine position to 40 mmHg when the arm is lifted. The lower pressure gradient explains why it is more difficult to work with the arm above the head than it is when the arms are at waist or heart level.

PRESSURE-VOLUME RELATIONSHIPS

Because veins are collapsible, their shape is determined by the transmural pressure. Transmural pressure is the difference between the pressure within the vein and the ambient tissue pressure. When the transmural pressure is low, veins assume a dumbell configuration, but as the intraluminal pressure rises, the cross section first becomes elliptical and finally circular (Figure 9-2). These changes in configuration,

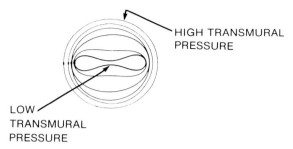

HIGH TRANSMURAL PRESSURE

LOW TRANSMURAL PRESSURE

Figure 9-2. Effect of various transmural pressures on the cross-sectional configuration of the venous lumen. Adapted by permission of the American Heart Association from Moreno et al: Mechanics of distension of dog veins and other thin-walled tubular structures. Circ Res 27:1069, 1970.

which are due primarily to "bending" of the venous wall with comparatively little increase in the venous circumference, are accompanied by a great increase in venous volume. After the vein becomes circular, further increases in pressure stretch the wall. Because the venous wall is rather stiff, a much greater change in pressure is required to produce a given change in volume when the vein is circular than is required when the vein is partially collapsed.

These points are illustrated graphically in Figure 9-3, which depicts a typical venous pressure-volume curve. When the subject is supine and transmural pressures are low, a small increase in venous pressure results in a large change in venous volume. However, when the subject is upright and transmural pressures are high, even a large increase in venous pressure has relatively little effect on venous volume. These observations are

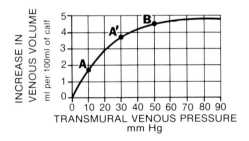

INCREASE IN VENOUS VOLUME
ml per 100ml of calf

TRANSMURAL VENOUS PRESSURE
mm Hg

Figure 9-3. Relationship of calf venous volume to transmural venous pressure. **A** Pressure and volume in normal supine limb; **A′** pressure and volume in a limb with venous obstruction; **B** pressure and volume when the transmural pressure has been artificially elevated to 50 mmHg. Reprinted with permission from Sumner DS: Strain gauge plethysmography in venous disease. In *Noninvasive Diagnostic Techniques in Vascular Disease,* second edition. Edited by EF Bernstein. St Louis, CV Mosby, 1982.

significant when one considers the effect of compression stockings on venous volume. The typical antiembolism stocking, which exerts 15 mmHg pressure, increases the "tissue pressure" from about 5 mmHg to 15 mmHg, and reduces the transmural pressure by about 10 mmHg. When the patient is supine, this reduction is transmural pressure markedly reduces venous volume, practically collapses the underlying veins, and speeds the velocity of venous blood flow. On the other hand, the same stockings have little effect on venous volume when the subject is sitting or standing.

Impedance plethysmography and other plethysmographic tests for deep venous thrombosis depend, in part, on the measurement of increases in calf volume that occur in response to the inflation (50 mmHg) of a pneumatic cuff wrapped around the thigh. After the cuff is inflated, venous outflow from the calf ceases until the venous pressure rises to 50 mmHg. The volume of the calf rises, until the rate of venous outflow equals the arterial inflow. In a normal limb, with a transmural venous pressure of 10 mmHg (point A in Figure 9-3) the increase in pressure to 50 mmHg (point B) results in a great increase in calf volume. When there is deep venous obstruction, the pressure within the calf veins is elevated (point A′) and there is relatively little increase in volume when the cuff is inflated to 50 mmHg (point B).

EDEMA FORMATION

Edema formation is one of the most consistent signs of an elevated peripheral venous pressure. According to the Starling hypothesis, as blood traverses the capillary, fluid escapes into the interstitial spaces on the arteriolar end and is resorbed on the venular end (Figure 9-4). On the arteriolar end, the sum of the intracapillary pressure (P_c) and the osmotic pressure of the interstitial fluid (π_{IF}) exceeds the sum of the interstitial fluid pressure (P_{IF}) and the osmotic pressure within the capillary (π_c), resulting in a net gradient favoring the motion of fluid out of the capillary. On the venular end, the drop in intracapillary pressure (P_c) reverses the gradient. At the center of the capillary, the forces are balanced, so that overall there is little fluid loss to the lymphatics.

Standing, however, increases the arteriolar, capillary, and venular pressures by 80 mmHg to 100 mmHg. The increased capillary pressure is no longer counteracted by the interstitial pressure and the osmotic pressure, resulting in a net loss of fluid into the interstitial tissues. In a normal individual, this tendency toward edema formation is circumvented by the venous pump mechanism, which acts to reduce venous pressure in the standing position.

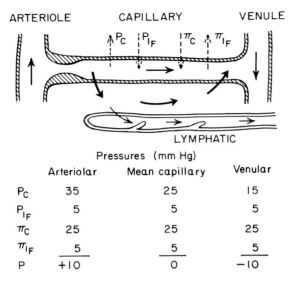

ARTERIOLE   CAPILLARY   VENULE

LYMPHATIC

Pressures (mm Hg)

	Arteriolar	Mean capillary	Venular
P_C	35	25	15
P_{IF}	5	5	5
π_C	25	25	25
π_{IF}	5	5	5
P	+10	0	-10

Figure 9-4. Diagram illustrating forces involved in fluid exchange across a capillary bed. *Solid arrows:* direction of fluid flow. *Dashed arrows:* direction of pressure gradients. Symbols are defined in the text. Reprinted with permission from Strandness DE Jr, and Sumner DS: *Hemodynamics for Surgeons.* New York, Grune & Stratton, 1975.

Venous thrombosis, by increasing venous pressure, causes edema to develop even when the patient is supine. In such situations, edema can be reduced by the application of elastic stockings, which increase the extravascular (interstitial) pressure, or by elevating the legs, which reduces the intravascular pressure in proportion to the decrease in hydrostatic pressure.

VENOUS DYNAMICS—AT REST

Respiration has a profound effect on venous flow patterns. Basically, blood returning from the legs must pass through two "closed" compartments, the abdomen and the thorax, before reaching the right atrium (Figure 9-5). During inspiration, the descent of the diaphragm increases the intraabdominal pressure ("P_{cv}") and reduces the intrathoracic pressure (P_{cv}). As a result, blood is propelled from the upper portion of the abdomen into the thorax. In contrast, inspiration impedes the flow of blood from the legs. The intraabdominal pressure rises, decreasing the pressure gradient from the periphery to the abdomen, and blood flow from the legs decreases, often to zero. With expiration, the intraabdominal pressure falls, blood flow from the legs to the abdomen increases,

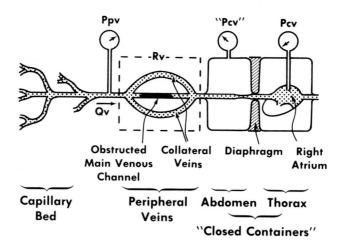

Figure 9-5. Factors influencing venous return from the legs. See text for discussion. Reprinted with permission from Sumner DS: The hemodynamics and pathophysiology of venous disease. In *Vascular Surgery*. Edited by RB Rutherford. Philadelphia, WB Saunders, 1977, pp 147–163.

and flow from the abdomen to the thorax decreases. These fluctuations in venous flow are readily detected with the Doppler flowmeter or the phleborheograph at all levels of the leg (see Chapters 11 and 12).

Venous obstruction, due to thrombi in the leg veins or extrinsic compression, may affect peripheral venous pressure (P_{pv}).

$$P_{pv} - P_{cv} = Q_v R_v \tag{9-2}$$

$$P_{pv} = Q_v R_v + P_{cv} \tag{9-3}$$

In these formulas, Q_v represents the venous outflow and R_v, the resistance of the peripheral veins. It is evident from Formula 9-3 that a rise in the venous resistance (R_v) would cause the peripheral venous pressure to increase. The magnitude of the increase in venous pressure depends on the extent of the venous thrombosis and the adequacy of the collateral circulation. It is also clear from formula 9-3 that cardiac failure, by increasing the central venous pressure (P_{cv}), would increase peripheral venous pressure.

Formula 9-2 can be rewritten to explain how an increase in peripheral resistance affects the pattern of blood flow from the legs:

$$Q_v = \frac{P_{pv} - ``P_{cv}"}{R_v} \tag{9-4}$$

With the increased resistance imposed by a thrombus or extrinsic compression, the peripheral venous pressure (P_{pv}) rises to a level far in excess of the intraabdominal pressure ("P_{cv}"). Therefore, the variations in intraabdominal pressure that accompany respiration have little effect on the overall pressure gradient ($P_{pv} - $ "P_{cv}"), and the fluctuations in venous flow that are normally appreciated with the Doppler or phleborheograph are reduced or abolished. In other words, flow becomes more continuous. This is one of the key diagnostic signs of venous obstruction.

VENOUS DYNAMICS—WITH EXERCISE

The return of blood flow from the legs against the force of gravity is facilitated by the muscle pump mechanism. The muscles of the leg—particularly those in the calf—act as the power source and the veins, as the bellows. Although the superficial veins take part, the deep veins—especially the intramuscular sinusoids—play the major role. The presence of valves is necessary to ensure the efficient action of the entire mechanism.

At rest, the veins simply collect the blood from the capillaries and transmit it passively to the heart, the blood being propelled only by the dynamic pressure gradient created by the contraction of the left ventricle (Figure 9-6). In normal extremities, contraction of the calf muscles

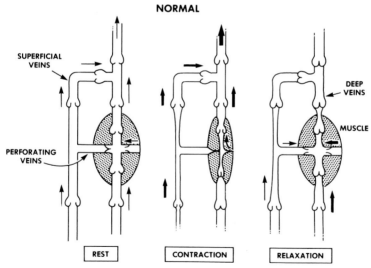

Figure 9-6. Dynamics of the muscle pump mechanism in a normal limb. Reprinted with permission from Sumner DS: Venous dynamics—varicosities. Clin Obstet Gynecol 24: 743–760, 1981.

forces blood upward in both the superficial and deep veins. Valves in the perforating veins and those distal to the calf muscles are closed, preventing the reflux of blood. When the calf muscles relax, a potential space is created in the deep veins, and blood is "sucked" from the superficial veins into the deep veins through the perforators. The more peripheral veins also empty into the veins of the calf. Closure of the valves in the proximal portions of the deep veins reduces the length of the blood column so that it no longer extends from the heart to the ankle, but only for a few centimeters between valves. The effect of this action is to reduce the peripheral venous pressure.

Figure 9-7 illustrates the effect of exercise on pressure measured in a foot vein of a normal subject. With the subject standing quietly, the

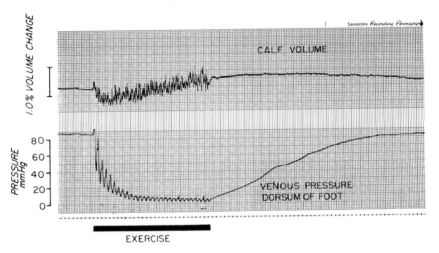

Figure 9-7. Effect of exercise on venous pressure in a normal limb. Calf volume is initially reduced but then increased as the muscle changes configuration. Reprinted with permission from Strandness DE Jr, Sumner DS: *Hemodynamics for Surgeons*. New York, Grune & Stratton, 1975.

pressure was about 88 mmHg. After a few calf muscle contractions, the pressure fell to about 5 mmHg. After the cessation of exercise, venous pressure rose very slowly to preexercise levels, the depleted veins being filled only through inflow from the capillaries.

Incompetence of the superficial venous valves impairs the normal function of the muscle pump. Patients with primary varicose veins have incompetent femoral valves and incompetent valves in the greater saphenous vein (Figure 9-8). Walking again forces blood cephalad in both the superficial and deep veins, but when the leg relaxes, blood falls down the

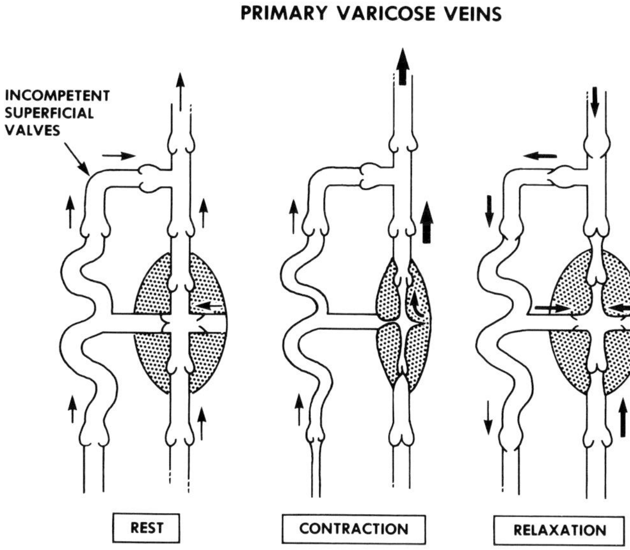

PRIMARY VARICOSE VEINS

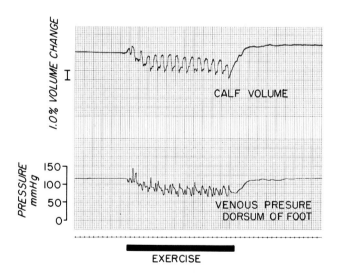

Figure 9-8. Dynamics of the muscle pump mechanism in a limb with primary varicose veins. Reprinted with permission from Sumner DS: Venous dynamics—varicosities. Clin Obstet Gynecol 24: 743–760, 1981.

Figure 9-9. Effect of exercise on venous pressure in a limb with primary varicose veins. Note that the calf volume and venous pressure rapidly return to preexercise levels after cessation of exercise. This is caused by reflux of blood down the saphenous vein. Reprinted with permission from Strandness DE Jr, Sumner DS: *Hemodynamics for Surgeons*. New York, Grune & Stratton, 1975.

superficial veins and reenters the deep system via the perforating veins. In effect, this creates an inefficient circular motion of a portion of the blood. In addition, the long uninterrupted column of blood from the heart to the ankle in the superficial veins keeps the venous pressure high. Walking reduces the venous pressure only 30–50 mmHg, depending on the severity of the venous incompetence (Figure 9-9).

The to-and-fro motion of blood in the superficial veins that characterizes limbs with varicosities is illustrated in Figure 9-10. As this figure indicates, the volume of blood refluxing down the veins is far greater than that forced up the veins during calf muscle contraction.

In cases of chronic venous insufficiency, the physiology is even more abnormal. Not only are the valves in the superficial, deep, and perforating veins incompetent, but also there is a variable element of venous obstruction (Figure 9-11). Because of the deep venous obstruction, blood

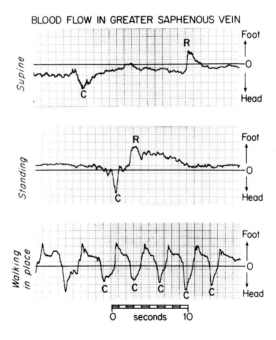

Figure 9-10. Blood flow in the greater saphenous vein of a patient with varicose veins. With calf muscle contraction (C) blood flows cephalad, but with relaxation (R) blood refluxes down the leg. Recordings were made with a Doppler flow detector. Reprinted with permission from Strandness DE Jr, Sumner DS: *Hemodynamics for Surgeons*. New York, Grune & Stratton, 1975.

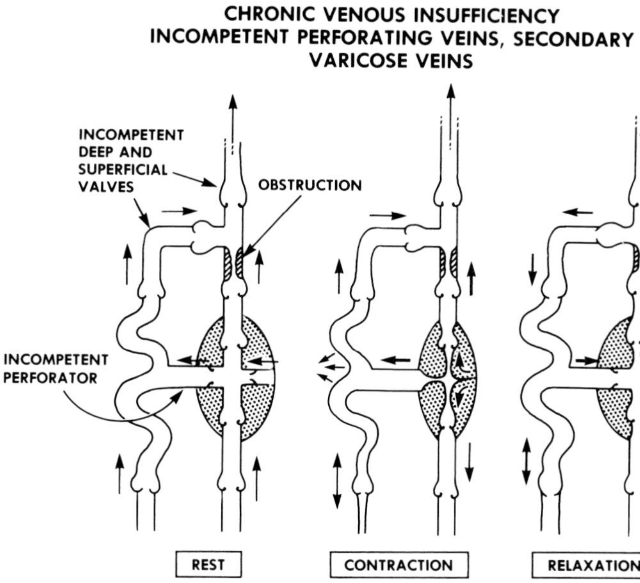

**CHRONIC VENOUS INSUFFICIENCY
INCOMPETENT PERFORATING VEINS, SECONDARY
VARICOSE VEINS**

Figure 9-11. Dynamics of the muscle pump mechanism in a postphlebitic limb. Reprinted with permission from Sumner DS: Venous dynamics—varicosities. Clin Obstet Gynecol 24: 743–760, 1981.

may flow out of the deep veins into the superficial veins through incompetent perforators—even at rest. In other words, the superficial veins function as collaterals from the obstructed deep veins. This outward flow through the perforators is accentuated during muscle contraction. Moreover, muscle contraction tends to force blood distally toward the foot, owing to both the incompetence of the deep valves and the impediment to cephalad flow created by the venous obstruction. With muscle relaxation, blood refluxes down both the superficial and the deep veins, creating a column of blood in both systems that extends from the heart to the ankles. The effect of all of this is to create an inefficient circular flow of blood and to prevent the calf muscle pump from reducing the peripheral venous pressure. In fact, in the more severe cases, walking actually increases the peripheral venous pressure.

Because of the increase in venous pressure, there is an exudation of fluid and red cells into the subcutaneous tissues. This fluid becomes organized, resulting in induration of the tissues and eventual ulceration. Changes are often most marked in those tissues that receive the high pressure outflow from the incompetent perforating veins.

COMMENT

The complexities of the venous circulation are receiving increasing attention—attention that is well deserved because of the magnitude of the clinical problems presented by venous disease. In no small part, this is due to the ready availability and simplicity of the newer noninvasive diagnositc methods, including the Dopper flow detector and various forms of plethysmography. These methods, which are discussed in subsequent chapters, permit the clinician to detect abnormal physiology, to evaluate its severity, and to localize the sites involved.

BIBLIOGRAPHY

1. Dodd H, Cockett FB: *The Pathology and Surgery of the Veins of the Lower Limb*. Edinburgh, Churchill Livingstone, 1976.
2. Ludbrook J: *Aspects of Venous Function in the Lower Limbs*. Springfield, Illinois, Charles C Thomas, 1966.
3. Strandness DE Jr, Sumner DS: *Hemodynamics for Surgeons*. New York, Grune & Stratton, 1975.
4. Sumner DS: The hemodynamics and pathophysiology of venous disease. In *Vascular Surgery*. Edited by RB Rutherford. Philadelphia, WB Saunders, 1977, pp 157–163.
5. Sumner DS: Venous dynamics—varicosities. Clin Obstet Gynecol 24:743–760, 1981.

CHAPTER 10

The Diagnosis and Assessment of Venous Disorders in the Office and Laboratory

Terry N. Needham

The clinical assessment of venous disorders of the limbs is less well defined than that for the arterial system. The hemodynamics are more complex (see Chapter 9), and there are no palpable pulses and no bruits (unless there is an A/V fistula). Venography gives structural, not functional, information, and for this noninvasive assessment is helpful. This chapter discusses the indications, the limitations, and the physiologic basis of these noninvasive examinations of the veins.

The advantages of noninvasive techniques are that the equipment is transportable, the tests are quite objective and repeatable, and they can be done in the office or laboratory by the clinician or technician. These tests are used in the following two categories of venous disorders:

1. Deep venous thrombosis, to make the diagnosis and to avoid unnecessary venography, hospitalization, and anticoagulant therapy.
2. Chronic venous insufficiency, to detect or confirm it and to differentiate between insufficiency of the deep or superficial venous systems; the management of deep venous insufficiency and superficial venous insufficiency differ, particularly if there is obstruction of deep veins and venous outflow is via superficial collateral channels.

Noninvasive tests also can be used to assess the results of surgery, to follow the course of patients with outflow obstruction or valvular incompetence, and to measure the efficacy of support hose or bandaging.

Damage to venous valves is a common sequel to deep or superficial venous thrombosis, and the resulting valvular incompetence can cause severe symptoms. Control of the superficial varices, or incompetent perforators, can improve venous function and encourage the healing of venous ulcers, even when the deep system remains incompetent. The various treatments—including elastic support, injection sclerotherapy, and surgery— attempt to correct the abnormal physiology by, for example, reducing the "dead space" into which the calf muscles pump blood, improving venous emptying, and lowering the elevated ambulatory venous pressure, thereby relieving symptoms and reducing the incidence of ulceration (Table 10-1). Lowering the ambulatory venous pressure should improve the rate of healing of ulcers and reduce the probability of recurrence.

The noninvasive techniques most commonly used to detect venous thrombosis are Doppler ultrasound,[1,2] impedance[3,4] and volume plethysmography[5,6] (see Chapters 11–13), and, less commonly, the ^{125}I fibrinogen uptake test (FUT).[7] In addition, thermography[8] (which requires equipment), strain-gauge plethysmography[9] and levels of β thromboglobulin[10] (both of which are largely supplanted), and ^{99}Tc plasmin[11] and Doppler imaging[12] (neither of which are in general use) have all been described.

Chronic venous insufficiency can be assessed by Doppler ultrasound[13] and by strain-gauge,[14] volume,[15] and photoplethysmography[16] (see Chapters 13 and 14), which can detect significant obstruction to outflow and

Table 10-1. The Incidence of Venous Ulceration (Active or Healed) Related to Ambulatory Venous Pressure (AVP)[a]

AVP mmHg	Incidence of Ulceration
<45	0
45–50	5%
50–59	15%
60–69	50%
70–79	75%
>80	80%

[a] Reprinted with permission from Nicolaides AN, Shull K, Fernandes é Fernandes, J, et al: Ambulatory venous pressure: new information. In *Investigation of Vascular Disorders*. Edited by AN Nicolaides and JST Yao. Edinburgh, Churchill Livingstone, 1981, pp 488–494.

valvular incompetence of the superficial, perforating, and deep venous systems. The most widely used methods are described in Chapters 11–14, and in a manual of noninvasive techniques.[17]

DIAGNOSING VENOUS INSUFFICIENCY

DOPPLER ULTRASOUND

Venous insufficiency is valvular insufficiency. The sites of clinical importance are the saphenofemoral and saphenopopliteal junctions and the popliteal vein. Incompetence in the leg veins is detected with the patient standing because reflux is greater and is heard more easily. The leg under examination should be relaxed with weight supported on the other leg. Reflux is elicited by the Valsalva maneuver. Augmentation can be heard proximal to common femoral, saphenofemoral, and popliteal levels with compression maneuvers. Directional Doppler instruments also detect reversed flow. (In our hands, Doppler ultrasound has been unreliable in detecting incompetent perforating veins, and we prefer venous photoplethysmography for this purpose.) Refer to the following chapter for a detailed discussion of the venous Doppler examination.

Examining the Saphenofemoral Junction

The patient stands facing the examiner and holds onto a table to prevent movement and leg-muscle contraction. Holding the probe over the common femoral artery at the crease of the groin, the examiner should angle the probe at 45 degrees and listen over the vein just medial to the artery. Flow may be so slow while the patient stands relaxed that nothing is heard, or a faint signal, phasic with respiration, may be heard. To confirm the position of the probe, the examiner squeezes the thigh or calf, eliciting a brisk signal from the blood that is forced up toward the heart. Repeating this maneuver, the examiner adjusts the position of the probe to obtain a maximal signal from the center of the vein.

During coughing or Valsalva maneuvers or after release of calf or thigh compression, no sound is heard unless there is reflux. If reverse flow and reflux away from the heart is audible, it is loud and clear, lasting one to four seconds. A faint, brief reverse signal is sometimes heard in normal legs, but it is of no clinical importance.

The examiner repeats the maneuver, but now occludes the saphenous vein 5–10 cm below the groin to prevent reflux. If reverse flow is not audible, then any reflux first heard was indeed saphenous. If reflux persists during saphenous occlusion, it signifies incompetence of the superficial femoral vein.

Examining the Popliteal Vein and the Saphenopopliteal Junction

The patient stands facing away from the examiner and holding onto a table or rail for steadiness and to ensure that no muscle contraction propels blood upward to confuse the examination. The examiner applies the Doppler probe at a 45-degree angle at the popliteal skin crease and listens for the popliteal artery and vein. Figure 10-1 shows the reversal of flow on release (tracing is below the zero baseline) that denotes reflux.

The technique for detecting reflux has been validated with ambulatory venous pressure measurements in normal volunteers, patients with primary varicose veins, and others with postphlebitic syndrome. The interpretation of reflux has been confirmed also by descending and ascending venography and by calf-volume plethysmography and photoplethysmography. Criteria for diagnosis of the various varicose vein syndromes are presented in Table 10-2.

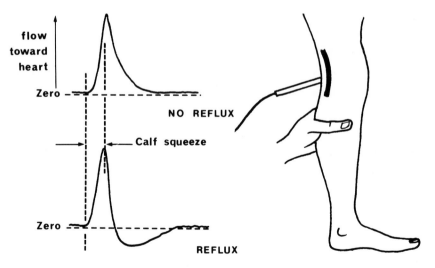

Figure 10-1. Doppler probe at level of popliteal vein with hand positioned ready to compress the calf. *Upper Doppler velocity tracing:* augmented flow toward heart when calf is compressed, and no reflux (flow below zero line) on release. *Lower tracing:* augmented flow when calf is compressed, but on release the flow falls below zero line, indicating reflux through an incompetent valve.

Table 10-2. Diagnostic Criteria for Superficial and Deep Venous Incompetence

Site of Incompetence	Directional Doppler Reflux	Effect of Superficial Venous Tourniquet
Saphenofemoral junction	Saphenofemoral reflux	High thigh tourniquet stops reflux and prevents filling of varicosities.
Saphenopopliteal	Popliteal reflux	Tourniquet just below the knee abolishes reflux and prevents filling of varicose veins.
Midthigh perforating		Low thigh tourniquet prevents filling of varicosities.
Deep venous valves	Popliteal reflux	No effect of superficial venous occluding tourniquets on popliteal reflux or on varicose veins.
Calf perforators	Not ideal for diagnosis of incompetent calf perforating veins	Tourniquet below the knee has no effect on varicosities.

AMBULATORY VENOUS PRESSURES

Ambulatory venous pressures are objective quantitative tests for the diagnosis and assessment of venous insufficiency, particularly the important clinical differentiation of deep and superficial venous valvular insufficiency, and for the objective measurement of its severity (Figure 10-2).

Measurement of ambulatory venous pressures, however, is an invasive technique unsuitable for routine clinical use. Two noninvasive methods are helpful in this regard, photoplethysmography and calf-volume plythysmography.

PHOTOPLETHYSMOGRAPHY

Photoplethysmography (PPG) has proved effective in the objective evaluation of chronic venous insufficiency. PPG cannot yet be calibrated accurately to measure blood flow, but it does detect changes in the blood content of the skin capillaries that reflect the changes in ambulatory venous pressure in health and disease.

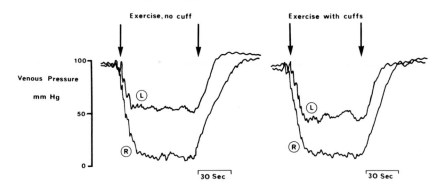

Figure 10-2. The effect of exercise on the ambulatory venous pressure in a normal limb (*right*) and in a limb with deep venous insufficiency (*left*). Note that the application of a cuff inflated to control the superficial venous system has not significantly affected venous pressure or refilling time.

The PPG probe is positioned with double-sided sticky tape on the lower calf just above the medial malleolus. The dorsum of the foot has been used for this purpose, but there is evidence that its use can give false-negative results because of the occasional presence of a competent valve distal to the ankle.[18] The output from the PPG is traced on a strip-chart recorder (Figure 10-3).[18] The technique utilizes the measurement of refilling time following exercise, as with the strain-gauge plethysmograph for calf-volume plethysmography. "Normal" refilling times vary from 18 seconds to 25 seconds according to the posture of the patient and the effectiveness of the exercise, and so it is important to establish normal and abnormal values for each laboratory's standard technique. We have found that refilling time measured with PPG has a nonlinear relationship to ambulatory venous pressure, and that although it differentiates between deep and superficial venous insufficiency, it is not possible to grade the severity within each group. The superficial venous tourniquet below the knee relieves superficial venous incompetence, as demonstrated in Figure 10-3.

CALF-VOLUME PLETHYSMOGRAPHY

Changes in calf volume during exercise may be used for the diagnosis of valvular incompetence of the superficial and deep veins. Calf-volume plethysmography (SPG) for this purpose is performed with mercury, or an alloy, in silastic strain-gauge tubes. The method is quantitative and can be as accurate as determinations of venous pressure.[14]

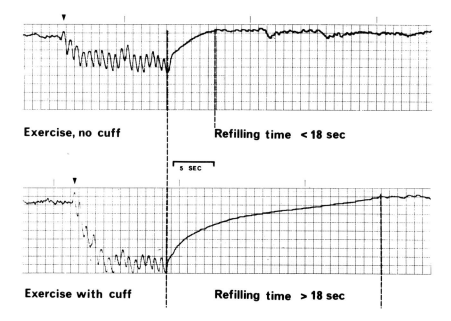

Exercise, no cuff   **Refilling time < 18 sec**

5 SEC

Exercise with cuff   **Refilling time > 18 sec**

Figure 10-3. PPG recordings from standing patient showing short refilling time (< 18 sec) at end of exercise (*upper tracing*), which is normalized (> 18 sec) by the application of a cuff at the knee inflated to occlude the superficial veins. Therefore, this leg demonstrates superficial venous incompetence. *Arrows:* onset of exercise. Compare with Figure 10-2.

Strain-gauge recordings are similar to those from a photoplethysmograph, but they exhibit a shorter refilling time. Following exercise, a competent venous system refills only from the arterial bed, and this requires at least 12 seconds. Venous incompetence allows reflux to refill the veins quickly, and so the refilling time is much shorter than normal. Deep venous insufficiency can be differentiated from superficial venous insufficiency by comparing refilling times before and after the application of a cuff inflated to occlude the superficial veins just below the knee. The cuff prevents reflux via the superficial system. Deep venous insufficiency is present when the refilling time is unaltered by the inflation of the superficial venous occlusion cuff. A combination of deep venous insufficiency and superficial venous insufficiency is suggested by a refilling time which lengthens following application of a tourniquet cuff, but which remains less than the normal 12 seconds. This method gives false-negative results if there is an incompetent perforating vein below the strain gauge, but this problem can be avoided either by moving the strain gauge more distally or by using photoplethysmography.

Diagnosing Deep Venous Thrombosis

Doppler Ultrasound

Clots in iliac, femoral, or popliteal veins affect the flow of blood, and these alterations modify the normal Doppler signal elicited over these veins. With experience, the user hears and recognizes these changes, and this is a convenient bedside or office test.

The signs of venous obstruction noted in acute deep venous thrombosis may persist to some extent during the chronic phase; extensive, abnormal, collateral circulation may be noted, as well as signs of the valvular incompetence that always occurs after a deep venous thrombosis.

Obstruction in the iliac veins encourages suprapubic collaterals, which empty the limb via the opposite iliac system. With the patient semi-recumbent, collateral venous flow can be heard and its source detected by compression maneuvers over the pubis. The common femoral vein in the normal limb is examined first and compared with the affected leg. The signal from the normal limb may be enhanced on pubic compression while that from the affected side is diminished or abolished. The patient must be relaxed and should not hold his breath during the period of compression. The pubic collateral may be present even though sufficient recanalization permits phasic venous sounds at the groin. High-pitched or continuous signals (not phasic with respiration) mean recent thrombosis with poor collateral circulation.

The following chapter discusses in detail the diagnosis of deep venous thrombosis by Doppler ultrasound.

Impedance Plethysmography

Thrombi in iliac, femoral, or popliteal veins decrease the capacity of these veins and impair venous outflow. Impedance plethysmography (IPG) measures the increase in limb volume induced when a suitable cuff is inflated to produce temporary venous occlusion, and it records the rate of decrease in leg volume upon sudden deflation.

The patient should be comfortable, with the limb relaxed and positioned above heart level (Figure 10-4). It may help to turn the patient slightly toward the side being examined. The normal limb shows considerable increase in volume (venous capacitance) when the cuff is inflated 45–55 cm H_2O and a rapid outflow on deflation (Figure 10-5, upper

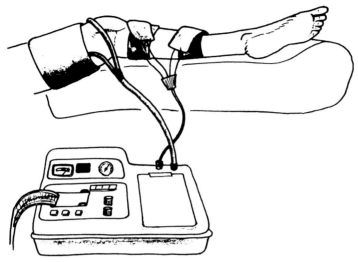

Figure 10-4. Lower limb positioned for recording an impedance plethysmogram. Note that the knee is flexed slightly and the leg rotated externally.

recording). Venous capacitance and venous outflow both decrease in the presence of obstructing thrombi in the major veins (Figure 10-5, lower recording). Although venous capacitance is reduced in the presence of venous thrombosis, it is related also to the initial volume of the calf or forearm. Outflow is the product of resistance proximal to the cuff and the volume of venous blood distal to the cuff. Thus, outflow is expressed as a function of venous capacitance, and relationships have been established that permit discrimination of the leg[3] or arm[4] having recent thrombosis. Figure 10-6 shows a scoring sheet suitable for the lower limb.

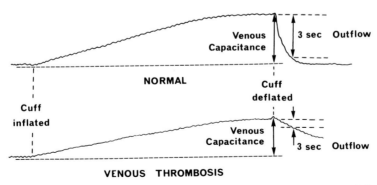

Figure 10-5. Impedance plethysmograms showing normal (*upper recording*) and abnormal (*lower recording*) relationships of venous capacitance and outflow.

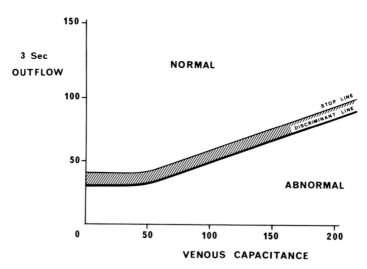

Figure 10-6. Scoring sheet for impedance plethysmography.

To avoid false-positive examinations, or when the results fall into the "gray area" close to the discriminant, the test should be repeated several times (Figure 10-6). If the findings are indeterminate, exercise by repeated plantar flexion and dorsiflexion of the foot induces hyperemia and may increase venous capacitance.

IPG is very accurate in detecting thrombosis of the iliac, femoral, and popliteal veins. Like the Doppler venous examination, IPG does not detect minor thrombi in calf veins, but according to most authorities these do not require anticoagulants or hospital treatment. When doubt exists, a phlebogram can resolve the question.

VOLUME PLETHYSMOGRAPHY

There are two methods of volume plethysmography for the detection of venous thrombosis. The first method is the phleborheograph (see Chapter 12).[5] Small changes in volume are recorded via sensitive pneumatic cuffs and recorders. Changes phasic with respiration are diminished or abolished distal to a calf-vein obstruction and are detected by the phleborheograph.

The second method uses a combination of one thigh, one foot, and three calf cuffs in two modes.[6,19] Following several rapid inflations of the foot cuff,[6] an increase in volume will be detected distal to a venous obstruction, whereas the normal limb will show no change. In addition, the cuff on the lower calf can be inflated similarly to record changes in the volume of the foot. Normal limbs experience a transient reduction in volume, but in obstructed limbs this reduction is absent or diminished.

STRAIN-GAUGE PLETHYSMOGRAPHY

Strain gauges around the fullest part of the calf are useful for recording the volume changes, as in impedance and volume plethysmography. Venous outflow by itself can be used to diagnose venous obstruction,[9] or venous outflow can be related to venous capacitance.[14,18] In our laboratory a venous outflow of less than 55 ml/100 ml/min is associated with obstruction.[14] Nix and Barnes express venous outflow during the first 3 seconds following deflation of the occluding cuff as a percentage of venous capacitance. Outflow percentages less than 50%–60% suggest venous obstruction above the knee.[17]

The effective use of any of these plethysmographic techniques in the diagnosis of deep venous thrombosis is assisted by measuring the highest value of venous capacitance. Many potentially false-positive examinations can be avoided by ensuring that the patient is positioned correctly and is relaxed and warm. Vasoconstriction from coldness, muscle tension, and apprehension causes errors.

SCANNING WITH ISOTOPICALLY LABELLED FIBRINOGEN AND PORCINE PLASMIN

This method is used mainly to compare the effectiveness of methods for preventing deep venous thrombosis. For the ^{125}I fibrinogen uptake test (FUT), labelled fibrinogen is injected into the patient and the leg scan detects its uptake into a new or established thrombus. Uptake is relatively slow, requiring at least 24 hours before a thrombus is labelled and detected reliably. Nevertheless, the FUT remains the most widely used method for the early detection of a thrombus, even before a deep venous thrombosis becomes symptomatic or detectable by other methods. The FUT also may demonstrate that a thrombus is extending.

To prevent the undesirable uptake of ^{125}I by the thyroid, the gland must be saturated with sodium iodine before the tracer is administered, and a daily oral dose of 100 mg potassium iodine must be maintained for the following three weeks.

The leg scanning is performed with legs elevated 20–30 degrees to prevent venous pooling, and the radioactivity is measured at points approximately 2 inches apart, from the ankle along the back of the calf to the knee, and thence to the groin following the usual path of the femoral vein. Usually, we measure 5 or 6 points below the knee and 6 or 7 above. The number of counts at each position along the leg are expressed as a percentage of the counts over the heart. An examination is regarded as positive when there is an increase of more than 20% over 24 hours at any one measurement site, or when there is a consistent difference of more than 20% between adjacent sites.

^{99}Tc PLASMIN

This technique is similar to the FUT, but measurements can be made one hour after administration of the isotope because plasmin interacts with a thrombus more rapidly than fibrin. In addition, it has the advantages that the thyroid gland does not need to be "blocked," and that the patient receives a lower dose of radiation. Counts are compared between the same levels in each leg. A difference of more than 10% is regarded as abnormal, but bilateral deep venous thromboses with the same uptake are likely to give a false-negative result.

The longer half-life of 60 days of ^{125}I permits the convenience of commercial sources of labelled fibrinogen, whereas the plasmin labelled with ^{99}Tc, the half-life of which is six hours, must be labelled daily, requiring two hours to prepare and the facilities of the medical physics (or similar) department. These inconveniences have probably limited its widespread use. Both labelled compounds will interact with an established thrombus, and this characteristic is particularly valuable for following the course of a patient with persisting deep venous thrombosis or for the patient with a previous history of deep venous thrombosis who exhibits fresh symptoms. Both detect a new thrombus in limbs that previously suffered from deep venous thrombosis—a situation in which tests are sometimes unreliable.

ISOTOPE VENOGRAPHY

Venography using a radioisotope instead of a contrast medium is useful for screening patients with suspected obstruction in the pelvic veins—an area where radioisotope uptake tests are unreliable, particularly following hip surgery. Human albumin micropheres (HAM) are labelled with ^{99}Tc and injected bilaterally into foot veins.[22] The course of the radioactivity is detected with a gamma camera positioned over the abdomen, giving a thromboscintigram of the larger veins. Although the definition is not as good as that of a contrast venogram, it is sufficient to show major filling defects and collateral circulation. This technique is used by medical physics or similar departments more than by vascular laboratories.

CONCLUSIONS

Clinical diagnosis of venous disorders, particularly deep venous thrombosis, has not proved adequate. Venography is invasive, expensive, and thrombogenic, and these facts have encouraged the use of other techniques. Nevertheless, all three diagnostic methods (clinical, venographic, and noninvasive) are complementary. Because the noninvasive approach does not neglect the patient's history and physical examination, the results of noninvasive tests can be more easily interpreted and false-positive examinations avoided. We prefer the simple Doppler examinations, although they require great attention to detail and are not learned easily. Nevertheless, they are the basis of noninvasive assessment and should be thoroughly familiar to vascular diagnosticians. These and other adjunctive methods are discussed in more detail in Chapters 11–14.

REFERENCES

1. Sumner DS: Diagnosis of venous thrombosis by Doppler ultrasound. In *Venous Problems*. Edited by JJ Bergan, JST Yao. Chicago, Year Book, 1978, pp 159–185.
2. Kupper CA, Shugart RE, Burnham S: Errors of Doppler ultrasound examination in diagnosis of deep venous thrombosis. Bruit 3 (December): 15–19, 1979.
3. Wheeler HB, Patwardhan NA, Anderson FA: The place of occlusive impedance plethysmography in the diagnosis of venous thrombosis. In *Venous Problems*. Edited by JJ Bergan, JST Yao. Chicago, Year Book, 1978, pp 145–158.
4. Gray B, Keifer T, Cudzilo S, et al: Evaluation of impedance phlebography of the upper extremity. Bruit 5 (December):22–25, 1981.
5. Cranley JJ, Canos AJ, Mahalingam K: Diagnosis of deep venous thrombosis by phleborheography. In *Venous Problems*. Edited by JJ Bergan, JST Yao. Chicago, Year Book, 1978, pp 187–205.
6. Lepore TJ, Savran J, Van De Water J, et al: Screening for lower extremity deep venous thrombosis: an improved plethysmography and Doppler approach. Am J Surg 135:529–534, 1978.
7. Nicolaides AN, Hobbs JT: The I-125 fibrinogen test: development and current status. In *Investigation of Vascular Disorders*. Edited by AN Nicolaides, JST Yao. London, Churchill Livingstone, 1981, pp 369–376.

115

8. Cooke ED: Thermography. In *Investigation of Vascular Disorders*. Edited by AN Nicolaides, JST Yao. London, Churchill Livingstone, 1981, pp 416–442.

9. Hallbook T, Gothlin J: Strain-gauge plethysmography and phlebography in the diagnosis of deep vein thrombosis. Acta Chir Scand 137:37–44, 1971.

10. Ludlam CA, Bolton AE, Moores B: A new, rapid method for the diagnosis of deep venous thrombosis. Lancet 2: 259–260, 1975.

11. Olson CG: TC99 plasmin: development and current status. In *Investigation of Vascular Disorders*. Edited by AN Nicolaides, JST Yao. London, Churchill Livingstone, 1981, pp 443–451.

12. Day TK, Fish PJ, Kakkar VV: Detection of deep vein thrombosis by Doppler angiography. Br Med J 1:618–620, 1976.

13. Barnes RW: Doppler ultrasonic diagnosis of venous disease. In *Noninvasive Diagnostic Techniques in Vascular Disease*. Edited by EF Bernstein. St Louis, CV Mosby, 1978, pp 344–350.

14. Fernandes e Fernandes J, Horner J, Needham TN, et al: Ambulatory calf volume plethysmography in the assessment of venous insufficiency. Br J Surg 66:327–330, 1979.

15. Thulesius O, Norgren L, GJores JE; Foot volumetry: A new method for the objective assessment of oedema and venous function. VASA 2:325–331, 1973.

16. Abramowitz HB, Queral LA, Flinn WR, et al: The use of photoplethysmography in the assessment of venous insufficiency. A comparison to venous pressure measurement. Surgery 86:434–441, 1979.

17. Nix ML, Barnes RW: *Noninvasive Peripheral Vascular Laboratory. Diagnostic Techniques*. Richmond, Medical College of Virginia, 1980.

18. Peterson LK: Photoplethysmography. Presented at the International Vascular Symposium. London, 1981.

19. Mutton T, Love BJ, Wilson C: The effect of leg and cuff position on accuracy of screening for deep venous thrombosis with the pulse volume recorder. Bruit 5 (September): 16–18, 1981.

20. Miles CR, Nicolaides AN; Photoplethysmography: principles and development. In *Investigation of Vascular Disorders*. Edited by AN Nicolaides, JST Yao. London, Churchill Livingstone, 1981, pp 501–515.

21. Nicolaides AN, Fernandes JF, Zimmerman H: Doppler ultrasound in the investigation of venous insufficiency. In *Investigation of Vascular Disorders*. Edited by AN Nicolaides, JST Yao. London, Churchill Livingstone, 1981, pp 478–487.

22. Dean RH: Isotope venography. In *Venous Problems*. Edited by JJ Bergan, JST Yao. Chicago, Year Book, 1978, pp 227–237.

CHAPTER 11

DOPPLER DIAGNOSIS OF DEEP VENOUS THROMBOSIS

Lee Nix

Venous Doppler examination for deep venous thrombosis has proven to be the most simple, rapid, inexpensive, and accurate noninvasive method in use in our laboratory. This extremely subjective testing procedure requires four to six months of practice for the examiner to reach a high level of accuracy. In addition, the examiner must have a basic understanding of the anatomy and physiology of the deep venous system and understand how the superficial system relates to the venous blood flow (see Chapter 9). Instruction in venous Doppler techniques is followed by four to six months of practice (four to five examinations per week) with contrast venographic follow-up to compare results. By examining all patients suspected of deep venous thrombosis, rather than only those whose disease has been confirmed venographically, the examiner in training becomes more broadly experienced and familiar with both normal and abnormal studies. In combination with venographic monitoring, this training regimen documents the increasing accuracy of the examiner. In our institution the radiology department requests that a venous Doppler examination be performed prior to venography.

A key factor in understanding the venous Doppler examination is the knowledge that this testing modality evaluates the venous system for obstruction rather than thrombosis. Venous Doppler examination is a physiologic assessment of flow. Obstruction in the system can be the result of intrinsic thrombosis or extrinsic compression of the vein. It is essential that the examiner have an in-depth understanding of the anatomic and physiologic factors that can cause abnormalities and affect the interpretation and application of the results of the venous Doppler examination. It is well established that the venous system is frequently anomalous, and the presence of a biphed system can produce a false-negative test. The presence of multiple deep veins in the calf makes diagnosis of isolated deep calf-vein thrombosis difficult. Despite these limitations, it is possible for an experienced examiner to differentiate those patients with normal venous flow from those with venous obstruction in a high percentage of cases. A highly skilled examiner is essential for consistent success with this examination. The examiner must interact with the patient and his environment in each testing situation, and only with a high level of awareness can the examiner handle such problems as cellulitis, respirators, congestive heart failure, pregnancy, and the like. Interpretation of results is an integral part of the examination process. Validation of Doppler result by comparison to venographic result is essential in each individual center because of the subjective nature of this noninvasive test. Comparison of the physiologic test (Doppler) to the morphologic test (venography) is the ultimate method of validation and a valuable means of understanding accuracy and error.

TECHNIQUE

The technique of the venous Doppler examination is based on an evaluation of audible venous flow in the resting limb and on the response of that flow to compression of the limb, both proximal and distal to the Doppler probe. A 5-MHz, hand-held Doppler probe with stethoscope earphones is used for the venous examination. (For demonstrations and teaching, the probe may be coupled to a portable speaker.) The broader, deeper penetration of a 5-MHz instrument seems to locate the low-flow (and, therefore, low-pitched) venous sounds better than the 8–10 MHz pencil-like probes used for arterial and cerebrovascular examinations, although some technologists do prefer an 8–10 MHz probe. The venous signal is located by finding the appropriate arterial signal (a louder, multiphasic sound) and then angling the Doppler probe to find the adjacent venous signal.

ANALYZING QUALITY OF FLOW

The five basic flow qualities evaluated in each segment of the venous system are spontaneity, phasicity, augmentation, competence, and pulsatility.

118

Spontaneity

Spontaneity is the audible presence of a spontaneous venous signal. The examiner listens at or near the normal location of the vein and notes the presence or absence of an audible signal. Limb-to-limb comparison of signals is useful, with the warning that increased arterial flow (as in cellulitis) increases venous flow signals.

Phasicity

Normal venous sounds are in phase with the respiratory cycle, unlike the pulsatile arterial signals that are cyclic with each heart beat. Venous flow decreases during inspiration because the inferior vena cava is compressed by the descent of the diaphragm. The loss of phasicity in the spontaneous venous signal usually indicates an obstruction in the venous system between the area examined and the diaphragm.

Augmentation

"Augmentation" refers to the audible increase in venous flow in response to compression distal to the area being examined (Figure 11-1), and to the increase in flow after release of proximal compression (Figure 11-2). Normally, if there is no obstruction in the venous system, there should be a significant increase in pitch (velocity) of the venous signal with distal compression of a limb. Obstruction either abolishes augmentation or allows only a small increase in flow. It is important to compare the quality (or degree of) augmentation on the right and the left to detect the less obvious changes resulting from a nonobstructive thrombus. Nonobstructing thrombi are recognized by careful comparison of the flow signals and their response to compression maneuvers.

Competence

"Competence" refers to the ability of the normal venous valves to prevent retrograde flow. Competent valves do not allow retrograde flow when the limb is compressed proximal to the Doppler probe. The flow stops with proximal compression and, after release of the compression, augmentation of flow is heard. Incompetent valves, on the other hand, do allow retrograde flow, which is heard during proximal compression. Venous incompetence of the deep veins is usually the result of old thrombosis or trauma.

Pulsatility

Leg veins normally do not have a pulsatile quality, but in conditions of fluid overload—congestive heart failure and dialysis (either transfusion

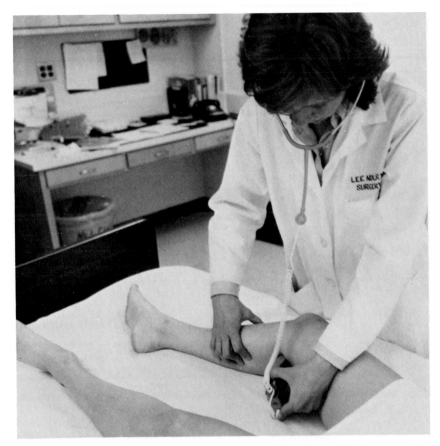

Figure 11-1. Doppler examination for deep venous thrombosis: distal compression maneuver. Examiner listens at the popliteal vein, compressing the calf and listening for augmentation of the popliteal venous sound.

or peritoneal), for instance, or in some patients undergoing intravenous fluid replacement—venous sounds in the leg may be pulsatile. Pulsatility in the leg veins is not an indication of obstruction or thrombosis in the venous system.

EXAMINING THE LOWER EXTREMITY

The patient is examined in the supine position with the head of the bed elevated about 60 degrees and the foot of the bed flat. This position allows for a slight natural pooling in the venous system of the legs. The

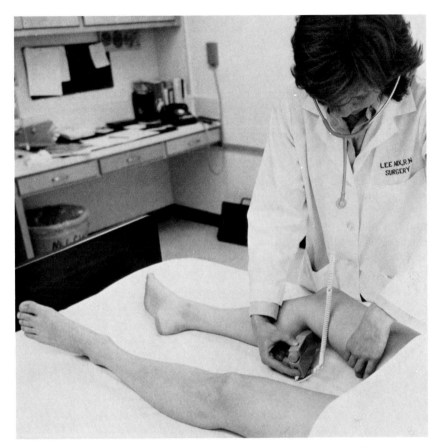

Figure 11-2. Doppler examination for deep venous thrombosis: proximal compression maneuver. Examiner listens at the popliteal vein, compressing above the knee and listening for reflux during compression and for augmentation of flow on release of compression.

examination usually proceeds in the following order, assuming that the right leg is suspected of harboring deep venous thrombosis:

Left posterior tibial vein
Left greater saphenous vein (at ankle)
Right posterior tibial vein
Right greater saphenous vein
Left common femoral vein
Left superficial femoral vein
Left popliteal vein
Right common femoral vein

Right superficial femoral vein
Right popliteal vein

The leg is relaxed, slightly flexed, and externally rotated to prevent both muscular and mechanical compression of the deep venous system behind the knee.

The Doppler examination begins in the posterior tibial vein just posterior to the medial malleolus. The examiner locates the arterial signal and searches the adjacent area for a spontaneous venous signal, which usually is posterior to the posterior tibial artery. Posterior tibial venous signals often are not audible in patients on bed rest or in those with cool extremities, but can be located by compressing the foot and eliciting augmentation. Calf-vein thrombosis is suggested by decreased flow into the calf following release of calf compression. Listening carefully, the examiner compares posterior tibial veins of the right and left legs. Next, the examiner listens to the greater saphenous vein (superficial system) at the ankle just anterior to the medial malleolus to detect increased superficial venous flow, which sometimes results from obstruction of deeper veins in the calf.

To find the common femoral venous signal, the examiner locates the common femoral arterial signal (initially by palpation, then with the Doppler) and then slightly angles the Doppler probe medially. The common femoral venous signal should always be audible unless there is acute or chronic iliofemoral deep venous obstruction. The common femoral vein is assessed for the five basic qualities of flow previously discussed. Competence of the common femoral and superficial femoral valves is assessed by asking the patient to perform a Valsalva maneuver or by gently compressing the abdomen.

The superficial femoral vein is located about four inches down from the common femoral vein. The superficial femoral vein is normally heard with the superficial femoral artery, as they overlie one another anatomically. The superficial femoral artery and vein are deep, and the penetration of the 5-MHz probe seems especially helpful here. The venous signal is assessed for the five qualities of flow.

Popliteal venous signals are usually found just lateral to the popliteal arterial signal. The patient may be examined in the supine position with the knee flexed and the hip externally rotated, or the patient may be prone with feet elevated on a pillow. Once more the venous signal is evaluated for the five basic qualities of flow. Care should be taken to compress the leg five or six inches above the Doppler probe to be certain a valve is present; otherwise reflux will not signify incompetence.

For a means of scoring and interpreting the examination of a lower extremity, see Table 11-1.

Table 11-1. Scoring and Interpreting the Doppler Venous Examination of Lower Extremities[a,b]

Diagnosis	Flow Quality	Findings				
		CFV	SFV	PV	PTV	GSV
Normal	Spontaneous	+	+	+	±	±
	Phasic	+	+	+	±	±
	Augmented	+	+	+	+	+
	Competent	+	+	+	+	+
	Nonpulsatile	+	+	+	±	±
Calf-vein thrombosis	Spontaneous	+	+	±	0	+
	Phasic	+	+	±	0	+
	Augmented	+	+	±	0	+
	Competent	+	+	±	0	+ (chronic)
Femoropopliteal venous thrombosis	Spontaneous	+	0	0	±	±
	Phasic	+	0	0	0	±
	Augmented	0	0	0	±	+
	Competent (chronic)	+	0	0	±	+
Iliofemoral venous thrombosis	Spontaneous	0	±	±	±	±
	Phasic	0	0	0	0	±
	Augmented	0	±	±	±	+
	Competent (chronic)	0	±	±	±	+

[a] Reprinted with permission from Barnes RW, Russell H, Wilson MR: *Doppler Ultrasonic Evaluation of Venous Disease.* Iowa City, University of Iowa Press, 1975.

[b] *CFV* common femoral vein; *SFV* superficial femoral vein; *PV* popliteal vein; *PTV* posttibial vein; *GSV* greater saphenous vein. *Symbols:* + = present, ± = variable or decreased, 0 = absent.

EXAMINING THE UPPER EXTREMITY

Deep venous thrombosis of the upper extremities is becoming of more concern with the increasing use of central venous lines for patient treatment and monitoring. Upper extremities are examined at the brachial, axillary, subclavian, and jugular venous segments, and each venous signal is evaluated for the aforementioned five qualities of flow—spontaneity, phasicity, augmentation, competence, and pulsatility. Venous signals in the upper extremities are usually pulsatile because of the closer proximity to the heart, and normally they are phasic as well. Competence is evaluated by having the patient perform a Valsalva maneuver.

The brachial, axillary, and subclavian venous signals normally are spontaneous, phasic with respiration, and somewhat pulsatile with the heartbeat. In the presence of subclavian or axillary venous thrombosis, the venous signals may be absent or continuous and nonphasic. With axillary or subclavian venous thrombosis, proximal continuous flow may be heard in the cephalic vein, which lies in the groove between the deltoid and pectoralis major muscles anterior to the shoulder joint. Normally the internal jugular venous signal is higher in pitch and more continuous, as well as somewhat pulsatile. An absent jugular venous signal suggests jugular venous thrombosis. Bilateral absence of both the jugular and the subclavian venous signals suggests superior vena cava thrombosis.

RESULTS

The results of a review of patients comparing their venous Doppler examination and contrast venogram are shown in Table 11-2. The venous Doppler examination proved to be extremely sensitive, correctly identifying 53 of 54 patients with an abnormal contrast phlebogram. The specificity was 85% with 12 false-positive Doppler examinations. This reflects both the ability of the venous Doppler examination to detect venous obstruction and its fallibility in differentiating extrinsic compression from intrinsic thrombosis. Common causes of extrinsic compression are intraabdominal tumor, pregnancy, and occasionally severe edema, or the anterior compartment syndrome. The negative predictive value of the Doppler examination was 99%, and its positive predictive value was 82%.

CONCLUSIONS

The venous Doppler examination has been shown to be a sensitive test for the diagnosis of deep venous thrombosis. An experienced technologist can perform the examination in about ten minutes at the bedside or in

Table 11-2. Comparison of Doppler Examination and Contrast Phlebography in the Diagnosis of Deep Venous Thrombosis (Lower Extremity)

Doppler Examination	Contrast Phlebogram	
	Normal	Abnormal
Normal	68	1
Abnormal	12	53

124

the laboratory. Because the venous Doppler examination is subjective, it requires considerable experience of the examiner to achieve maximal accuracy. Nevertheless, with sufficient practice the technologist may employ this instrument with skill and versatility to detect both obstruction and valvular incompetence in the superficial, communicating, and deep veins of the lower and upper extremities.

BIBLIOGRAPHY

1. Barnes W, Russell HE, Wilson MR: *Doppler Ultrasonic Evaluation of Venous Disease.* Iowa City, University of Iowa Press, 1975.
2. Strandness DE Jr, Ward K, Krugmire R Jr: The present status of acute deep venous thrombosis. Surg Gyn Obstet 145:433–445, 1977.
3. Sumner DS, Baker DW, Strandness DE Jr: The ultrasonic velocity detector in a clinical study of venous disease. Arch Surg 97:75–80, 1968.
4. Sumner DS, Lambeth A: Reliability of Doppler ultrasound in the diagnosis of acute venous thrombosis both above and below the knee. Am J Surg 138:205–209, 1979.

CHAPTER 12

PHLEBORHEOGRAPHY
IN THE DIAGNOSIS
OF DEEP VENOUS THROMBOSIS

John J. Cranley

The diagnosis of superficial thrombophlebitis, phlegmasia alba dolens, and phlegmasia cerulea dolens can usually be made by physical examination alone. For many years, however, the common kind of deep venous thrombosis has presented problems of diagnosis. A limb that appears to be entirely normal, clinically, may harbor potentially lethal clots, while a limb with all the symptoms and signs typical of thrombosis in the deep system may be shown radiologically to have a patent venous tree. The clinical diagnosis is approximately 55% accurate by phlebography,[1] suggesting that objective noninvasive methods have a vital role to play in establishing the true diagnosis in limbs with and without thrombosis, if needless hospitalization, anticoagulation, and phlebography are to be avoided.

In 1971, spurred by our interest in the work of Wheeler,[2] we developed a new concept for diagnosing deep venous thrombosis of the lower extremity and pelvis. In the first phase of our study, a standard polygraph was used, but early in 1973 a modified, simplified instrument called the phleborheograph (PRG) was developed. Its name describes its primary function, that is, tracing the moving currents within the veins. The results obtained with the polygraph and the PRG are identical. The PRG differs from other noninvasive modalities for diagnosing deep venous thrombosis by being based on segmental volume changes that can be accurately measured.[3-11]

The current model uses state-of-the-art electronic equipment. A technician can be taught to perform the test with approximately two weeks' training, and an interested physician can learn to interpret the tracings in approximately three days. Economical to operate and sparing of the physician's time, the phleborheographic test is highly accurate and well tolerated by patients. It has, in fact, become the standard clinical test for thrombophlebitis of the deep venous system in our institution.

PHYSIOLOGIC PRINCIPLES

REDUCTION OF RESPIRATORY WAVES IN DEEP VENOUS THROMBOSIS

Normal breathing produces a rhythmic increase and decrease in the volume of the lower extremity that is recorded as an oscillation on the tracing, which is synchronized with the wave recorded from another recording cuff around the chest. Present in all normal extremities, these respiratory waves result from alterations in the volume of the limb produced by the mechanical effects of the respiratory movements of the thorax and diaphragm. These waves produce the changes heard over a major vein when using the Doppler velocity detector. Acute deep venous thrombosis reduces or suppresses the sounds as heard on Doppler examination. Similarly, during the acute thrombotic period, the tracings of the respiratory waves are significantly diminished or obliterated. Developing collateral circulation causes absent respiratory waves to reappear within two weeks and increases those that were merely reduced. Postthrombotic waves can be distinguished by their smaller-than-normal elevation and rounder-than-normal contour.

That the waves travel down the limb via collateral veins is suggested by the absence of waves in tracings from the thigh of a patient with isolated femoroiliac thrombophlebitis and by their presence in tracings from the same limb in the unobstructed leg veins. At times, the waves in the lower extremity are larger when the patient lies on his left side than when he is supine. This is sometimes true when he lies on his right side also. We have no ready explanation for these phenomena. In some instances, after massive venous thrombosis, the respiratory waves are permanently suppressed and the collateral circulation remains minimal.

INTERFERENCE WITH BLOOD OUTFLOW
IN RESPONSE TO RHYTHMIC COMPRESSION

Similar to active muscle contraction on walking, intermittent compression of the normal extremity propels blood proximally toward the heart. Deep venous thrombosis impedes this outflow. A recording cuff proximal to the site of compression transmits the momentary blockage of blood when venous thrombosis (or extraluminal compression) bars its exit. Reacting to this impediment, the baseline of the volume recorder rises. (The baseline remains level when no obstruction is present.) The rise in baseline localizes the site of thrombosis. If the thigh tracing exhibits a stepwise rise on calf compression, the level of obstruction to the deep veins lies above the thigh cuff. Rarely, external compression is at fault. Otherwise, intraluminal compression is present.

When obstruction exists at or above the recording cuffs, compression of the foot raises the baseline tracings from the leg. A rise in baseline is unequivocal evidence of venous obstruction.

COMPRESSION OF THE CALF

This maneuver has two effects: (1) blood is propelled up the unobstructed extremity, and (2) blood is siphoned out of the normal foot. With calf compression, a recording cuff on the foot reveals a fall in baseline. Absent or less-than-normal foot emptying together with a rise in baseline and obliterated respiratory waves indicate acute deep venous thrombosis. We retain this maneuver because it permits detection of a normal tracing at a glance; it is, however, more conducive to artifacts than rhythmic compression at other sites of transmission or respiratory waves from the chest.

INDICATIONS

The basic function of the PRG is the detection of deep venous thrombosis. Three commonly encountered clinical applications of the technique involve the following:

1. *The patient with a hugely swollen limb.* A normal PRG unequivocally rules out clots in the deep veins.

2. *The patient with or without clinical symptoms.* A tracing considered to be abnormal means emergency admission to the hospital for anti-coagulation therapy. The sole exception to this rule is the patient with a history of massive deep venous thrombosis (alluded to above) whose deep system has not recanalized and whose venous collateral circulation remains minimal.

3. *The patient with calf tenderness.* A normal PRG is interpreted as possible, very early nonocclusive acute deep venous thrombosis. This patient is treated expectantly, with repeat PRGs in two or three days, or until the remission of symptoms.

In the patient with established deep venous thrombosis, serial PRGs may be obtained to follow the development of collateral circulation. As an alternative to prophylactic anticoagulation, patients at high risk of developing venous thrombosis may be monitored by serial tracings.

TECHNIQUE

POSITIONING PATIENT AND CUFFS

The current model PRG (Grass Instrument Company, Quincy, Massachusetts) provides state-of-the-art electronics, which ensure efficient and consistent clinical performance. There are now six channels on the console (Figure 12-1), making it possible to apply all the pressure cuffs at once, to calibrate them simultaneously, and to run the test without interruption. The patient lies quietly in bed with the lower extremities approximately 10 degrees below heart level and with the knee slightly flexed while the cuffs are applied. Cuff 1 is placed around the thorax, so that all the changes in a limb are recorded synchronously with respiratory movements. The respiratory tracing monitors abnormal or involuntary, apprehensive intakes of breath that may occur on application of pressure, causing a sudden rise in baseline that otherwise might wrongly be interpreted as significant. The cuff of the second channel is placed on the thigh just above the knee. Three cuffs are placed on the leg, one each on the upper portion, the midleg, and at the ankle. The sixth cuff is placed on the foot.

Channels 1–4 record only volumetric changes, while the fifth and sixth channels may be used to record volumetric change or to apply pressure

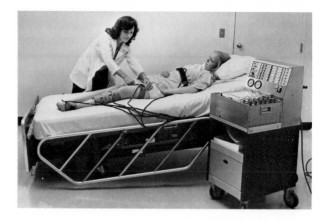

Figure 12-1. Console of phleborheograph. Six channels make it possible to apply at once all pressure cuffs to the lower extremity of the patient, who lies quietly in bed with limbs approximately 10 degrees below heart level and with knee slightly flexed while the cuffs are applied.

to the limb. Thus, when the sixth cuff is being used to apply pressure to the foot, the fifth cuff, as well as all the others above it, are recording volumetric changes. Similarly, when the fifth cuff is being used to apply pressure to the calf, the sixth cuff records volumetric changes in the foot. All of the cuffs are currently available blood-pressure cuffs. The strap of the chest cuff has been lengthened to permit its use around the epigastrium. The cuff encircling the upper thigh also has been lengthened. Currently, the cuff used on the foot is twice as wide as the others.

OPERATING THE PRG

After the cuffs have been applied, an automatic inflation sequence is activated, filling the cuffs to 10 mmHg to ensure a snug coupling between cuff and limb. A monitor lamp and a pressure gauge on the instrument panel indicate the inflation process, and an additional lamp is illuminated when proper recording pressure has been reached. A paper speed of 2.5 mm/sec is usually selected for venous studies. For pulse tracings, a 25 mm/sec paper speed is used.

Calibration is volumetric. When the calibrating button is depressed, 0.2 cc of air is removed from each recording cuff. Amplification is adjusted so that the 0.2 cc of air brings about a 2 cm downward deflection of the recording pen. By calibrating before each recording, one can accurately compare the magnitude of the respiratory waves, the emptying of the foot, and the amplitude of the digital pulses even when tests are performed at different times or on different subjects.

There are two recording modes. With the selector switch on *Run A,* the sixth cuff is used to apply pressure to the foot while the other cuffs record volume changes. During the first period of the tracing, the technician merely observes the respiratory waves, then presses the *COMPRESS* button to deliver three short bursts of air to the sixth cuff. Currently, we apply 100 mmHg for approximately 0.5 second at intervals of 0.5 second. The amount delivered is monitored by a pressure gauge on the instrument panel as well as at the source in the instrument. Approximately half of this pressure is lost in the airway; thus only 50 mmHg pressure is delivered to the foot. The patient experiences no discomfort, nor is the pressure sufficient to dislodge a clot. In the normal subject, the baselines of the tracings of the limb remain level despite application of pressure to the foot (Figure 12-2, left panel). In the patient with deep venous thrombosis, however, compression of the foot causes congestion of blood in the limb and raises the baseline of the tracing (Figure 12-2, right panel).

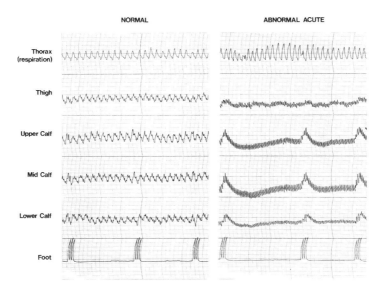

Figure 12-2. Run A: foot compression. *Left:* normal tracing. The baselines of the tracings remain level despite application of pressure to the foot. *Right:* abnormal tracing. In the patient with deep venous thrombosis, compression of the foot cuff causes congestion of blood in the limb, raising baseline.

Upon completion of Run A, the cuffs are deflated and the mode switch moved to *Run B*. The cuffs are reinflated and the instrument is recalibrated. At this time, when the *COMPRESS* button is pressed, pressure is applied to the lower calf. In this instance, 50 mmHg is used as the source pressure, and approximately 30 mmHg is delivered to the patient's calf. Compression of the calf raises the baseline of the proximal tracings when there is obstruction of venous outflow. In addition, calf compression normally produces some degree of foot emptying, which is diminished or obliterated by deep venous thrombosis (Figure 12-3).

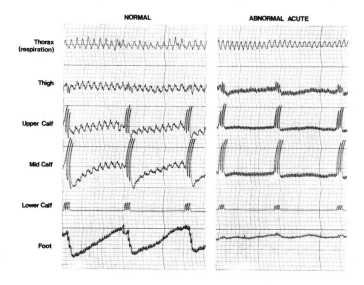

Figure 12-3. Run B: calf compression. *Left:* normal tracing. Baseline remains level in the normal extremity. *Right:* abnormal tracing. Compression of the calf raises baseline of the proximal tracings if venous outflow is obstructed.

A six-position *FUNCTION* switch on each phleborheograph amplifier adjusts the frequency response of the system to amplify the recording as desired. The *RESP* position enables the technician to filter out pulse waves and record only respiratory waves.

The *PRG* position provides the frequency response required to record pulses and respiratory waves. In the *PULSE* position, respiratory waves are filtered and amplification is automatically increased fivefold to permit detailed observation of the pulse contour.

Two dc positions are provided to facilitate unidirectional or bidirectional Doppler velocity recording.

The *ECG* position provides the high-frequency response needed for recording the electrocardiogram, should that be desired. A special ECG amplifier can be obtained to facilitate the ECG recording.

OTHER USES OF THE PRG

With a finger oncometer, the PRG can be used as a digital plethysmograph. This mechanism measures the amplitude of the digital pulses and relates them to the size of the enclosed finger by the water-displacement method. It also can measure blood flow by the venous-occlusion method. In the pulse position, the PRG may be used to permit the analysis of pulse waves visually and the measurement of amplitude volumetrically. A mercury-in-rubber or indium gallium strain-gauge tracing also can be made. The digital pulse may be recorded using a photoelectric transducer. The equipment may also be utilized to measure maximal venous outflow.

The maximum calibrated sensitivity of the phleborheograph in the PRG mode is 0.25 ml for full-scale pen deflection, or 50 mm. In the pulse mode, sensitivity is increased to 0.05 ml full scale. With sensitivity controls at maximum, the overall system sensitivity can be increased approximately 0.15 ml full scale in the PRG mode and 0.03 ml full scale in the pulse mode. Circuitry is also provided to facilitate the PRG's connection to tape recorders and computers.

RESULTS

More than 22,000 extremities were studied by the PRG, 714 of which also had a phlebogram (Table 12-1). The problem of an equivocal tracing is usually resolved by repeating the test in one or two days. Errors in interpretation have been determined by comparison with a phlebogram. Technical errors have virtually been eliminated. Inherent false negatives have remained approximately 5% throughout the 10-year period of the instrument's availability and have, with few exceptions, involved small clots below the knee. In a group of 57 patients with thrombi limited to the infrapopliteal area, 12 (21%) false-negative tests have occurred. False positives, on the other hand, are not easily explained. It is certain, however, that the extended knee can occlude the popliteal vein, and we believe that in some patients the femoral vein may be obstructed by

Table 12-1. Correlation of Phlebographic and Phleborheographic
Findings in 714 Extremities

Misdiagnosis	Type of Error	Number of Extremities
False negatives	Total errors	21/272 (7.7%)
	Equivocal error	2/272 (0.7%)
	Interpretive error	6/272 (2.2%)
	Inherent error	13/272 (4.7%)
False positives	Total errors	23/442 (5.2%)
	Equivocal error	3/442 (0.7%)
	Technical error	5/442 (1.1%)
	Interpretive error	4/442 (0.9%)
	Inherent error	11/442 (2.5%)

flexing the thigh. In young athletic adults, compression of the veins by muscle mass may result in a false-positive tracing. But some false positives defy explanation. We have come to accept an abnormal tracing as evidence of compression of the veins due to some cause that eludes our perception.

DISCUSSION

Without doubt, the greatest impediment to the development of phleborheography is the fact that the technique is new and must be learned. The test is technician-sensitive, and thorough training is imperative. The technician learns to recognize abnormal patterns, then maneuvers the patient to various positions, observing whether the tracing reverts to normal. If is does, the test is considered normal. If thrombosis is present, no amount of positional maneuvering succeeds in producing a "normal" tracing. Most patients can be examined in 30 to 45 minutes, although acutely ill, disabled, or uncooperative persons may require more time. An experienced physician can immediately interpret 80% of tracings, but the remaining 20% call for close scrutiny.

The PRG measures two variables: (1) the presence or absence of obstruction in the deep venous system and (2) collateral venous circulation as indicated by the presence, absence, or size and contour of the respiratory waves. If there is obstruction, without respiratory waves, the process is acute. If there is obstruction, combined with visible respiratory waves, the process is subacute. If there is obstruction in the presence of larger-than-normal respiratory waves, the process is usually chronic.

Serial tracings show the gradual transition from acute occlusion to development of the chronic state or to dissolution of the thrombi.

CHRONIC DEEP VENOUS THROMBOSIS

Caution and good clinical judgment are needed to diagnose the chronic state. For example, the day after ligation of the femoral vein (not for venous thrombosis), the PRG will show obstruction and large respiratory waves, indicating excellent collateral circulation. The tracing reflects the actual state, although the occlusion is certainly not chronic.

Another caveat concerns the PRG's inability to detect a clot that does not actually obstruct the flow of blood. Thus, the thrombus may partially but not completely occlude a small segment of a vein, such as the popliteal or femoral. Normal respiratory waves are present, but the incomplete blockage may raise the baseline. This does not represent chronic occlusion, but rather an acute early lesion. The test, repeated in a day or so, now shows the absence of respiratory waves, signifying that the partially occluding thrombus has propagated. The patient has been in no jeopardy. A mural thrombus over which blood continues to flow will, in our opinion, lyse. Furthermore, it is questionable that a thrombus is clinically significant until the vein is occluded, after which the soft jellylike clot forms on the head of the thrombus.

Tracings from limbs with chronic occlusion of the popliteal or femoral veins have been negative at times. If indicated, chronicity can be detected radiologically by the presence of many collateral veins around the obstruction, by clot retraction, by irregularity (tree-barking) of the vein walls, or, occasionally, by clinical history.

ACUTE THROMBOSIS SUPERIMPOSED ON CHRONIC OCCLUSION

The terms "acute" and "chronic" are clinical judgments, made by the physician; the PRG is merely capable of recording obstruction or its absence and either large or small respiratory waves. A combination of fresh clot and old obstruction poses some difficulty in diagnosis. In the post-thrombotic limb, the respiratory waves are so large that they may still appear to be within normal limits even when their size is reduced by the obstruction of a fresh clot. An acute episode may be suspected on the basis of an increase in existing symptoms or because new symptoms appear in a chronically insufficient extremity. The physician should follow the patient.

135

PULMONARY EMBOLISM

In our practice, we have observed four instances of a pulmonary embolism following a normal PRG. Three other instances have been reported to us. In three of our patients, the embolus was fatal. The critical factor common to all seven cases is the time interval between the normal PRG and the lodgement of the embolus. In five patients, it was between 8 and 12 days, and in the remaining two it was 6 days. Propagation may be rapid, so that clot in the soleal veins or in the named leg veins may progress to the popliteal and from there progress to the femoral in two or three days. Retrospective analysis has convinced us that some patients had the pulmonary embolism before the PRG was taken. If a large clot breaks off totally, leaving an empty vein behind, a normal PRG is to be expected. The problem of undiagnosed pulmonary embolism is not limited to the PRG. Proved clots in the lung are known to occur in a patient whose phlebogram shows a patent venous tree from ankles to the vena cava.

SOURCES OF ERROR IN INTERPRETATION

Technical errors account for most false-positive tests. The flow of venous blood is being interfered with by a mechanism not determinable at the moment. The false negatives, in addition to infrapopliteal thrombi, are chronic occlusions of the main venous trunks with development of large collateral vessels and, on occasion, a test conducted under contraindicated conditions. For example, a patient on a respirator who has deep venous thrombosis will have a PRG tracing with visible respiratory waves.

The phlebogram, the so-called "golden standard" by which all other modalities are judged, is not infallible. Biplanar views are essential. For example, one patient had an abnormal PRG and a normal-appearing phlebogram in which the pelvic veins were visualized in the anteroposterior position. A lateral view, however, showed nearly complete compression of the right common iliac vein.

CONCLUSIONS

With increasing familiarity, we have come to rely on the phleborheograph for diagnosing deep venous thrombosis. It also broadened our interpretation of the physiologic signals of health and disease in the deep venous system.

REFERENCES

1. Haeger K: Problems of acute deep venous thrombosis. Angiology 20:219–223, 1969.
2. Mullick SC, Wheeler HB, Songster GF: Diagnosis of deep venous thrombosis by measurement of electrical impedance. Am J Surg 119:417–422, 1970.
3. Cranley JJ, Gay AY, Grass AM, et al: A plethysmographic technique for the diagnosis of deep venous thrombosis of the lower extremities. Surg Gynecol Obstet 136:385–394, 1973.
4. Cranley JJ: Phleborheography. In *Vascular Surgery*, Volume 2: *Peripheral Venous Disease*. Hagerstown, Harper & Row, 1975, pp 79–95.
5. Cranley JJ, Canos AJ, Sull WJ, et al: Phleborheographic technique for diagnosing deep venous thrombosis of the lower extremities. Surg Gynecol Obstet 141: 331–340, 1975.
6. Cranley JJ, Canos AJ, Sull WJ: The diagnosis of deep venous thrombosis. Fallibility of clinical symptoms and signs, Arch Surg 111:34–36, 1976.
7. Cranley JJ, Canos AJ, Mahalingam K: Noninvasive diagnosis and prophylaxis of deep venous thrombosis of the lower extremities. In *Venous Thrombosis: Prevention and Treatment*. Edited by JL Madden, M Hume. New York, Appleton-Century-Crofts, 1976, pp 131–153.
8. Cranley JJ, Canos AJ, Mahalingam K: Diagnosis of deep venous thrombosis by phleborheography. In *Venous Problems*. Edited by JJ Bergan, JST Yao. Chicago, Year Book, 1978, pp 187–205.
9. Cranley JJ, Canos AJ, Mahalingam K; Diagnosis of deep venous thrombosis of the lower extremity by phleborheography. In *Noninvasive Diagnostic Techniques in Vascular Disease*. Edited by EF Bernstein. St Louis, CV Mosby Co, 1978, pp 351–358.
10. Cranley JJ: Air plethysmography in venous disease: the phleborheograph. In *Noninvasive Diagnostic Techniques in Vascular Disease*. Edited by EF Bernstein. St Louis, CV Mosby Co, 1978, pp 148–156.
11. Cranley JJ: Phleborheography. In *Practical Noninvasive Vascular Diagnosis*. Edited by RF Kempczinski, JST Yao. Chicago, Year Book, 1982, pp 305–321.

CHAPTER 13

VENOUS PLETHYSMOGRAPHY

Robert W. Barnes, John Middleton, and D. Glenn Turley

Plethysmography (literally, to record an increase) is an instrumental method of evaluating those changes in the dimension of a portion of the body that occur with each heartbeat or in response to temporary occlusion of venous return (with a pneumatic cuff, for instance, as in venous occlusion plethysmography).[1] Plethysmography permits the documentation of four types of physiologic information: (1) recording of pulse waveform contours, (2) measurement of systolic blood pressure of the limbs or digits, (3) recording of blood volume changes in the extremity, and (4) quantification of arterial inflow or venous outflow from the extremity. The latter two techniques have been used to detect and to quantify abnormal venous hemodynamics associated with acute deep venous thrombosis and chronic venous insufficiency of the superficial, perforating, and deep veins.

There are several different types of plethysmographs, which vary according to the type of transducer they use—water,[2] strain gauge,[3] impedance,[4] air,[5] or photoelectric.[6] The water plethysmograph has been used for many years by physiologists, but the technique is complicated and the equipment bulky, so the method is unsuitable for routine clinical use. The other four types of plethysmographic transducers are effectively used to study patients with acute or chronic venous disease. The more common methods will be reviewed in this chapter.

VENOUS OUTFLOW PLETHYSMOGRAPHY

TECHNIQUE

The patient is studied in the supine position with the legs elevated above atrial level. This is readily achieved by elevating the foot of the hospital bed. The patient's lower extremity must be appropriately positioned— the knee and hip flexed and the hip externally rotated—to prevent narrowing of the major deep veins in a hyperextended extremity. The feet should be at least 25–30 cm above atrial level.

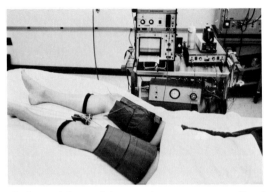

Figure 13-1. Technique of determining maximum venous outflow by strain-gauge plethysmography.

The two plethysmographs most commonly used for measuring venous outflow are the impedance (IPG)[4] and the strain-gauge (SPG)[7] plethysmographs. The impedance electrodes (IPG-200, Codman Shurtleff, Inc., Randolph, Massachusetts) are applied with a contact gel and the proximal and distal bands are separated on the calf by a distance of approximately 6 cm. The strain gauge should be placed around the maximum girth of the calf. For the strain-gauge technique, the calf should be elevated off of the bed, although the method also can be performed in a manner similar to impedance plethysmography, with the calf resting on the bed. A pneumatic cuff with large inlet and outlet ports is placed on the thigh and connected to an automatic cuff inflator (D. E. Hokanson, Inc., Issaquah, Washington) or to a hand-held manometer with an extra large outlet port. The plethysmographic transducer is connected to a recorder via an amplifier. The gauge is balanced and calibrated. With two-channel instruments (SPG-16, MedaSonics, Inc., Mountain View, California), venous outflows may be measured on both legs simultaneously (Figure 13-1).

The thigh pneumatic cuff is inflated to a pressure of 30–50 mmHg to occlude temporarily venous return. The resultant increase in calf circumference is recorded. The thigh cuff remains inflated for approximately two minutes or until the circumference of the calf stabilizes, at which point it is rapidly deflated and the resultant decrease in calf circumference or volume recorded. The test should be repeated at least once or, if an abnormal test is found, several times in order to establish whether or not the result was falsely positive. Every effort should be made to minimize muscle contraction, pain, straining, or other physiological factors that might lead to a false-positive result.

DIAGNOSTIC CRITERIA

The diagnostic criteria for impedance plethysmography have been generated by several institutions with large experience in this technique.[8,9] Diagnostic techniques usually involve plotting an outflow value based on the capacitance (maximal change in calf impedance during cuff inflation) versus the outflow at three seconds after cuff deflation. A discriminant line with appropriate ranges incorporating standard deviations of normal values has been generated.[9] Plots of outflow values that fall below the standard range of normal are considered evidence of deep venous thrombosis at or above the level of the knee. Again, it is important that the technologist perform repeat examinations, taking into account appropriate positioning and patient management in order to minimize false-positive results.

The IPG test is not sensitive to isolated calf-vein thrombosis or to incomplete obstruction of the major deep veins. Furthermore, chronic venous insufficiency with recanalization of deep veins or with the development of prominent collateral venous channels may result in a false-negative examination.

The diagnostic criteria for maximum venous outflow depends on the technique and on the variables of the pneumatic cuff, the size of the outflow tubing, the position of the patient, and the number of legs studied at one time. The maximum venous outflow and cc/min per 100 cc of calf tissue may be calculated from the tangent line drawn to the initial (steepest) portion of the outflow curve.[7] A new automatic self-balancing strain-gauge plethysmograph (SPG-16, MedaSonics) makes it possible to calculate rapidly the maximum venous outflow. Attempts to relate venous outflow at three seconds to the incremental volume during cuff inflation (expressed as a percentage) does not result in a study as accurate as the measurement of maximum venous outflow. In our laboratory, the lower limit of normal for maximum venous outflow is approximately 25 cc/min per 100 cc of tissue, but normal values should be established for each laboratory under the condition of the study in that particular unit.

RESULTS

The sensitivity of venous outflow measurements by impedance or strain-gauge plethysmography have been reported to equal or exceed 90%. Such reports only relate to phlebographically proven disease that involves the major deep veins at or proximal to the popliteal veins. Isolated calf-vein thrombosis cannot be detected reliably by these techniques. The incidence of false-positive results depends on the prevalence of other conditions that may mimic venous thrombosis—ruptured Baker's cyst, subfascial hematoma, marked edema of other etiology, and extrinsic venous compression by malignancy, for example. Such conditions may extrinsically compress the venous system and result in falsely positive venous outflow determinations. Technically, such abnormal values are not falsely positive if one considers the fact that venous obstruction does exist in such patients; the test has been designed to detect acute deep venous thrombosis, however, and so the abnormalities associated with mimicking conditions must be considered falsely positive. The likelihood that another condition may be confused with venous thrombosis should alert the physician to establish the diagnosis phlebographically.

VENOUS VOLUME PLETHYSMOGRAPHY

TECHNIQUE

Venous volume plethysmography involves techniques that assess altered venous hemodynamics on the basis of volumetric changes in the extremity due to respiratory or pneumatic-compression maneuvers. The technique that typifies this form of venous plethysmography is phleborheography, as developed by Cranley (see Chapter 12).[10] The technique actually consists of multisegmental air plethysmography, with pneumatic cuffs placed on the thigh, on the calf at three levels, and on the foot, with an additional recording transducer on the chest to monitor respiratory movements. The patient is studied in the supine position, with the head of the bed elevated and the legs in a dependent position to permit pooling of deep

141

venous blood in the extremity. The pneumatic cuffs on the extremity record changes in limb volume associated with quiet respiration and in response to rapid, repeated compression of a cuff on the foot or calf.

DIAGNOSTIC CRITERIA

The phleborheographic method involves three separate steps. The initial recording is made with the patient breathing quietly. Limb volume normally fluctuates with each respiration, increasing during inspiration and decreasing during expiration. In this manner the plethysmograph qualitatively records those changes that may be documented by Doppler ultrasonic evaluation of venous flow velocity. In the presence of deep venous thrombosis proximal to the recording cuffs, the respiratory waves are attenuated or absent.

The second phase of the study is to record changes in segmental leg volume during and immediately following rapid repetitive inflation of the pneumatic cuff on the foot. Normally, such foot compression accelerates venous blood flow up the leg, but in an unobstructed venous system the limb volume does not significantly increase, so there is no rise in the baseline of the multisegmental recordings. In the presence of deep venous thrombosis proximal to the recording cuffs, though, foot compression increases limb volume and raises the baseline of the recordings at the various levels distal to the venous obstruction.

The third part of the test involves recording after rapid sequential inflation of the calf cuff. Calf compression normally results in no significant rise in baseline of the recording cuffs proximal to the calf, but the distal cuffs on the lower leg and foot should document a decrease in volume associated with emptying of the distal venous system by the calf compression. Normally, the recovery time to baseline is many seconds. In the presence of calf-vein thrombosis, though, there is an attenuation of the decrement of distal leg and foot volume. In chronic venous insufficiency, calf compression may result in little or no decrease in foot volume, and the recovery time is more rapid because of the reflux of calf venous blood through incompetent deep veins.

RESULTS

Phleborheography permits the most accurate assessment of acute deep venous thrombosis of the major veins of the leg, including major calf venous disease as well as venous obstruction of all major deep veins proximal to this site. Its accuracy has exceeded 95% in the experience of Cranley.[9] As in venous outflow plethysmography, the incidence of false positives is usually related to concomitant obstructive diseases.

Phleborheography is somewhat more challenging to perform than standard venous outflow plethysmography and, once again, proper positioning of the patient and attention to technical details are necessary for maximal accuracy. Nevertheless, the method is very versatile for assessing patients with not only acute deep venous thrombosis, but also chronic venous insufficiency. In the latter situation, respiratory waves may return, although a rise in baseline may be noted in response to the cuff compression maneuvers. Likewise, abnormality of foot venous volume recovery may be noted following calf compression.

Cranley offers a detailed discussion of phleborheography in Chapter 12.

VENOUS REFLUX PLETHYSMOGRAPHY

TECHNIQUE

Patients with chronic venous insufficiency due to primary or secondary varicose veins or to postthrombotic (postphlebitic) venous stasis disease may be studied by strain-gauge, photoplethysmographic (PPG), or water (foot volumetry) techniques.

Patients may be studied in the supine position by strain-gauge plethysmography, as originally reported by Barnes et al.[11] The technique is similar to that of venous outflow plethysmography except for the fact that the thigh cuff is inflated during temporary arterial occlusion induced by a proximal thigh tourniquet. Inflation of the distal thigh cuff translocates the underlying venous blood in a distal direction at a rate proportional to the degree of incompetence of the deep venous valves. The technique is somewhat uncomfortable and cumbersome and has been replaced by more simple methods of assessing venous incompetence in the upright patient during active muscle exercise.

A strain gauge may be placed around the calf with the patient in the sitting (Figure 13-2) or standing position.[12] With the gauge connected to the recorder, the patient is asked to contact the calf muscles by active plantar-flexing of the foot or by actually walking on a treadmill. The resultant changes in calf circumference reflect the integrity of the musculovenous pump of the calf. The test may be repeated with a rubber tourniquet applied to the leg just below or just above the knee to prevent

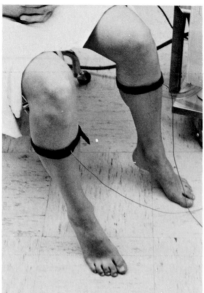
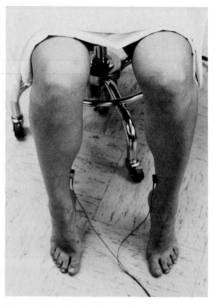

Figure 13-2. Quantifying venous reflux by strain-gauge plethysmography.

Figure 13-3. Technique of determining venous reflux by photoplethysmography.

reflux of blood through incompetent superficial (varicose) veins.

Venous reflux photoplethysmography on the other hand, is performed with the patient in the sitting position (Figure 13-3).[13] The PPG electrodes are attached to the skin on the medial aspect of the lower left leg with double-faced clear plastic tape. The transducers are connected to the recorder by the amplifier, which is placed in the venous (dc) mode. The transducers are balanced and the recording adjusted so that the pen stylus is near the top of the recorder. The patient is asked to contract the calf muscle by plantar-flexing of the feet on five successive occasions while the skin blood content of the lower leg is recorded with the PPG. The test is repeated with rubber tourniquets applied immediately below each knee to prevent reflux in incompetent superficial veins. The recording is continued until the tracing returns to baseline.

Foot volumetry may be performed by placing the foot and lower leg in a water plethysmograph, which accurately records the total volume of the submerged portion of the limb.[14] The patient then actively contracts the calf muscles by bending the leg at the knee and ankle on several successive occasions. The volume of the lower leg and foot is recorded during and immediately after the calf-muscle contraction.

DIAGNOSTIC CRITERIA

Venous reflux plethysmography using a strain gauge permits assessment of the integrity of the deep musculovenous pump of the calf. Normally, the calf circumference decreases by at least 2% following contraction of the calf muscle, and it takes an average time of 10 seconds or longer for the calf circumference to return to baseline. Very strong calf-muscle contractions may lead to marked postexercise hyperemia, however, shortening recovery time significantly. In patients with chronic venous insufficiency of the deep veins, the postexercise decrement in calf circumference is reduced and recovery time is accelerated. Importantly, marked peripheral venoconstriction or hypovolemia may result in false-positive results. Furthermore, any condition leading to increased blood flow, such as inflammation, infection, hyperthyroidism, and the like, may accelerate venous return and shorten the recovery time.

Venous reflux PPG normally demonstrates a significant decrease in skin blood content following calf-muscle contraction, the recovery time varying between 10 and 60 seconds (Figure 13-4). The marked variability

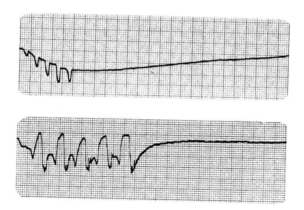

Figure 13-4. Venous reflux PPG tracings from normal (*top*) and postthrombotic (*bottom*) extremities.

in recovery time reflects the effects of skin temperature, ambient temperature, proximity to active inflammation, and other conditions that influence skin blood flow. Nevertheless, patients with venous valvular incompetence of the perforating or superficial veins may have accelerated recovery times of less than 10 seconds. In addition, the drop in skin blood content during calf-muscle exercise may be attenuated or absent.

Indeed, in patients with marked postthrombotic venous insufficiency of the deep and perforating veins, the skin blood content may actually increase following calf-muscle exercise. Such patients are particularly prone to markedly slow rates of healing of chronic venous stasis ulcers. Venous reflux PPG may be falsely positive in patients suffering from active ulcers with surrounding hyperemia of the skin. In addition, any local inflammation such as lymphangitis or superficial thrombophlebitis may result in a rapid recovery time.

PPG may differentiate incompetent perforating from isolated superficial varicose veins (primary varicose veins). In deep or perforator venous incompetence, the abnormal venous reflux remains despite the application of a superficial tourniquet; if the tourniquet normalizes the venous reflux curve, however, isolated superficial venous insufficiency is implied.

Foot volumetry, using the water plethysmograph, may document similar abnormalities of deep and superficial hemodynamics. Technique has been well outlined by Norgren.[14] Abnormalities of venous emptying of the foot and lower leg in response to calf compression and rapid venous refilling time may be noted in patients with chronic venous insufficiency. The technique is somewhat more cumbersome than that described for SPG or PPG, but the method is quite quantitative and provides meaningful information about abnormal venous hemodynamics in chronic venous disease states.

RESULTS

The sensitivity and specificity of these methods of detecting abnormal venous reflux vary with the technique, but they achieve an overall accuracy of about 90%. The prevalence of false-positive results relates to the frequency with which other conditions mimic chronic venous insufficiency.

In a series of 64 limbs studies by both strain-gauge and photoplethysmography, we have documented abnormalities by both tests in all 15 patients with chronic venous stasis disease.[15] Only two of the 15 limbs showed evidence of abnormal venous outflow. These data tend to suggest that most patients with venous stasis disease suffer abnormal cutaneous manifestations on the basis of venous valvular insufficiency, as opposed to venous outflow obstruction. In seven extremities with secondary varicose veins, SPG indicated that deep venous hemodynamics were altered in five extremities, and PPG indicated that hemodynamics were abnormal in six extremities. None of five limbs with primary varicose veins had abnormal deep venous hemodynamics by SPG, but the PPG was abnormal in three extremities. In 37 limbs with pain and/or edema, deep venous abnormalities were noted by SPG in 23, and cutaneous alterations were found by PPG in 21 limbs. Only two extremities had abnormal venous outflow by SPG.

Thus, the combination of SPG and venous reflux PPG permits qualitative and quantitative documentation of altered venous dynamics in terms of both outflow obstruction and venous valvular incompetence. Such information may lead to improved understanding of altered physiology in patients with chronic venous insufficiency.

CONCLUSIONS

Venous plethysmography provides an objective, versatile, and accurate method of defining those alterations that may result from acute or chronic venous disease, namely venous outflow obstruction and venous reflux through incompetent venous valves. Impedance or strain-gauge plethysmography provides the most accurate means of quantifying abnormal venous outflow in acute deep venous thrombosis. Venous volume plethysmography, using the phleborheograph, provides very sensitive determination of altered venous hemodynamics in acute deep venous thrombosis; it also serves to assess some patients with chronic venous insufficiency. Combinations of strain-gauge and photoplethysmography lead to useful measures of venous reflux in deep, perforating, and superficial veins. This information, along with measurements of maximum venous outflow, may provide the most versatile means of establishing altered hemodynamics in patients with chronic venous insufficiency.

REFERENCES

1. Landowne M, Katz LN: A critique of the plethysmographic method of measuring blood flow in the extremities of man. Am Heart J 23:644–675, 1942.
2. Brodie TE, Russell AE: On the determination of the rate of blood flow through an organ. Proc Physiol Soc Lond XLVII–XLIX, 1905.
3. Whitney RJ: The measurement of changes in human limb volume by means of a mercury-in-rubber strain gauge. J Physiol 109:5, 1949.
4. Wheeler HB, Pearson D, O'Connell D, et al: Impedance phlebography. Technique, interpretation and results. Arch Surg 104:164–169, 1972.

5. Dohn K: Experience with surgical treatment of the post-thrombotic disease. J Bone Joint Surg 34B:528–529, 1952.
6. Hertzman AB: The blood supply of various skin areas as estimated by the photoelectric plethysmograph. Am J Physiol 124:328–340, 1938.
7. Barnes RW, Collicott PE, Mozersky DH, et al: Noninvasive quantitation of maximum venous outflow in acute thrombophlebitis. Surg 72: 971–979, 1972.
8. Wheeler HB, O'Donnel JA, Anderson FA, et al: Bedside screening for venous thrombosis using occlusive impedance phlebography. Angiology 26:199–210, 1975.
9. Hull R, Van Aken WG, Hirsh J, et al: Impedance plethysmography using the occlusive cuff technique in the diagnosis of venous thrombosis. Circulation 53:696–700, 1976.
10. Cranley JJ, Canos AJ, Sull WJ, et al: Phleborheographic technique for diagnosing deep venous thrombosis of the lower extremities. Surg Gynecol Obstet 141:331–339, 1975.
11. Barnes RW, Collicott PE, Mozersky DJ, et al: Noninvasive quantitation of venous reflux in the postphlebitic syndrome. Surg Gynecol Obstet 136:769–773, 1973.
12. Holm JS: A simple plethysmographic method for differentiating primary from secondary varicose veins. Surg Gynecol Obstet 143: 609–612, 1976.
13. Barnes RW, Collicott RE, Hummell BA, et al: Photoplethysmographic assessment of altered cutaneous circulation in the post-phlebitic syndrome. Proc Assoc Adv Med Instrum 13:25, 1978.
14. Norgren L: Functional evaluation of chronic venous insufficiency by foot volumetry. Acta Chir Scand [suppl. 444]:1–48, 1974.
15. Cox D, Nix L, Thornhill B: Plethysmography in chronic venous insufficiency. Bruit 4 (December):35–38, 1980.

CHAPTER 14

PHOTOPLETHYSMOGRAPHY IN THE EVALUATION OF CHRONIC VENOUS INSUFFICIENCY

Donna R. Blackburn, Linda K. Peterson, and James S. T. Yao

Chronic venous insufficiency affects a vast number of people. It has been estimated that over 0.5% of the population of the United States suffers from chronic venous insufficiency, and this causes a loss of 2,000,000 working days per year.[1] Manifestations of chronic venous insufficiency include varicose veins, leg pains, stasis dermatitis, brawny hyperpigmentation, and ulceration.

Until recently, there has been no objective means of assessing the severity of chronic venous insufficiency. Doppler ultrasonic techniques are useful in detecting deep venous valvular incompetence at the femoral and popliteal levels, for instance, but they cannot quantitate the degree of venous insufficiency. Photoplethysmography, on the other hand, can.

The use of photoplethysmography to record cutaneous blood content was first described by Barnes and colleagues.[2] They found that the time it takes for cutaneous blood to refill at the ankle level after exercise differed markedly between normal and postphlebitic limbs. Since that time, photoplethysmography has been found to correlate with venous pressure and to assess accurately dysfunction of the venous valves and the muscular pump, which returns blood to the heart.

Portions of this chapter appeared in modified form in Abramowitz HB, Queral LA, Flinn WR, et al: The use of photoplethysmography in the assessment of venous insufficiency: a comparison to venous pressure measurements. Surgery 86:434–441, 1979, and in Kempczinski RF, Yao JST (editors): *Practical Noninvasive Vascular Diagnosis*. Chicago, Year Book Medical Publishers, 1982.

INSTRUMENTATION

The photoplethysmograph (PPG; MedaSonics Model PA 13 Photo Pulse Plethysmograph) consists of a transducer, an amplifier, and a strip-chart recorder (Figure 14-1). The PPG transducer emits infrared light from a light-emitting diode into the adjacent tissue, and back-scattered light is detected by an adjacent photodetector (Figure 14-2). The signal is filtered, the output voltage dc coupled, and the cutaneous blood content in the capillary network displayed on a strip-chart recorder as a continuous line. A shift in baseline represents changes in the opacity of the underlying tissue as a result of changes in the blood content of the skin. The skin blood content is correlated with venous pressures, which are a function of arterial inflow and venous outflow and/or reflux, and which are objective measurements. Although the PPG does not quantitate flow, information is derived from changes in cutaneous opacity before, during, and after exercise.

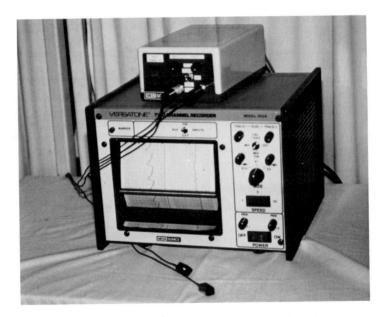

Figure 14-1. Photoplethysmography unit consisting of transducers, amplifier, and two-channel strip recorder. Reprinted with permission from Flinn WR, Queral LA, Abramowitz HB, et al: Photoplethysmography in the assessment of chronic venous insufficiency. In *Investigation of Vascular Disorders.* Edited by AN Nicolaides, JST Yao. London, Churchill Livingstone, 1981.

150

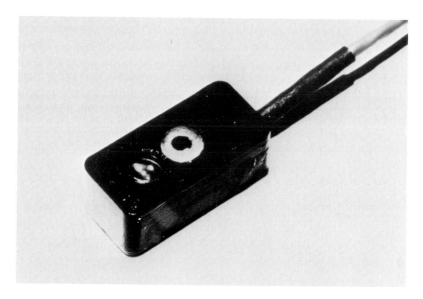

Figure 14-2. Close-up of photoplethysmograph transducer showing the light-emitting diode and adjacent photodetector.

TECHNIQUE

The examination is performed with the patient seated and with the legs in a dependent, non-weight-bearing position (Figure 14-3). The PPG transducer is applied to the skin above and slightly behind the medial malleolus with double-stick transparent tape (Figure 14-4). Because this is frequently the site of skin ulceration, it may be necessary to position the transducer at an alternate site—the forefoot or the pad of the great toe, for example. Care should be taken not to place the transducer directly over a large subcutaneous varicose vein, a major pedal artery, or an area of joint motion. It may be necessary to reposition the transducer to avoid arterial pulsation, to prevent drift, and to establish a smooth, stable resting baseline.

Once this resting baseline is achieved on the recorder, the instrument is zeroed mechanically. The patient is instructed to dorsiflex and plantar-flex his feet vigorously five times and then to relax his legs completely. Adjustment of the gain may be necessary to ensure that the tracing remains within the boundaries of the strip-chart recorder. In patients who are unable to exercise the leg sufficiently, the calf muscle may be compressed by the technologist.

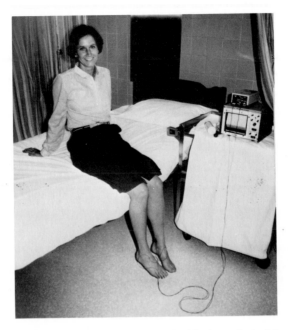

Figure 14-3. The PPG examination is performed with the patient sitting, the legs in a dependent, non-weight-bearing position.

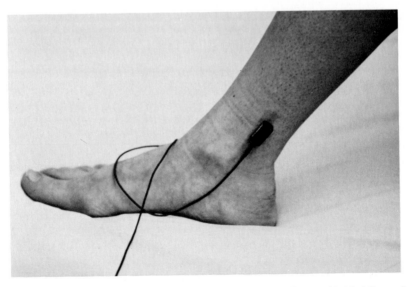

Figure 14-4. Usual placement of the PPG transducer is slightly above and behind the medial malleolus. The transducer is secured with double-stick cellophane tape.

CALCULATING THE REFILLING TIME

The venous refilling time is defined as the number of seconds required for the PPG curve to reach and maintain a stable endpoint for a period of five or more seconds. The refilling time is measured from the point at which exercise ceases to the return to the stable endpoint (Figure 14-5). The test is repeated three to five times on each limb and the refilling times averaged to express the final PPG refilling time.

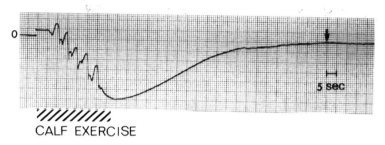

Figure 14-5. Venous refilling time is measured from cessation of calf exercise to the return of a stable baseline (*arrow*). Refilling time in this case is 110 seconds. Reprinted with permission from Flinn WR, O'Mara CS, Peterson LK, et al: The use of photoplethysmography in the assessment of chronic venous insufficiency. In: *Practical Noninvasive Vascular Diagnosis.* Edited by RF Kempczinski, JST Yao. Chicago, Year Book, 1982, pp 323–240.

INTERPRETATION

The normal physiologic response to leg-muscle exercise is a rapid reduction of venous volume and pressure. When the venous valves are competent, capillary refilling is primarily a function of arterial inflow and is, therefore, relatively slow. The normal response is a PPG refilling time of 25 seconds or longer.

When the venous valves are incompetent and resting venous hypertension is present, the refilling time is shortened because venous reflux causes congestion. Refilling time depends on valvular integrity and arterial inflow; it is long in the normal limb and short in the postphlebitic limb. Incompetent venous valves, in either the large deep veins (femoral, popliteal) or the tibial veins or perforators at calf level, cause abnormal venous refilling. Venous refilling time is shortened also in patients with long or short saphenous vein insufficiency. PPG refilling time is less than

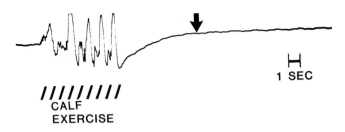

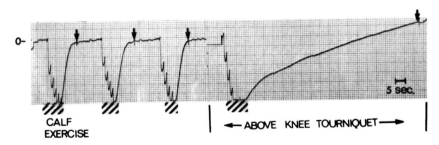

Figure 14-6. PPG curve of a patient with venous insufficiency. PPG refilling time is eight seconds (*arrow*).

20 seconds in cases of superficial or deep venous valvular incompetence. In severe venous insufficiency, venous refilling occurs in less than 10 seconds (Figure 14-6).

In order to assess the contribution of the superficial veins to the overall venous hemodynamics of the leg, a tourniquet is applied above the knee and inflated to 50 mmHg to occlude the greater saphenous venous flow. The standard PPG examination is then repeated. If the tourniquet corrects the physiologic abnormality, the abnormality is primarily the result of saphenous or other superficial vein insufficiency, and the PPG refilling time will normalize (over 25 seconds) with the above-knee tourniquet in place (Figure 14-7).

In a previous report, we studied 58 limbs (18 normal, 40 with deep or superficial venous insufficiency) to establish the diagnostic criteria. PPG and direct venous pressure measurements were compared and correlated well (0.931).[3]

Figure 14-7. PPG curves. The first three curves are abnormal, with refilling times of eight seconds. With an above-knee tourniquet in place, the refilling time normalizes, indicating superficial venous insufficiency. Reprinted with permission from Flinn WR, Queral LA, Abramowitz HB, et al: Photoplethysmography in the assessment of chronic venous insufficiency. In *Investigation of Vascular Disorders*. Edited by AN Nicolaides, JST Yao. London, Churchill Livingstone, 1981.

CONCLUSIONS

Photoplethysmography is an objective, useful screening and diagnostic test for venous insufficiency of the legs. It is simple, reproducible, and correlates very well with direct measurements of venous pressure. If the venous refilling time is normal, venous insufficiency is not the cause of the patient's symptoms. A normal venous refilling time with a tourniquet in place above the knee indicates superficial venous incompetency and differentiates between primary and secondary varicose veins. It also suggests a good result from stripping of superficial varicose veins. Abnormal, prolonged PPG refilling time with the above-knee tourniquet in place indicates deep venous incompetence. These patients will not realize complete relief of their symptoms with superficial vein stripping, and probably will need elastic support after their operations.

REFERENCES

1. Browse NL, Burnarnd KG: The postphlebitic syndrome: a new look. In *Venous Problems*. Edited by JJ Bergan and JST Yao. Chicago, Year Book, 1978, pp 395–404.
2. Barnes RW, Collicott RE, Hummell BA, et al: Photoplethysmographic assessment of altered cutaneous circulation in the post-phlebitic syndrome. Proc Assoc Adv Med Instrum 13:25, 1978.
3. Abramowitz HB, Queral LA, Flinn WR, et al: The use of photoplethysmography in the assessment of venous insufficiency: a comparison to venous pressure measurements. Surgery 86:434–441, 1979.

Part III

NONINVASIVE DIAGNOSIS OF CAROTID OCCLUSIVE DISEASE

CHAPTER 15

THE ANATOMY AND PATHOPHYSIOLOGY OF EXTRACRANIAL ATHEROSCLEROTIC CEREBROVASCULAR DISEASE

Richard A. J. O'Connor

The brain is supplied by two pairs of arteries, the large carotid arteries anteriorly and the vertebral arteries (so called because they are so close to the vertebral column) posteriorly. All four arteries enter the skull at the base of the brain and are connected in the arterial circle of Willis, a unique safety device that permits arterial blood to cross from one side to the other, in case of need, or from front to back or back to front. When one inflow artery is narrowed or occluded, flow increases via other inflow arteries to maintain pressure and flow within the circle. This collateral circulation is also assisted by inflow to the circle through the orbit. When needed, arterial blood reaches the circle of Willis from the face by traversing the orbit in reverse direction. In unusual circumstances, blood in the circle of Willis can leave the brain and flow down the vertebral artery—the so-called "vertebral steal."

Next follows a detailed description of the anatomy, particularly as it affects the signs, symptoms, and noninvasive diagnosis of cerebrovascular disease.

ANATOMY OF THE CEREBROVASCULAR CIRCULATION

Four large arteries arise from the aortic arch to supply the arms and the head (Figures 15-1 and 15-2). The first branch is the innominate, which lies behind the junction of the clavicle and the sternum. It rapidly divides into the right common carotid and right subclavian arteries. The left

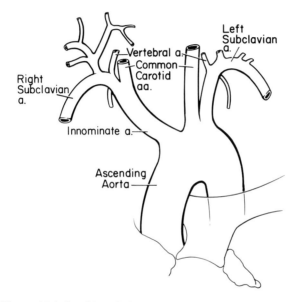

Figure 15-1. Brachiocephalic arteries arising from the aortic arch.

common carotid and subclavian arteries arise separately from the arch and quickly pass posteriorly behind the left sternoclavicular joint. The common carotid arteries pass up the neck anteriorly and have no branches. The subclavian arteries arch laterally above the clavicle and pass posteriorly behind the scalenus anticus muscle and over the first ribs en route to the arms. Here, above the clavicles, the subclavian arteries are accessible to the stethescope, and the Doppler probe can record the Doppler velocity tracings. The principal branches of the subclavian arteries in the neck are the vertebral arteries, which supply the posterior part of the brain. The other branches are the internal mammary, the thyro-cervical, and the transverse cervical arteries, all of which form abundant

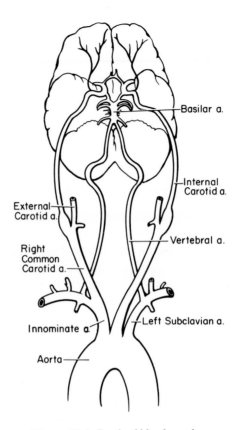

Figure 15-2. Cerebral blood supply.

collateral bypass pathways around subclavian arterial occlusions.

As Figure 15-3 indicates, the vertebral arteries pass upward for a short distance in the neck and then enter the foramen of the sixth cervical vertebra, continuing upward to enter the skull through the foramen magnum and uniting there with the opposite vertebral artery to form the midline basilar artery. The branches in the cervical portion of the vertebral arteries are muscular and spinal. The basilar artery is midline and, therefore, signs of vertebrobasilar insufficiency are usually bilateral. The basilar artery terminates in the two posterior cerebral arteries that supply the visual areas in the occipital lobes of the brain. Prior to this point, the branches of the basilar artery are to the cerebellar and pontine region (Figure 15-3). As long as one vertebral artery is intact, the basilar artery is usually well perfused and no symptoms occur.

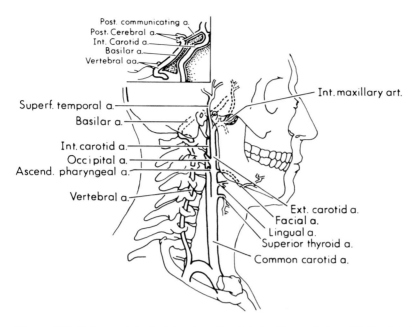

Figure 15-3. Extracranial arterial system. Reprinted with permission of D. Bandyk, MD.

The common carotid arteries ascend within the carotid sheaths adjacent to the internal jugular vein, which lies laterally, and to the vagus nerve, which lies posteriorly (Figure 15-3). At about the level of the larynx, the common carotid bifurcates into the internal and external branches. The level of the bifurcation varies among individuals and may be quite low or, sometimes, high.

The internal carotid artery goes deep and lies medial, close to the wall of the pharynx (Figures 15-2 and 15-3), and is divided into the following four portions: cervical, petrous, cavernous, and intracranial. There are no branches in the neck. The first major branch, the ophthalmic artery, arises from the cavernous segment. Small, less important branches arise in the cavernous and petrous portion. The internal carotid terminates in the anterior cerebral artery, supplying the frontal lobes; the middle cerebral artery supplies the parietal lobe laterally and the posterior communicating branch (Figure 15-3).

When the internal carotid is narrowed, the external carotid artery is an important source of collateral circulation. Its branches are divided into the following four groups (Figure 15-3): (1) anterior branches: superior thyroid, lingual, and facial; (2) posterior branches: occipital and auricular;

(3) ascending branches: pharyngeal; and (4) terminal branches: superficial temporal and internal maxillary. The branches of most importance to the collateral circulation of the brain are the occipital, facial, superficial temporal, and internal maxillary arteries.

COLLATERAL CIRCULATION

Blood flow in the subsidiary channels of the circulatory network provides a defense against narrowing or occlusion of the main arteries. These collateral pathways begin to function when needed, particularly in response to a blood pressure differential across the site of an occlusion. The decrease in blood pressure distal to the occlusion is transmitted through the next major branch of the occluded primary artery, opening anastomotic channels between the branch artery and the adjacent artery and initiating retrograde flow into the branch artery distal to the occluded artery. When successful, the collateral flow refills and maintains the circulation in the occluded artery. The intracranial collaterals of most importance are the circle of Willis and the persistent trigeminal and persistent hypoglossal arteries, embryologic vessels which occasionally remain patent (Table 15-1).

Table 15-1. Collateral Pathways of Clinical Significance

Intracranial Collaterals	Extracranial-Intracranial Collaterals
Circle of Willis	Ophthalmic artery
Persistent trigeminal artery	Occipital artery
Persistent hypoglossal artery	Spinal anastomosis
	Meningeal branches from carotid siphon
	Caroticotympanic artery

THE CIRCLE OF WILLIS

The circle of Willis is a unique anatomic structure that connects the arterial inflow from four principal sources—the two internal carotid arteries and the two vertebral arteries—via the basilar artery (Figure 15-4).

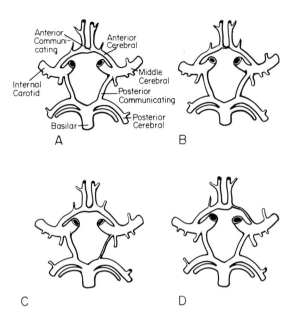

Figure 15-4. The circle of Willis with some of its variations. **A** Normal, **B** hypoplasia (anterior communicating), **C** hypoplasia (posterior communicating), **D** hypoplasia (anterior cerebral).

Under normal circumstances there is some crossover. When needed, though, blood crosses from one side to the other or from front to back to maintain both flow and pressure within the circle, thus providing the major source of collateral circulation. The circle of Willis has many anatomic variations, and the normal configuration exists in only 50% of cases. Figure 15-4 shows some of the basic variations, which may limit collateral flow.

BRANCHES OF THE EXTERNAL CAROTID ARTERY

Second only to the circle of Willis as a source of collateral flow is the group of vessels connecting the extra- and intracranial circulation. These branches of the external carotid artery are small, and they cannot enlarge quickly enough to prevent infarction from a sudden, major occlusion, but they do gradually increase the flow in the circle as they enlarge over a period of time. As Table 15-1 indicates, these extracranial collaterals include the superficial temporal branches of the external carotid, the facial artery, the internal maxillary artery, the occipital artery, the meningeal branches of the external carotid artery, and the caroticotympanic artery. The superficial temporal branches and the facial artery are the most important and can be examined by noninvasive techniques. The other potential pathways are not very important; they carry little blood and are seen only in very detailed arteriograms.

COMMON PATTERNS OF COLLATERAL CIRCULATION

With Occlusion of the Vertebral Arteries

Occlusion of one vertebral artery occurs occasionally. When it does, the unobstructed vertebral artery provides enough collateral flow to supply the basilar artery. With narrowing of both vertebral arteries, the posterior communicating arteries of the circle of Willis bring collateral flow

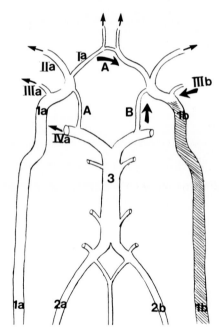

Figure 15-5. Circle of Willis with collateral blood flow after occlusion of internal carotid artery (*1b*) as shown by the large arrows: *IIIb*, ophthalmic artery reverse flow from branches of external carotid artery; *A*, anterior communicating artery brings blood from other side of circle; *B*, posterior communicating artery brings blood from vertebrobasilar system. *Inflow arteries: 1a, b,* internal carotid arteries; *2a, b,* vertebral arteries; *3,* basilar artery; *A, B,* posterior communicating arteries. *Outflow branches: Ia,* anterior cerebral artery; *IIa,* middle cerebral artery; *IIIa, b,* ophthalmic arteries; *IVa,* posterior cerebral artery.

posteriorly from the internal carotid arteries. In such cases, arteriograms may reveal the following minor pathways: (1) communications with the occipital branch of the external carotid artery via the muscular branches, (2) vertebral-to-vertebral communications, and (3) communications between the ascending cervical and the distal vertebral arteries.

With Occlusion of the Internal Carotid Artery

When the internal carotid is occluded, blood flow is maintained through the intracranial collaterals (mainly the other arteries that feed into the circle of Willis) and through the intra- and extracranial collateral system via the orbit of the eye (Figure 15-5).

The branches of the external carotid entering the orbit provide the main extracranial source of collateral circulation, reversing flow in the ophthalmic artery and perfusing the internal carotid artery (Figure 15-5B). The ophthalmic artery (Figure 15-6) is the first intracranial branch of the internal carotid. It runs anteriorly to supply the orbit by several small branches that anastomose with the frontal, supraorbital, infraorbital, and facial branches of the external carotid. Normally, flow via these branches is out of the orbit (Figure 15-6A). With stenosis or occlusion of the internal carotid artery, however, flow reverses in these vessels, which enlarge and contribute significantly to intracranial circulation (Figure 15-6B). The examiner can detect reversal of flow in these arteries by listening above the orbit with the directional Doppler. Compression of the source of the collateral (i.e., the facial or the superficial temporal arteries) audibly decreases the periorbital Doppler signals (see Chapter 18). The remaining meningeal and caroticotympanic branches are of minor clinical significance.

ARTERIAL PATHOLOGY

The main cause of stroke is cerebral or carotid atherosclerotic occlusive disease. Lesser causes of local arterial disease include arterial tortuosity kinking, fibromuscular dysplasia, trauma, aneurysms, and inflammatory arteriopathies.

Atherosclerosis begins with abnormal lipid deposits and degeneration of the subendothelial layer of the lining of the arteries, which interferes with the function of endothelial smooth muscle and leads to proliferation. Next, fibrosis develops and the intimal lining of the artery thickens.

165

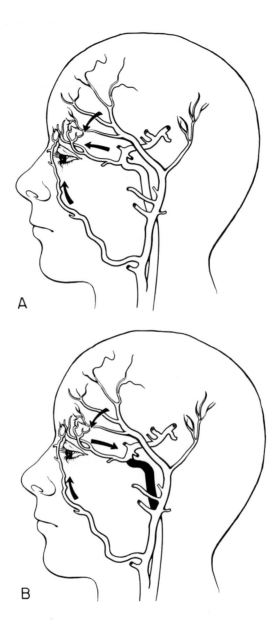

Figure 15-6. Periorbital circulation. **A** Normal periorbital flow. *Middle arrow:* ophthalmic artery. *Lower arrow:* facial artery. *Upper arrow:* branches of superficial temporal artery. **B** Reversal of periorbital flow with occlusion of internal carotid artery. *Middle arrow:* reversed flow in ophthalmic artery. The internal carotid artery is thrombosed and occluded up to ophthalmic branch.

Finally, the interaction of platelet and clotting factors in the arterial lesions leads to thrombosis.

In more detail, atherosclerosis progresses from fatty streaks and deposits to the formation of fibrous plaques, and there is increased proliferation of both smooth muscle cells and fibrous connective tissues, with extracellular lipid deposits finally leading to complicated, thick plaque with ulceration, necrosis, and calcification. Although the atherosclerotic process is generalized, the worst arterial lesions are localized, primarily at sites of turbulence and mechanical stress, such as branches and large arterial bifurcations (Figure 15-7).

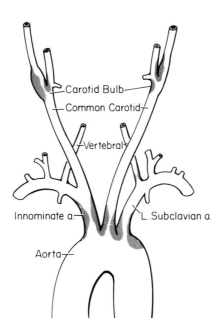

Figure 15-7. Common sites of atherosclerotic plaques and stenoses.

The major pathologic findings are narrowing of the arterial lumen and ulceration of the surface of the plaque. These ulcers may be classified as minimal, large, or compound. Stenosis and ulcer usually coexist, but the atherosclerotic process is unpredictable and variable, progressing in stages punctuated by episodes of sudden narrowing, caused by subintimal hemorrhage or microemboli from ulcerated plaques, to, finally, complete occlusion with or without thrombosis. (Figure 15-8 shows the

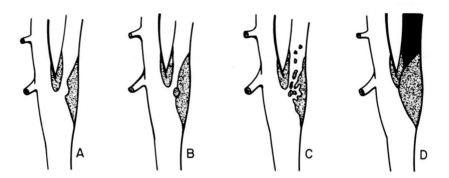

Figure 15-8. Atherosclerotic changes at the bifurcation of the carotid artery: **A,** stenosing plaque with ulceration; **B,** stenosing plaque with platelets on surface; **C,** emboli from ulcerating plaque; **D,** thrombosis with complete occlusion.

pathologic changes typical of the carotid bifurcation.) If an artery becomes completely occluded, the outcome is influenced by several factors, including the adequacy of the collateral circulation, the duration of the ischemia, the site of the infarction (some are in the "silent area" and cause no symptoms), and the general status of the cardiovascular system.

As atherosclerotic lesions enlarge, their central portions may soften and rupture through the intimal surface, discharging debris into the blood stream (Figure 15-8C). This process can cause transient ischemic attacks (TIAs), strokes, visual disturbances, and other significant neurologic problems. Furthermore, what remains of the ulcer may serve as a site for platelet aggregation or thrombus formation. If loosely attached, thrombi can be swept into the blood stream as emboli. Occasionally, a soft atheroma may hemorrhage, suddenly worsening the stenosis or occluding the artery acutely (Figure 15-8D).

These atheromatous lesions characteristically occur at arterial bifurcations (Figure 15-7). The most common sites of such lesions are the origins of arteries from the aortic arch, the proximal subclavian artery, the vertebral artery, the carotid bifurcation, the carotid syphon, the origin of the anterior cerebral artery, and along the course of the basilar artery. The ratio of extracranial to intracranial lesions is two to one.

The carotid bifurcation, especially in the proximal portion of the bulbous internal carotid, is the most frequent site of atherosclerosis and a common source of strokes. Ulceration may occur without significant stenosis and must be suspected whenever TIAs, amaurosis fugax (transient monocular blindness), or strokes suggest embolization. The ulcerated surface may develop mural thrombosis that completely occludes the internal carotid. If collateral circulation is established, the extent of the thrombus is limited by active blood flow into the cavernous portion of the internal carotid artery. Thrombosis does not extend into this segment. A similar mechanism prevents the extension of the thrombus proximal to the nearest arterial branch, limiting thrombosis to certain arterial segments. A thrombus may extend, however, if collateral circulation is inadequate.

The neurologic syndromes and clinical manifestations of cerebral ischemia are determined by the location, severity, and duration of cerebral ischemia. The clinical syndromes of most importance to vascular surgeons and noninvasive technologists are classified below. Syndromes resulting from thromboses of small or terminal arteries are not discussed here.

CLINICAL SYNDROMES OF CEREBROVASCULAR INSUFFICIENCY

STROKE

Stroke (sometimes referred to as cerebrovascular accident) is defined as a permanent neurologic deficit. Strokes vary in severity from mild, residual, permanent deficits to hemiplegia, aphasia, and coma. They are subdivided into *acute stroke, stroke in evolution* (which is unstable, with symptoms waxing or waning, and the outcome of which is still in doubt), and *completed stroke* (a stable neurologic defect neither progressing nor improving). The reversible ischemic neurologic defect (RIND) is usually considered a stroke because brain tissue has been damaged, even though complete recovery occurs after twenty-four hours. When recovery is complete in less than 24 hours, the event is classified as a TIA.

TRANSIENT ISCHEMIC ATTACK

A TIA is a localized neurologic defect from which the patient recovers within 24 hours. TIAs are characteristically sudden, brief (lasting only about 10 to 15 minutes), and often repetitive. TIA symptoms are classi-

Table 15-2. Localizing Symptoms of Cerebral Ischemia

Territory	Symptom
Carotid (hemispheric)	Unilateral paresis
	Unilateral paresthesia/anesthesia
	Aphasia
	Monocular disturbances
Vertebrobasilar	Vertigo
	Ataxia
	Bilateral visual blurring
	Diplopia
	Bilateral paresthesia/anesthesia
	Drop attacks
Nonlocalizing	Dizziness
	Syncope
	Dysarthria
	Headache
	Confusion

fied as carotid territory (i.e., hemispheric), vertebrobasilar territory, or nonlocalizing, as Table 15-2 indicates. Figure 15-9 and Table 15-3 also provide guides to localizing signs and symptoms. As their brief duration and characteristically complete recovery suggest, there is no brain damage.

Microemboli cause TIAs with specific clinical signs and symptoms (Figure 15-9). The TIA episodes are frequently repetitive, with the same signs and symptoms suggesting that the embolus from a particular site passes in the blood stream to the same site. Blood flow may be laminar, and blood passing certain sites uniformly flows into specific branches in the brain or eye.

Carotid Territory Ischemia: Hemispheric Symptoms

Carotid territory ischemia involves the anterior two-thirds of the brain, while vertebrobasilar insufficiency, discussed below, involves the posterior brain. The signs and symptoms of carotid territory ischemia are

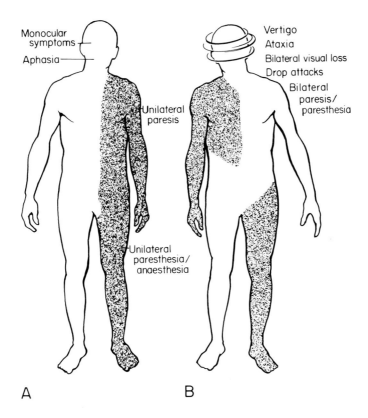

Figure 15-9. Ischemic brain syndromes: **A**, hemispheric, carotid territory signs and symptoms; **B**, vertebrobasilar symptoms. Adapted from an original painting by Frank H. Netter, MD, and reprinted with permission from Fields WE: Ciba Clinical Symposia, volume 26, number 4, 1974.

regional and usually multiple (Table 15-3). Amaurosis fugax and other ocular ischemic symptoms are described separately below.

The duration and the manner in which symptoms occur offer valuable clues to the mechanism of ischemia. Microemboli from atheromatous plaques or ulcers temporarily retard blood flow in the terminal artery branches, producing TIAs. A typical TIA would present with transient unilateral paresis or weakness of one arm or leg or both, resulting from an embolus to the motor cortex. Similar emboli can cause transient sensory losses to the face or extremities. Transient partial or complete monocular blindness, on the other hand, is commonly the result of microembolization to the retina.

Table 15-3. Localizing Ocular Symptoms and Signs of Cerebral Ischemia

Territory	Symptom or Sign
Carotid	Amaurosis fugax
Retinal	Asymptomatic atheromatous emboli (cholesterol, platelet, fibrin, calcific, or fibrinoid emboli)
	Reduced ophthalmic arterial pressure
	Monocular retinal vascular changes
	Retinopathy or infarction of acute occlusion
	Chronic hypoxia from reduced perfusion
Vertebrobasilar	Bilateral visual blurring
	Episodic diplopia
	Isolated homonymous hemianopia

These symptoms and the frequent operative findings of atherosclerosis in the related internal carotid artery suggest a cause-and-effect relationship for other TIAs. Loss of function of the entire leg and arm occurs less frequently with embolic TIAs. Although some severe TIAs result from small arterial emboli, these patients usually have severe stenosis at the carotid bifurcation. Their TIAs are hemodynamic, the result of low flow when, for example, a short run of rapid heart action prevents filling of the heart and decreases its output. The nonlocalizing symptoms of dizziness, syncope, dysarthria, headache, and confusion are symptoms also caused by low flow to the brain. TIAs from microembolization also occur in patients with "low flow" TIAs when both stenosis and ulceration are present.

Microembolization or impaired perfusion produce characteristic episodes of ocular symptoms and findings, including amaurosis fugax, which usually lasts for a period of several minutes and which may or may not be associated with contralateral limb symptoms. Amaurosis may involve all or part of the visual field. The emboli may be of atheromatous, cholesterol, platelet aggregate, fibrin, or calcific material. Some emboli are loose aggregates of platelets or fibrin that disperse and leave no permanent damage. Ophthalmologists have seen an embolus arrive in the retinal artery, stop temporarily at the first branch, and then fragment or slide over and move on to the next branch. Such emboli may partially or completely stop blood flow to a segment of the retina, impairing one-quarter to one-half of the visual field. They usually break up and are

172

washed distally, giving multiple showers of emboli and transient symptoms. Stenosis of the ophthalmic artery may reduce ophthalmic arterial pressure and cause retinal vascular changes, neovascularization, or infarctions. Central retinal artery thrombosis causes blindness and the severe retinopathy of acute occlusion. Chronic ocular hypoxia may result from reduced perfusion via the ophthalmic artery (Table 15-3).

Vertebrobasilar Insufficiency

The mechanisms of vertebrobasilar insufficiency are less well understood. They are less often embolic and frequently the result of low flow or low pressure in the circle of Willis. Vertebral artery plaques or occlusions are much less common than carotid atheromata. The vertebral arteries are smaller and carry less blood, and occlusion of one vertebral artery causes no symptoms when collateral flow from the other vertebral artery or from the circle of Willis is available. Indeed, vertebrobasilar insufficiency is unusual unless collateral flow is limited by an associated carotid stenosis, and correction of the carotid stenosis is sufficient to restore flow and pressure in the circle and to relieve the symptoms.

The symptoms of vertebrobasilar insufficiency are bilateral motor or sensory deficits, ataxia, bilateral cranial nerve signs or symptoms (e.g., vertigo, double vision, etc.), or bilateral visual blurring caused by ischemia of the occipital lobes and visual cortex (Table 15-2). Symptoms may sometimes be provoked by rotation or extension of the neck. "Drop attacks" are sudden attacks of muscular weakness during which the patient drops to the floor. They are dramatic, but rare, and are said to signify episodes of brain-stem ischemia. They occur without loss of consciousness and are followed by rapid recovery. Without significant intracranial vascular disease, lesions of the vertebral artery rarely cause symptoms unless there is stenosis of the carotid artery. Improvement after carotid endarterectomy hinges on the postoperative improvement of collateral flow to the posterior circulation. The ocular signs of vertebrobasilar disease include episodes of bilateral blurring, diminished vision, and diplopia (Figure 15-9 and Table 15-2).

Nonlocalizing Symptoms

Finally, nonlocalizing symptoms, including dizziness, syncope, dysarthria, headache, and confusion, may indicate insufficient total cerebral perfusion. They are often the only manifestations of serious extracranial vascular disease. The reversible nature of these chronic signs may be recognized only in retrospect following surgical restoration of blood flow to the hemispheres. The distinction between senility, the result of various types of brain damage, and the low-flow syndrome is very diffi-cult to make.

THE "SUBCLAVIAN STEAL" SYNDROME

This syndrome is a manifestation of vertebrobasilar insufficiency, whereby the arm "steals" blood from the brain, reversing the flow from the verte-bral into the subclavian artery. The classic symptoms are vertigo, weak-ness, and syncope, particularly after exercise of the arm. Because the origin of the subclavian artery is occluded, the pressure in the arm is lower than that in the circle of Willis. Therefore, flow reverses in the vertebral artery so that it fills the distal subclavian artery to supply the arm. The vertebral artery is one of the major subclavian collaterals to supply blood to the arm. A significant difference (i.e., $\geq$ 20–30 mmHg) between the two arms suggests the possibility of the "steal" phenomenon.

CHRONIC CEREBRAL ISCHEMIA

Patients with chronic cerebral ischemia exhibit fluctuating confusion, loss of memory, impaired mentation, and/or motor deterioration. Their symptoms are difficult to classify and to distinguish from the senility that results from various types of brain damage.

THE ASYMPTOMATIC BRUIT

This is a murmur audible over the carotid bifurcation, with no accom-panying symptoms. It is heard with the stethescope at the mid-carotid region near the angle of the jaw. It is usually well localized and disap-pears quickly as one listens inferiorly. It is not a diagnosis, only a reason for further evaluation to determine its source and significance. Ninety percent of such bruits arise from the internal carotid arteries and the carotid bifurcation. The rest are of external carotid origin or from other more uncommon lesions.

Auscultation of the neck should now be part of a routine physical examination, especially in patients over the age of 40. Murmurs appear when stenosis is 50%, but diminish or disappear when severe stenosis markedly decreases flow. Detection of a carotid bruit in an asymptomatic patient signals the need for noninvasive examination to determine its source and severity, as well as the possible presence of potentially serious cerebrovascular disease.

CONCLUSIONS

It is estimated that more than half of all strokes result from extracranial, usually correctable, atherosclerotic lesions of the carotid, vertebral, or other brachiocephalic arteries. Alert physicians, nurses, and technologists can diagnose and locate obstructing lesions with the aid of noninvasive and angiographic techniques. The extracranial arteries are accessible, and surgical techniques can remove or bypass these lesions to prevent emboli and/or restore flow and to prevent strokes. The following chapters discuss the diagnosis of such lesions by noninvasive means.

BIBLIOGRAPHY

1. Abrams HL: *Angiography,* volume 2. Boston, Little, Brown, 1971.
2. Alksne JF: Arterial collateral circulation of the nervous system. In *Collateral Circulation.* Edited by DE Strandness. Philadelphia, WB Saunders, 1969.
3. Baker WH: *Diagnosis and Treatment of Carotid Artery Disease.* Mount Kisco, New York, Futura, 1979.
4. Bandyk D: *Extracranial Arterial Disease: Anatomy and Clinical Presentation. Noninvasive Diagnostic Methods.* Seattle, University of Washington, 1980.
5. Barker WF: *Peripheral Vascular Disease.* Philadelphia, WB Saunders, 1975.
6. Field WS: *Aortocranial Occlusive Vascular Disease (Stroke).* CIBA Clinical Symposia 26:11, 1974.
7. Fields WS, Bruetnan ME, Weitel J: Monographs in the surgical sciences. In *Collateral Circulation of the Brain.* Baltimore, Williams and Wilkins, 1965.
8. Fields WS, North RR, Hass WK, et al: Joint study of extracranial arterial occlusion as a cause of stroke. I. Organization of study and survey of patient population. JAMA 203:153, 1968.
9. *Gray's Anatomy,* edition 35. Philadelphia, WB Saunders, 1973.
10. Hershey FB, Calman C: *Atlas of Vascular Surgery,* Second edition. St Louis, CV Mosby, 1967.
11. Hoyt, EF: Ocular symptoms and signs. In *Extracranial Cerebrovascular Disease: Diagnosis and Management.* Edited by EF Wylie, WK Ehrenfield. Philadelphia, WB Saunders, 1970.
12. Hutchinson EC, Acheson EJ: *Strokes: Natural History, Pathology & Surgical Treatment.* Philadelphia, WB Saunders, 1975.

13. Mungas JE, Baker WH: Amaurosis fugax. Stroke 8:232, 1977.

14. Rutherford RB: *Vascular Surgery*. Philadelphia, WB Saunders, 1977.

15. Thompson JE, Talkington CM: Carotid endarterectomy. Ann Surg 185:1, 1976.

16. Thompson JE: Cerebrovascular insufficiency. In *Peripheral arterial disease, Volume IV: Major Problems in Clinical Surgery*. Philadelphia, WB Saunders, 1975.

CHAPTER 16

COMPREHENSIVE NONINVASIVE EVALUATION OF EXTRACRANIAL CEREBROVASCULAR DISEASE

Ghislaine O. Roederer, Yves Langlois, and D. E. Strandness, Jr.

The relationship between stroke and extracranial atherosclerotic carotid disease is now well established.[1,2] The devastating, often irreversible consequences of stroke warrant and justify the necessity of detecting the disease prior to the ischemic event. Although contrast arteriography is still considered the mainstay in the evaluation of suspected carotid arterial disease, it may not be the method of choice. The risk, cost, and discomfort associated with this invasive procedure[3] preclude its widespread use, limiting its application mainly to those patients in whom operation is being considered. These considerations alone suggest the need for a safe, widely applicable, easily repeatable, and accurate noninvasive method of evaluating carotid disease. Such methods would be applicable to a large group of patients not only for purposes of screening, but also to evaluate the natural history of carotid bifurcation disease in various patient populations.

It is now recognized that the atherosclerotic plaque should be defined in terms of its location, morphology, physiologic effects, and clinical behavior over time. Clearly, no one diagnostic test is capable of providing such detailed information. For this reason, a variety of tests have been developed to examine different parameters. These methods are classified into two broad categories, namely indirect and direct. The indirect tests, which are used to estimate the physiologic effects of the disease, include pulse-delay (fluid-filled) ocular plethysmography,[4,5] pressure (air-filled) oculoplethysmography,[6,7] and supraorbital directional Doppler examination.[8,9] Conversely, the direct tests rely on information obtained from the site of the disease itself and include phonoangiographic analysis of carotid bruits, both visually[4,5] and with spectral analysis,[10] Doppler velocity waveform analysis,[11-13] Doppler systems coupled to flow-map imaging,[14] B-mode scan imaging,[15] and, finally, combined B-mode imaging and Doppler systems, with or without spectral analysis of the signal.[16-18]

The ability of these methods to predict angiographically confirmed disease at the carotid bifurcation will be discussed. As a rule, the accuracy of a test is defined in terms of its sensitivity (ability to detect the presence of disease) and specificity (ability to recognize the absence of disease). These terms are independent of the relative numbers of true negative and true positive tests in the total population and therefore are more meaningful than the overall accuracy. The results of most noninvasive tests are expressed in the form of a binary decision with respect to a particular degree of arterial narrowing. The cutoff point varies among studies, however, making the comparison of techniques difficult. For this reason, the results reported in this chapter specify the criteria for a positive result for every technique described.

For unknown reasons, atherosclerotic disease at the carotid bifurcation is usually limited to the bulb and to the first few centimeters of the internal carotid artery. This unique feature of the disease, along with the superficial location of the bifurcation, make this site ideal for the use of direct methods. In the application of noninvasive methods, these are three types of information that are important to the physician: (1) the degree of stenosis, (2) the presence of occlusion, and (3) the presence or absence of ulcerated plaque. Each of these involve special consideration. Let us briefly review the pathologic aspects of the disease and its potential relation to symptoms:

Stenosis. Narrowing produced by plaque is generally considered in two categories—those that reduce flow versus those that do not. In the carotid system, flow reduction is thought to occur when the cross-sectional area of the arterial lumen is reduced to 25% of its original dimensions.[19] This equates with a 50% reduction in diameter. Therefore, all lesions that reduce total blood flow are termed hemodynamically significant.

Occlusion. Complete obstruction of the internal carotid artery is the most pathologically advanced lesion. Its occurrence results in two major physiologic changes. First, it stops flow in the occluded segment, creating a large pressure gradient between the patent segments adjacent to the obstruction. The patency of the common carotid is usually ensured by continuing flow in the external carotid. The reentry collateral channels in the distal segment prevent propagation of the thrombus. Second, an occlusion calls into play the collateral pathways available from the ipsilateral external carotid, the intracranial communicating vessels from the opposite carotid system, and, lastly, the vertebrobasilar system. Although very tight stenoses approximating a 90%–95% reduction in diameter may mimic the hemodynamic behavior of an occlusion, the distinction between severe narrowing and occlusion has important therapeutic implications.

Plaque Ulceration. Ulceration arises because of degenerative changes within the atherosclerotic plaque. The resulting loss of surface continuity of the intima favors the accumulation of platelet and fibrin thrombi that may then embolize to the brain. Emboli appear to take three forms: fibrin, platelets, or cholesterol fragments. Importantly, whether or not a plaque ulcerates is independent of the degree of narrowing.

Both embolization from ulcerated plaques and reduction in hemispheric blood flow caused by significant stenoses or occlusions appear to be mechanisms responsible for cerebral ischemia.[20-22] Two studies have demonstrated that 50% of patients presenting with cerebral ischemic symptoms do not have hemodynamically significant lesions,[23,24] however, indicating that the ideal noninvasive test must be able to detect plaques in all stages of development.

INDIRECT TESTS

There are two basic methods of assessing the distal effects of a lesion at the carotid bifurcation. These involve the use of plethysmographic systems and the periorbital Doppler examination, the principles and relative values of which are reviewed below. Chapters 17 and 18 discuss these indirect tests in detail.

PLETHYSMOGRAPHIC TECHNIQUES

There are currently two commonly used oculoplethysmographic techniques, the pulse-delay oculoplethysmographic system described by Kartchner and McRae[4,5] and the pressure oculoplethysmographic technique developed by Gee.[6,7] Both techniques are used to assess the contribution of the ipsilateral internal carotid artery to the eye via the ophthalmic artery.

Pulse-Delay Oculoplethysmography

Pulse-delay oculoplethysmography (K/M OPG) assesses ocular filling and pulse arrival times in the eyes.[4,5] It requires bilateral fluid-filled corneal suction cups that are held in place by a negative pressure of 40–60 mmHg. A volume change in each globe occurs with every heartbeat and generates a waveform. The rates of ocular filling are then compared electronically, and expressed as a differential tracing of the pulse wave. In addition, photoplethysmographs are applied to each earlobe to provide the basis for simultaneous recordings of the times the pulse arrives from the external carotid arteries. A delay in ocular filling suggests a flow-reducing lesion in the internal carotid artery on the side of the delay. To detect bilateral stenosis or occlusion of the internal carotid arteries, the ocular waveforms are compared with those detected from the ears. A delay in both ocular pulses, as compared with the ear pulses, indicates bilateral internal carotid disease.

This technique has the advantages of excellent patient acceptance, minimal side effects, and easy performance. Although the simultaneous use of carotid phonoangiography has improved the accuracy of K/M OPG, there are important diagnostic limitations: (1) only pressure-reducing stenoses are detected, (2) bilateral common carotid disease or disease in both external and internal carotid arteries is difficult to assess, and (3) high-grade stenoses are not differentiated from occlusions. In addition, there are important variables that may affect the results, [25] including ocular disease, changes in the properties of the vessel wall, intracranial atherosclerosis, and the adequacy of collateral circulation. One review showed the accuracy of the method to range from 59% to 92% for the detection of high-grade stenoses (>50%). Its sensitivity was reported to range from 52% to 73% and its specificity from 63% to 97%.[26]

Pressure Oculoplethysmography

The principle of pressure oculoplethysmography (OPG-Gee) for the measurement of retinal arterial pressure is similar to that of the brachial artery systolic pressure as measured by a sphygmomanometer. Small suction cups are placed on the sclera of both eyes and a negative pressure of 300–500 mmHg applied. The resulting increase in intraocular pressure is sufficient to obliterate ocular pulsations. The point at which ocular pulsations return, as the vacuum is slowly reduced, can be related to the systolic pressure in the retinal artery. A retinal systolic pressure difference of 5 mmHg between the eyes indicates very high-grade stenosis or occlusion. Furthermore, the comparison of ocular pulse amplitudes may be useful. Bilateral internal carotid stenoses can be identified by comparing the ocular-to-brachial-systolic-pressure ratio. Also, when OPG-Gee is performed in conjunction with low common carotid compression, the resulting retinal arterial systolic pressure correlates well with carotid stump pressure.

OPG-Gee is well tolerated by patients and carries a low rate of complication, but it cannot be performed in the presence of ocular disease. While many of the diagnostic limitations of this method are the same as those of K/M OPG, it appears that the sensitivity of this technique is best for the detection of lesions that reduce diameter by 75% or more. A review comparing OPG-Gee and angiography showed an overall accuracy of 80%–97% in the detection of lesions that reduced luminal diameter by more than 60%. By the same criteria, its sensitivity ranged from 82% to 88%, and its specificity was between 80% and 100%.[26]

PERIORBITAL DOPPLER EXAMINATION

This technique, originally developed by Brockenbrough et al.[27] and subsequently refined by Barnes et al,[9] assesses the flow dynamics in the medial frontal and supraorbital branches of the ophthalmic artery, which anastomose with those of the external carotid artery. Normally, blood flows out of the orbit via the branches of the ophthalmic artery (antegrade flow). In the presence of significant stenosis or occlusion of the extracranial internal carotid artery, flow in the branches of the ophthalmic artery may be reversed because of the development of collaterals provided for by the external carotid artery. This change in the direction of flow can be detected with a direction-sensing ultrasonic velocity detector. Such flow patterns are confirmed by diminution or reversal of flow upon compression of one or more branches of the external carotid artery. Furthermore, compression of the common carotid artery low in the neck identifies collateral flow from either the contralateral carotid or the intracranial circulation.

Because of the multiplicity of collateral pathways and their anatomic variability, this technique requires considerable skill and an understanding of the available arterial pathways. Because it relies on the development of collateral pathways to detect the presence of a lesion, those plaques that do not reduce flow will not be detected because they do not stimulate the development of collaterals. Again, this test cannot differentiate between very high-grade stenosis and occlusion. A total of 18 studies using the periorbital Doppler evaluation in the detection of disease were recently reviewed. The cutoff point for defining a significant stenosis varied from 40% to 75%. The median sensitivity was 77% (range: 17%–96%), and the specificity was 96% (range 69%–100%).[28]

DIRECT TESTS

Direct tests derive their information from the vessels comprising the carotid bifurcation. They may be classified into two categories. The first is based on the analysis of bruits and includes carotid phonoangiography[4,5] and phonoangiographic spectral analysis.[10] The second category includes a variety of ultrasonic methods. Chapters 17, 19, 20, 21, 22, and 23 discuss these direct tests in detail.

BRUIT ANALYSIS

Auscultation of the low, middle, and high neck is routinely performed during a clinical examination. However, the presence or absence of a bruit by stethoscopic examination is not a reliable indicator of the presence or absence of internal carotid disease. Ziegler et al. showed that 73% of 199 patients had a stenosis demonstrated by arteriography without an associated bruit.[29] In a study by David et al., 14% of 417 patients with asymptomatic bruits were judged normal by angiography.[30] Also, looking at the relationship between the presence of a bruit and age, Hammond and Eisenger showed that only 12% of the subjects over 60 years of age had a detectable bruit.[31] Clearly, the finding of a bruit alone is often inadequate in predicting its origin. Because of the problems associated with the audible interpretation of a bruit, methods have been developed to assist in defining the origin of the finding.

Carotid Phonoangiography

Carotid phonoangiography (CPA) involves the use of a microphone and an amplifier to enhance the bruit electronically. In addition, a visual display of the bruit's relation to the first and second heart sounds may be used to facilitate interpretation. Criteria based on the site of maximal amplitude and on the duration of the bruit within the cardiac cycle are used to localize and to estimate the degree to which the carotid artery is narrowed. Kartchner and McRae developed CPA to complement the use of the OPG.[4,5] These investigators developed a stenosis-flow scoring chart to grade disease at the carotid bifurcation according to the combined results of OPG and CPA. Although the simultaneous use of OPG and CPA by Kartchner and McRae improved the accuracy of both methods when used separately, others have not been able to confirm this.[25,32] (Refer to Chapter 17 for more information about CPA.)

Phonoangiographic Spectral Analysis

Spectral phonoangiography evaluates the residual diameter of the arterial lumen by a quantitative spectral analysis of bruits arising at the carotid bifurcation.[10,33] Arterial bruits occur when the pattern of flow becomes turbulent as a result of a stenosis. Turbulent flow produces a characteristic sound spectrum in which the amplitude rises to a given frequency and thereafter falls sharply with a characteristic slope as frequencies continue to rise (Figure 16-1). The frequency at which the fall-off occurs, also termed the "break frequency," bears a constant relationship to the residual diameter of the arterial lumen, as follows:

$$ d = \frac{100}{f_b} $$

where f_b = break frequency, d = residual diameter, and 500 = constant rate of flow for the carotid bifurcation.

In 31 out of 33 stenoses, Kistler et al. found that the results of phonoangiography and arteriography agreed to within 0.5 mm.[33] Knox et al. have confirmed the accuracy of the method, although not all detected bruits could be analyzed using this device.[34] Low-intensity bruits associated with mild or very severe stenoses may be difficult to interpret.

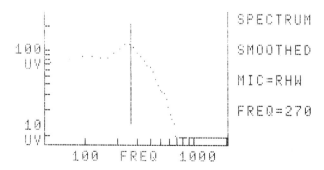

Figure 16-1. Bruit frequency spectrum. On the CRT display, the break frequency of the bruit is indicated by the vertical line.

Also, bruits arising in the external carotid are a potential source of error. Therefore, this technique is not ideal for screening, but may be of value when combined with other techniques. A potentially important application is the monitoring of disease progression in patients with bruits.

ULTRASONIC TECHNIQUES

Ultrasonic methods have been widely applied to the diagnosis of vascular disease in the form of Doppler, pulse-echo ultrasound, or a combination of the two. Doppler ultrasound provides information about particles in motion, such as red blood cells, whereas pulse-echo ultrasound generates an anatomic image based on the acoustic interfaces between tissues of different densities. The techniques based on both modalities combine a Doppler device and a pulse-echo imaging system. It must be noted, however, that flow imaging is also possible by electronic processing of the Doppler signal.

Ultrasonic Doppler Principles

The basic element of ultrasonic instrumentation is the transducer. This crystal is deformed slightly by an electric voltage applied to it, resulting in a mechanical pressure wave. This phenomenon, termed piezoelectricity, is the basis for the production of ultrasound. Similarly, a mechanical deformation of the crystal occurs upon contact with the returning ultrasound, which generates an electric voltage. Based on this property, the same transducer may function as a transmitter, a receiver, or both. It is the interface between two tissues of different acoustic impedance that causes the transmitted ultrasound to be reflected back with a strength proportional to the density difference between the two tissues.

Doppler ultrasound works on the basic principle that any moving object in the path of an emitted sound beam will shift the frequency of the emitted signal. In practice the frequency shift, Δf, is related to the velocity of blood as follows:

$$\Delta f = \frac{2 v f_0 \cos \Theta}{c}$$

where f_0 = transmitted frequency, v = velocity of red blood cells, c = velocity of sound in tissue, and Θ = angle of incident sound beam. (See Chapter 21 for a detailed account of Doppler physics, and Chapter 23 for a discussion of the physical phenomena associated with its clinical application.)

According to this equation, the frequency shift is linearly related to the emitted frequency. Most Doppler instruments used in clinical practice employ transmitting frequencies in the range of 2 to 10 MHz. Since tissue penetration is inversely related to the emitted frequency, high-frequency systems are most suitable for the examination of superficial arteries. Conversely, low frequencies are chosen for the evaluation of deeper vessels.

Doppler Instrumentation

Both continuous-wave and pulsed Doppler have been used for direct interrogation of the carotid bifurcation. The conventional continuous-wave Doppler uses separate transmitting and receiving transducers that operate continuously to detect flow at all points along the emitted sound beam. The signal thus obtained may contain information from more than one vessel along the path of the beam. The pulsed Doppler overcomes this disadvantage by detecting flow at discrete points along the beam. The pulsed device may employ a single transducer functioning as both a transmitter and receiver. The transducer emits short bursts of ultrasound, and a small portion of the time interval between bursts is allocated to the receiver function. Given the relatively constant velocity of sound in soft tissue, flow may be detected at different tissue depths by varying this time interval. The ability to sample flow at different depths is termed range gating, and the region in space where flow is detected is referred to as the sample volume. The size of the sample volume will be determined by pulse length, transducer configuration, and beam focusing (Figure 16-2).

Early work with continuous-wave Doppler provided nondirectional flow information only. As a result, the determination of forward and reverse flow components was not possible.[35-37] To overcome this serious limitation, quadrature phase separation was developed and is currently the most commonly used method to detect the direction of flow.[38.39]

Doppler Signal Processing

Audible interpretation of the directional Doppler signals is adequate for many simple applications, but it does have severe limitations. To provide a more informative method of displaying the Doppler signal, several alternatives to process the velocity signal have been developed. The most widely utilized are the zero-crossing detectors and frequency spectral analyzers. Inexpensive and easy to use, the zero-crossing frequency detector provides an analogue waveform of the Doppler signal, employing a frequency-to-voltage converter. The voltage output is proportional

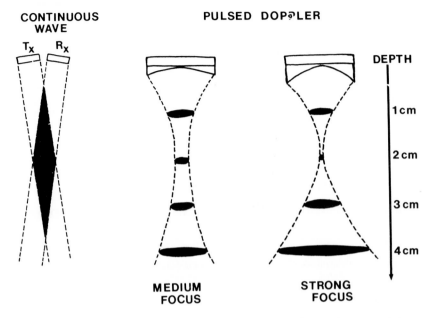

Figure 16-2. Sample volume concepts. Continuous-wave Doppler uses two separate transducers that operate continuously to detect flow at all points along the emitted sound beam. Pulsed-wave Doppler may utilize one transducer functioning intermittently as a transmitter and as a receiver. Flow may be detected at various tissue depths. The region in space where flow is detected is termed the sample volume. The size of the sample volume is determined by pulse length, transducer configuration, and beam focusing. Courtesy of DJ Phillips, University of Washington.

to the number of zero-crossings. This method has been shown to be highly dependent on the signal-to-noise ratio and on the amplitude of the return signal.[40, 41]

Spectral analysis is the method of choice for processing the Doppler signal (see, for instance, Chapter 20). First, it allows the visualization of artifacts that may be present in the waveform, such as background noise, signals arising from arterial wall motion or probe movements, and signals generated by the simultaneous recording from two different vessels. More importantly, the frequency analyzer displays the complete frequency and amplitude content of the Doppler signal. The spectral information is usually displayed with time on the horizontal axis, frequency on the vertical axis, and amplitude expressed as a function of a gray-scale intensity.

Early work with spectral analysis was performed using an off-line method, but this technique was time-consuming, and various methods for real-time spectral analysis have since been developed. These include multiple-band pass filters,[39,42,43] digital time-compression analysis,[37,44] and fast Fourier transform (FFT).[45] The commercially available FFT units provide a wide dynamic range and can operate on line to give a continuous display of frequency versus time with amplitude expressed as a function of the gray-scale intensity.

Clinical Applications

As previously mentioned, ultrasound has been employed in various instruments in the form of Doppler, pulse echo, or both. Depending on the type of Doppler used and the signal processing performed, the velocity information can be expressed in the form of an analogue waveform, a frequency spectrum, or a flow image. The pulse-echo mode, when used alone, provides only an anatomic image based on acoustic characteristics of tissue. Four diagnostic modalities based on these principles are discussed here: (1) velocity waveform analysis, (2) Doppler imaging systems, (3) pulse-echo imaging systems, and (4) duplex scanning with spectral analysis.

Velocity waveform analysis.   Each of the branches of the common carotid artery has distinct flow patterns. The flow in the external carotid artery is similar to other peripheral arteries in which flow during diastole reaches zero or transiently reverses. Flow in the internal carotid artery is relatively constant and never reaches zero. This is a reflection of the very low resistance of the intracranial bed. As the common carotid artery gives rise to two vessels of substantially different resistance, the flow within it assumes an intermediate pattern. Because it contributes 80% of its flow to the internal carotid artery, its flow pattern resembles that of a low-resistance vessel.[46] These patterns are readily recognized by both auditory interpretation of the Doppler signal and inspection of the velocity waveform.

Various features from the recorded waveforms have been utilized to assess the amount of disease at the carotid bifurcation. Planiol and Pourcelot, using a continuous-wave Doppler, defined a resistivity index from the common carotid artery as a means of predicting the extent of disease at the carotid bifurcation. This index is the ratio of the difference between the peak systolic and diastolic velocities, normalized by the peak systolic velocity. If this ratio is greater than 0.9, it is very likely that there is either a total occlusion or a more than 90% diameter reduction of the internal carotid artery.[11] In 1976 Gosling described the a/b ratio.[47] This feature uses the two characteristic systolic peaks seen in the Doppler-shifted frequency waveform. The diagnostic value of this ratio was first emphasized by Baskett et al.[48] and later by Prichard et al.[49] In 1977 Rutherford introduced a more complex multidiscriminant analysis of the common carotid waveform, using a continuous-wave device.[13] This analysis involved five parameters, was 100% accurate in differentiating normal from diseased arteries, and reached an 82% accuracy in discriminating between stenoses that reduced luminal diameter by more than and less than 50%.

Ultrasonic arteriography.   The addition of a position-sensing arm to the Doppler transducer made it possible to generate images of flow on a storage oscilloscope. Such flow-imaging systems use either continuous or pulsed Dopplers. These methods permit visualization and identification of the arteries of the neck, and in addition are capable of detecting regions of abnormal flow as the image is being generated.

Continuous-wave Doppler ultrasonic arteriography, introduced by Spencer et al.,[50] combines a position-sensing arm and a continuous-wave Doppler device with a storage oscilloscope. It employs 5-MHz transmitting and receiving crystals that operate continuously to produce an image of the carotid bifurcation and to permit the evaluation of flow patterns across the bifurcation. The direction-sensing capabilities of the Doppler allow the exclusion of venous signals so that only arterial flow contributes to the image. A tape recording of the signal is made for replay and auditory analysis of the flow characteristics. In an early report comparing the results of carotid imaging and angiography in 148 arteries, the accuracy of the method was 96% in the detection of stenoses greater than 50%.[50] There were five false-negative and one false-positive examination for critical stenosis. A more recent study by Weaver et al. showed a 52% accuracy in the detection of 50%–75% stenoses, increasing to 71% in the 76%–99% category of disease. In the detection of 0%–50% stenoses the test had no predictive value. A false-negative rate of 56% and a false-positive rate of 19% were also reported.[51]

A slightly different method, based on the same principles, was introduced by White and Curry.[52] This technique also involves a continuous-wave Doppler device, but differs in that the frequencies detected are expressed in the form of a color code on the ultrasonic image. Although these authors reported an 80% accuracy in the 75%–99% diameter reduction range, the distinction between normal arteries and mildly diseased arteries was still poor.

Pulsed Doppler ultrasonic arteriography (Figure 16-3), first introduced by Hokanson et al. in 1971,[14] employs a 4-mm piezoelectric crystal mounted on a position-sensing arm, a six-gate pulsed-Doppler ultrasonic flow

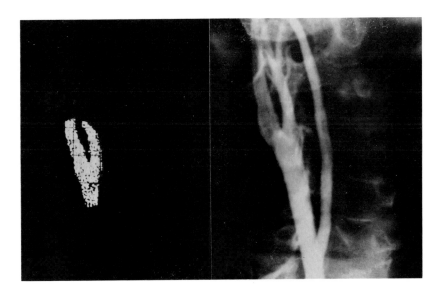

Figure 16-3. Pulsed-Doppler ultrasonic arteriogram of a normal carotid bifurcation (*left*) with corresponding contrast angiogram (*right*). Reprinted with permission from Strandness DE Jr: Doppler ultrasonic techniques in vascular disease. In *Noninvasive Diagnostic Techniques in Vascular Disease.* Edited by EF Bernstein. St Louis, CV Mosby, 1978, p 16.

detector, and a storage oscilloscope. Selecting 40% diameter reduction as the criterion for a positive test, Russell et al. reported an overall accuracy of 86%, a sensitivity of 90%, and a specificity of 84%. When the image was used to estimate the degree of stenosis, two types of errors were found: faulty identification of the vessels and underestimation of vessel narrowing when using only a single-plane view of the artery (projection errors). Furthermore, vessel calcification was found to be a source of problems in visualizing suspicious areas.[53]

The recent addition of spectral analysis, using the FFT method, maintained or improved the accuracy of the Hokanson device in each category of disease and allowed correct identification of the external and internal branches of the carotid bifurcation.[53] Also, in order to reduce misinterpretation caused by projection errors, a microcomputer was interfaced to the ultrasonic arteriograph to produce simultaneous anteroposterior and lateral views of the bifurcation along with transverse cross sections at selected points along the vessel. Using this modification, Miles et al. reported a 90% accuracy in detecting lesions that reduced luminal diameter by more than 40%. All lesions greater than 40% by angiography were identified with the computerized ultrasonic arteriograph, and 52 of the 61 arteries that were reduced by less than 40% were correctly identified.[54]

Chapters 21 and 22 discuss pulsed-Doppler ultrasonic arteriography in detail.

Pulse-echo (B-mode) imaging.   Ultrasound has found another clinical application in the form of pulse-echo, or B-mode, imaging. As previously described, the depth of a particular tissue interface is proportional to the time interval between the transmitted pulse and the echo received, because the velocity of sound is approximately constant in all soft tissues. This results in a linear display of echoes, representing the various tissue interfaces along the axis of the beam. A series of such linear displays yields a two-dimensional image, obtained by moving the transducer over the surface of the skin and by using position-sensing electronics to process the echoes. The strength of an echo is expressed in terms of brightness on an oscilloscope. "B-mode" refers to a type of representation using brightness modulation, and "B-scan" defines the B-mode technique that employs a moving transducer.

The use of this principle in the diagnosis of carotid disease led to the development of both the B-mode ultrasonic arteriograph, introduced by Mercier et al.,[15] and the duplex scanner, first described at the University of Washington.[16]

The B-mode ultrasonic arteriograph was developed in 1978 at the Stanford Research Institute.[15] In employs a 10-MHz focused mechanical scanner. Such high-frequency transducers, while lacking penetrance, have the physical advantage of markedly improved resolution for superficial vessels, such as the carotid bifurcation. First recorded on videotape, the B-mode images are subsequently photographed on Polaroid film for further review. Because the anatomic images generated are based on the acoustic interfaces between tissues of different densities, the vessel lumen appears sonolucent and the vessel walls yield prominent echoes as a result of higher acoustic reflectivity. If this technique is to be used in the detection of carotid disease, the identification of the vessel wall/lumen interface is of critical importance. Calcium, often present in conjunction with atherosclerotic plaques, inhibits the transmission of ultrasound. These calcified plaques can be identified by bright intraluminal echoes, accompanied by characteristic posterior shadowing. Further limitations are related to the inability of ultrasound to differentiate between substances of similar acoustic impedance. Because noncalcified plaques and thrombi have approximately the same acoustic impedance as blood, freshly occluded vessels and plaques containing soft, fatty

190

material may be undetected or misinterpreted by B-mode imaging alone.

Initial studies performed at the Mayo Clinic reported a close correlation between ultrasonic imaging and angiography in 13 of 21 vessels. Using the same B-mode prototype, Humber et al. reported a sensitivity of 82% and a specificity of 58% in predicting stenoses greater or less than 50% in 63 arteries. These investigators found the method to be relatively insensitive in its ability to grade stenoses, as evidenced by a 36% sensitivity in the detection and quantitation of stenoses greater than 50%.[55] The unreliability of B-mode imaging in identifying occlusions was evidenced in a report by Katz et al., using a commercially available unit. In this study only 6 of 21 (29%) occluded vessels were correctly identified.[56] Although the ability of B-mode scanning to detect ulceration has been suggested, insufficient data are available to substantiate this claim.

Although B-mode imaging of the carotid bifurcation has many advantages, it is misleading in the presence of soft plaques, calcification, and occlusions. Conversely, the use of a Doppler device alone is limited by its inability to identify the site and angle at which flow is sampled. A duplex scanning system, on the other hand, which combines a pulsed Doppler with a real-time B-mode imaging system, offers advantages over either method when used alone. With this combination, the pulsed echo is used to define the location and anatomy of the blood vessels and the pulsed Doppler is used to acquire blood flow velocity information at specific arterial sites. The rest of this chapter focuses on this device.

DUPLEX SCANNER

DESIGN

The concept of a duplex scanner was first described by Babter et al,[16] and the instrument itself (Mark V Scanner, Advanced Technology Laboratories, Bellevue, Washington) was developed at the University of Washington for clinical studies. It combines a single-gate pulsed Doppler with a B-mode imaging system (Figure 16-4). The scanhead contains three fixed 5-MHz transducers, imbedded in a rotating wheel, which generate a two-dimensional image of soft-tissue interfaces. The B-mode image is used to locate the carotid bifurcation and to recognize anatomic variations. The axis of the ultrasonic beam is indicated by a white line on the screen and the sample volume by a white dot along this line. Manual

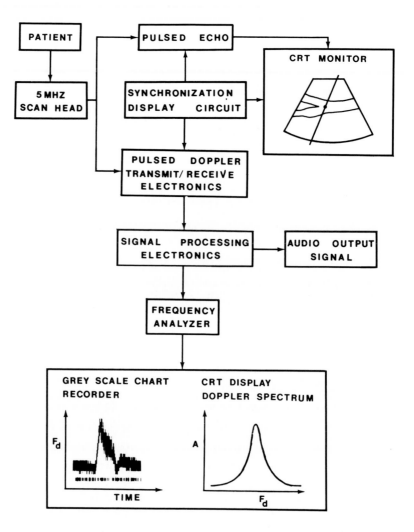

Figure 16-4. Block diagram of the ultrasonic duplex scanner.

controls mounted on the scanhead allow the examiner to adjust both Doppler angle and sample volume depth on the image display (Figure 16-5). This allows the examiner to place the sample volume in the center stream of the vessel of interest and to set a desirable Doppler angle with respect to the vessel axis. The examiner may then change to the Doppler mode using a foot switch. In this mode, the B-mode is electronically frozen and one of the transducers is used as the pulsed Doppler.

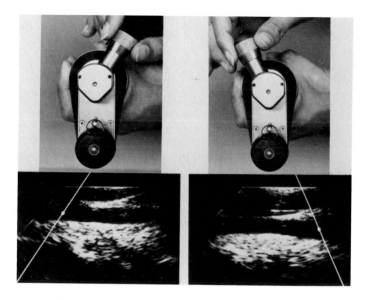

Figure 16-5. Controls for spatial adjustment of Doppler direction and sample volume depth. Courtesy of DJ Phillips, University of Washington.

As measured in our laboratory, the pulsed-Doppler sample volume measures approximately 3 cubic millimeters at an operating range of 25 mm. In addition to the auditory interpretation, the quadrature outputs of the pulsed-Doppler signal are sent to an on-line FFT spectral analyzer (prototype FFT spectrum analyzer, Honeywell Inc., Denver, Colorado). The analyzer provides 400 spectra per second with a frequency resolution of 100 Hz. The copy output of the directional mode-normalized Doppler spectrum is in the form of a time versus frequency gray-scale spectrum. The 10-kHz frequency range along the ordinate allows 7 kHz for forward flow and 3 kHz for reverse velocity components, with respect to the zero baseline. The intensity of the spectrum gray scale is proportional to the amplitude of the Doppler signal for each frequency during the analysis time.

METHOD OF EXAMINATION

The examination is performed with the patient supine and begins with a longitudinal scan of the extracranial carotid arteries on both sides. The anatomy of the bifurcation is visualized on the B-mode image. Using the

Doppler mode, the examiner then identifies the vessels by their characteristic audible flow signal. As the examination proceeds, both B-mode images and Doppler signals are recorded on videotape for later analysis and review. The sites routinely recorded include the low common carotid, the high common carotid at the bifurcation, the proximal and distal internal carotid artery, the external carotid artery, and, finally, any site along the bifurcation where high-velocity signals are detected during the longitudinal scan (Figure 16-6). Flow-reducing lesions, characterized by harsh, high-frequency signals, are easily detected using only auditory analysis of the signals. Flow disturbances secondary to minor stenoses ($<50\%$) and those which occur in the normal bifurcation, however, do not have these characteristic features and may be undetected by auditory interpretation alone. Real-time spectral analysis greatly improves the ability of this system to evaluate those stenoses that reduce luminal diameter by less than 50%.

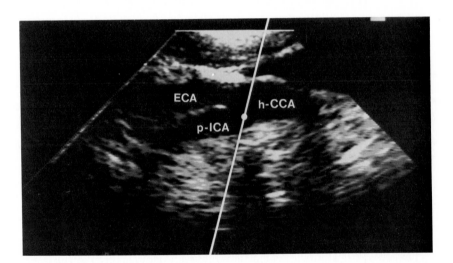

Figure 16-6. B-mode image of the carotid bifurcation. The vessel lumen appears sonolucent and the vessel walls yield prominent echoes because of their higher acoustic reflectivity. The position of the Doppler beam is indicated by a white line and the sample volume by a white dot. Note the 60° angle of the beam with respect to the vessel axis. The sites routinely recorded are the low common carotid (not shown), the high common carotid at the bifurcation (h-CCA), the proximal and distal internal carotid (p-ICA; d-ICA not shown), and the external carotid proximally (ECA). All high-velocity signals detected along the bifurcation are also recorded.

SPECTRAL ANALYSIS

Doppler spectral analysis is based on three basic hypotheses: (1) various degrees of arterial narrowing will produce predictable alterations of the velocity waveforms, (2) the information can be easily acquired using a Doppler system, and (3) specific features of the spectral waveform may be identified and quantified to determine the severity of disease.

Before focusing on the frequency content of the spectral waveforms, it is important to note that the envelope of the waveform can assist in identifying the vessel from which data are obtained. The external carotid artery has a multiphasic flow pattern similar to that of any peripheral artery. The internal and common carotid arteries, on the other hand, have higher mean flow because of the low resistance of the intracerebral circulation (Figure 16-7).

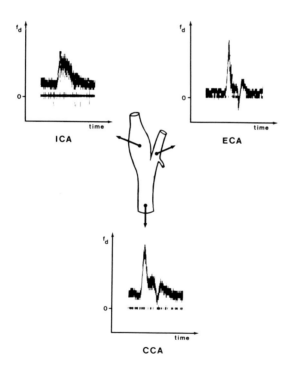

Figure 16-7. Spectrum from the external carotid artery (*ECA*) demonstrating multiphasic flow pattern characteristic of any peripheral artery. Spectra from the internal (*ICA*) and common carotid arteries (*CCA*) show high mean flow throughout the cardiac cycle, because of the low vascular resistance of the intracerebral circulation.

In the analysis of the content of the velocity spectrum, peak systolic velocity and spectral width are the two basic features used to evaluate the severity of disease (Figure 16-8). During systole, normal arterial flow is characterized by laminar movement of the red cells, which is seen on the spectrum as a narrow band of frequencies during systole with a clear window beneath the envelope. Intimal roughening secondary to a minimal lesion may interfere with this normally laminar pattern and give rise to disturbed flow without increasing peak velocity. On the spectrum, this abnormality is expressed as spectral broadening, which results from red cells moving randomly through the Doppler sample volume. In general, as the severity of the stenosis increases, the spectral broadening comes to occupy the entire window beneath the systolic envelope.[18] In stenoses that narrow the vessel lumen by more than 50% of their original diameter, the velocity of flow greatly increases in the narrow segment, pro-

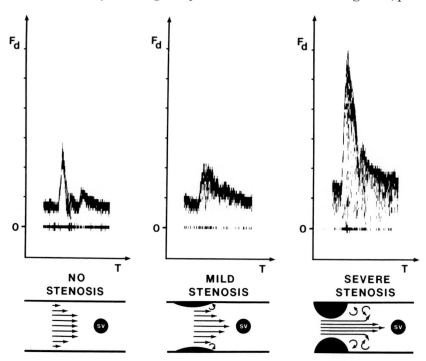

Figure 16-8. Center-stream flow from a normal artery is laminar and demonstrated on the spectrum (*left*) as a narrow band of frequencies during systole, with a clean window beneath the envelope. Turbulence caused by mild stenosis appears as spectral broadening on the frequency spectrum (*center*), without producing changes in the peak systolic velocity. High peak velocities and spectral broadening throughout the cardiac cycle characterize high-grade lesions. Also note the increase in end-diastolic velocity (*right*).

ducing higher peak systolic frequencies on the spectrum. Peak systolic velocity of the normal arteries ranges from 2 to 3 kHz, whereas vessels associated with severe narrowing show peak systolic frequencies well above 4 kHz. The combination of high peak systolic frequencies and spectral broadening throughout the entire cardiac cycle is characteristic of high-grade stenoses.

It must be emphasized, however, that the value of spectral analysis in grading the severity of disease depends on several important details. Because steep velocity gradients are present near the arterial wall, the sample volume must be placed in the center of the artery. This avoids errors in interpreting as disturbed flow the spectral broadening caused by such gradients. Similarly, when the size of the sample volume is equal to or larger than the diameter of the vessel, the entire range of velocities present across the artery is detected and displayed as spectral broadening.[57] Also, it is important to maintain a standard Doppler angle with respect to the vessel axis if the recorded peak frequencies are to be used in the analysis.

CLINICAL STUDIES AND RESULTS

Accuracy

Several reviews reporting our experience using duplex scanning and spectral analysis have been published.[18,58-60] To compare the accuracy of spectral analysis with angiography, the arteriograms were read by one radiologist and the carotid arteries classified according to the percentage of vessel narrowing: (1) normal, (2) 1%–15% diameter reduction, (3) 16%–49% diameter reduction, (4) 50%–99% diameter reduction, and (5) occlusion.

Correspondingly, the spectra were placed into one of these five classes according to criteria designated by the letters A through E: (A) normal: peak frequency below 4 kHz without spectral broadening; (B) less than 15% diameter reduction: peak frequency below 4 kHz, minimal spectral broadening in the decelerating phase of systole, and clear window below the acceleration phase of systole; (C) 15%–49% diameter reduction: peak systolic frequency above 4 kHz, spectral broadening throughout systole, and increased diastolic frequencies; and (E) total occlusion: absence of signal in the internal carotid artery and characteristic low diastolic flow in the common carotid.

The comparison between the duplex and angiographic results were expressed in terms of overall accuracy, sensitivity, specificity, and Kappa. The Kappa statistic, first introduced by Cohen in 1960,[61] provides a measure of agreement corrected for chance in two-way tables. The value of Kappa is equal to zero if the observed agreement is equal to that reached by chance alone. A perfect agreement reaches a maximal value of +1.

The initial studies using this spectral classification scheme reported a sensitivity of 98%,[58,59] but specificity was much less, ranging up to only 36%. This poor specificity was partly related to the transducer design and sample volume size.[57] At the time of these studies a 5-MHz, medium-focus transducer with a 9.5-mm diameter was used. At the 4-cm focal point, the size of the Doppler sample volume was 17 cubic millimeters. At the distance from the skin surface where carotid arteries usually lie, however, the effective sample volume size was 24 cubic millimeters. Consequently, the development of a transducer with a focal length of 2 cm and a sample volume size of 3 cubic millimeters permitted the detection of a more discrete region in space at the depth of the bifurcation. With this device, specificity increased to 50%, while sensitivity remained at 98%. The overall agreement corrected for chance (Kappa) also increased from 0.581 ± 0.046 to 0.682 ± 0.064.[59] Although these data represent improvement in specificity, further work was undertaken to improve it to a more acceptable level.

Because flow separation zones and eddies are known to occur at the carotid bifurcation as a result of the geometry of the bulb,[62,63] it became apparent that these flow disturbances contributed to our difficulty in differentiating normal arteries from those with minimal disease. With increasing experience, we have come to recognize the importance of using data from the low common carotid velocity waveform as a predictor of disease in the internal carotid bulb. Although poorly understood, this fact had also been noted by other authors.[13,48,49] A new feature derived from the common carotid waveform was evaluated and defined as the ratio of the peak frequency at systole (a) to the point of first zero slope after systole (b), normalized by the peak frequency at systole (Figure 16-9). A normal value for this ratio is greater than 0.5.[64]

The addition of this ratio to the previously used criteria led to a slight modification of the spectral classification scheme (Table 16-1). Figures 16-10 to 16-14 illustrate frequency spectra obtained from the common and internal carotid arteries for all five categories. Table 16-2 summarizes the latest results of duplex scanning and spectral analysis when this new feature is added.[65] A total of 336 sides were available for angiographic comparison. Two-hundred eighty-seven sides were correctly identified by duplex scanning for an overall accuracy of 85%. The ability to predict correctly the degree of stenosis was high in each category of disease: 84% of normal sides, 80% in the 1%–15% diameter reduction

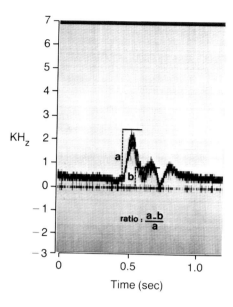

Figure 16-9. Normal low common carotid arterial velocity waveform. Peak systolic frequency (a) and maximum frequency at the point of first zero slope after systole (b) are used to calculate the $(a-b)/a$ ratio. A ratio above 0.5 is normal.

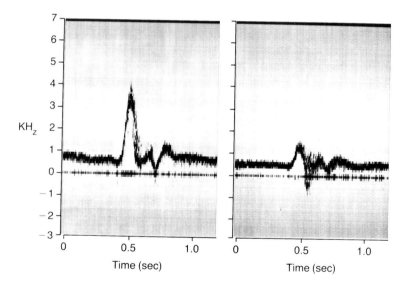

Figure 16-10. Typical normal common artery as defined by $(a–b)/a$ ratio (*left*) feeding a normal internal carotid artery (*right*).

Table 16-1. Categories of Internal Carotid Artery Disease

Class	Rating (% Stenosis)	Artery[a]	Diagnostic Criteria
A	Normal	CCA	Normal[b] CCA contour.
		ICA	No or minimal spectral broadening in decelerating phase of systole. Window still present.
B	Minimal disease (1%–15%)	CCA	Abnormal[b] CCA contour.
		ICA	Minimal or even no spectral broadening in decelerating phase of systole. Clear window.
C	Moderate disease (16%–49%)	ICA	Spectral broadening throughout systole. No window. Systolic peak <4 kHz.
D	Severe disease (50%–99%)	ICA	Systolic peak >4 kHz. Increased diastolic flow. Marked spectral broadening.
E	Occlusion	CCA	Flow to zero or reversed.
		ICA	No signal.

[a] CCA, common carotid artery; ICA, internal carotid artery.
[b] If the first zero slope after systole occurs *below* the midslope: normal. If the first zero slope after systole occurs *above* the midslope: abnormal.

Table 16-2. Accuracy of Duplex Scanning versus Angiography[a]

Angiography	Duplex					Total
	A	B	C	D	E	
Normal	47	9				56
1%–15%	4	49	8			61
16%–49%		14	62	4		80
50%–99%		1	7	91	1	100
100%				1	38	39
Total	51	75	77	96	39	336

[a] K ± SE(K) = 0.813 ± 0.024.

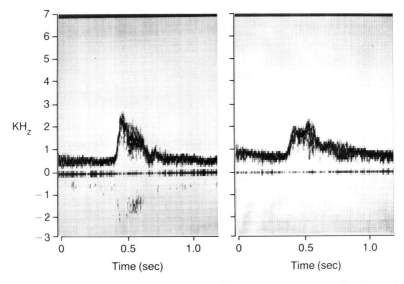

Figure 16-11. Typical abnormal common carotid artery spectrum, as defined by (a–b)/a ratio (*left*) feeding an internal carotid artery with mild disease (1%–15% diameter reduction) by angiography (*right*).

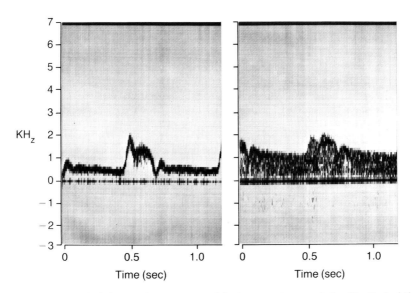

Figure 16-12. Typical abnormal common carotid artery spectrum as defined by the (a–b)/a ratio (*left*), feeding an internal carotid artery with moderate disease (16%–49% diameter reduction) by angiography (*right*). In the internal carotid artery signal, spectral broadening occurs throughout systole; peak systolic frequency is below 4 kHz.

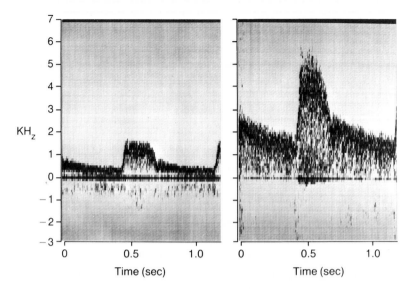

Figure 16-13. Typical abnormal common carotid artery spectrum, as defined by the (a–b)/a ratio (*left*), feeding an internal carotid artery with severe disease (50%–99% diameter reduction) by angiography (*right*). In the internal carotid signal, spectral broadening occurs throughout systole, and peak systole is well above 4 kHz.

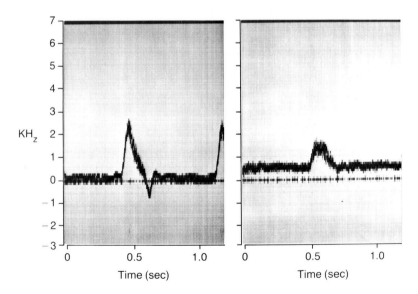

Figure 16-14. Spectrum from common carotid artery proximal to an internal carotid occlusion (*left*), and spectrum from the contralateral common carotid artery feeding a patent internal carotid (*right*).

category, 78% in the 16%–49% diameter reduction category, 91% in the 50%–99% diameter reduction category, and 97% of the occlusions were correctly classified. Hence the specificity increased to 84% and the sensitivity remained at 98%. The overall agreement corrected for chance was 0.813 ± 0.024.

In order to make the feature analysis more quantitative and objective, work is underway to develop a computer-based velocity waveform pattern recognition system. This method processes and further classifies the complex Doppler velocity signals into categories of disease according to computer-selected waveform parameters. The Doppler signals from the common carotid artery and from the proximal internal carotid artery at the site of maximal audible flow disturbance are recorded on audiotape along with the ECG. An average of 25 heart cycles is collected on tape and further processed by the FFT spectral analyzer. Both the digital output and the ECG R-wave timing information are recorded directly onto disc for storage. The computer selects and averages 20 suitable heartbeats to produce an ensemble-averaged spectrum. For each spectrum, the frequency of maximum amplitude, or mode, is computed along with the 3-db and 9-db levels above and below the mode (Figure 16-15).

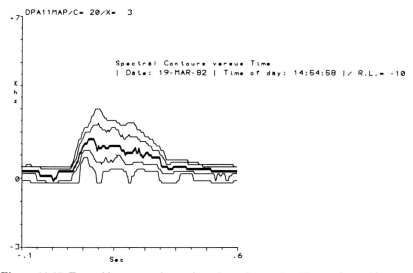

Figure 16-15. Ensemble-averaged waveform from the proximal internal carotid artery. Time axis extends from −100 msec to +600 msec relative to the R-wave. The center contour line represents the mode. Also represented are the 3 and 9 db lines both above and below the mode. Reprinted with permission from Langlois Y, Roederer GO, Chan AW, et al: Evaluating carotid artery disease: the concordance between pulsed Doppler/spectrum analysis and angiography. *Ultrasound in Medicine and Biology.* New York, Pergamon [in press, 1983].

The ensemble waveform thus generated is then analyzed by a software package developed at the University of Washington to perform pattern-recognition work.[66] Selected waveform parameters are weighted and used to arrive at a decision about the severity of disease. The waveform parameters, or "features," were selected by the computer as those allowing classification of a set of known vessels (training set) with the highest degree of accuracy when compared to arteriography (Table 16-3).

The pattern-recognition process goes through the following decision steps: (1) normal versus diseased; (2) if diseased, more or less than 50% diameter stenosis; and (3) if less than 50%, more or less than 20% diameter reduction. A total of 170 sides were prospectively submitted to the pattern-recognition program (Table 16-4).[67] Of the 29 normal arteries, 27 (93%) were correctly identified. Of the 54 lesions in the 1%–20%

Table 16-3. Features Chosen by the Automatic-Selection Algorithm

Decision	Feature Number	Definition	Site	Weight
Normal versus diseased	I.1	Ln (early diastolic mean flow/cos Θ)	PCCA	−43.8
	I.2	Ln (late diastolic mean flow/cos Θ)	PCCA	21.0
	I.3	Ln (mode of mean waveform DFT)	PICA	−16.7
	I.4	Postsystolic deceleration/cosΘ	PCCA	15.9
	I.5	First minimum in mean waveform DFT	PICA	10.7
Greater versus less than 50% stenosis	II.1	Ln (lower 3 db at systole + 100 msec)	PICA	2724
	II.2	Ln (first minimum in mean waveform DFT)	PICA	−2262
	II.3	Ln (upper 3 db/cos Θ at systole)	PICA	2724
	II.4	Postsystolic deceleration/cos Θ	PICA	1482
	II.5	Maximum overall 9 db frequency	PICA	444
Greater versus less than 20% stenosis	III.1	Ln (maximum overall 9 db frequency)	PICA	25.8
	III.2	Ln (area under systolic peak/cos Θ)	PCCA	−23.2
	III.3	Maximum overall 9 db frequency	PICA	−16.4
	III.4	Lower 9 db width at systole	PCCA	5.6
	III.5	Ln (mode of mean waveform DFT)	PCCA	−3.7

PCCA, proximal common carotid artery; *PICA*, proximal internal carotid artery, site of maximum turbulence; Θ, Doppler beam to vessel axis angle; *DFT*, discrete Fourier transform; *mean waveform*, waveform resulting from performing a weighted average of the five contour lines—it is an estimate of the mean (first moment) frequency at each point in the cardiac cycle; *Ln*, natural logarithm.

Table 16-4. Accuracy of Pattern Recognition by Computer versus Angiography[a]

Angiography	Computer				
	Normal	1%–20%	21%–50%	51%–99%	Total
Normal	27	2			29
1%–20%	4	44	6		54
21%–50%		5	29	3	37
51%–99%		1	8	41	50
Total	31	52	43	44	170

[a] Kappa = 0.769 ± 0.039.

category, 44 (81.5%) were correctly classified, as were 78% (29/37) of the lesions in the 21%–50% and 82% (41/50) of the lesions in the 51%–99% categories. The overall agreement corrected for chance was K ± SE(K) = 0.769 + 0.039.

Because these studies were performed to demonstrate the accuracy of our method as compared with contrast angiography, it was important to assess the validity of the arteriographic examination. In a study reported by Chikos et al.,[68] the level of agreement obtained by the same radiologist on dual reading of 128 arteriograms was K ± SE(K) = 0.711 ± 0.054, whereas two different antiographers reading the same 128 studies reached an agreement of K ± SE(K) = 0.568 ± 0.058.[60] A comparison of the various Kappa values obtained for each study clearly shows that ultrasonic duplex scanning with spectral analysis has reached the limit of arteriography (Table 16-5). Pattern recognition appears promising, and further improvements should make this method most suitable for documenting the progression of disease both before and after endarterectomy.

Value as a Screening Test

Duplex scanning with spectral analysis is an easily repeatable and accurate method of assessing atherosclerotic disease at the carotid bifurcation. Thus it is an excellent method of screening patients who are considered possible candidates for arteriography. While it is considered standard practice to arteriogram all patients with transient ischemic attacks, there are specific findings that, if known, would preclude the use of this invasive procedure. Patients with either a normal or a completely occluded

Table 16-5. Comparative Scale of Kappa Values

Kappa	Diagnostic Modality
1	[Perfect agreement]
0.813	Spectral analysis using the common carotid waveform
0.769	Computer pattern-recognition program
0.711	Intraangiographer agreement
0.682	Spectral analysis using a short focal length scanhead
0.581	Spectral analysis using a medium focal length scanhead
0.568	Interangiographer agreement
0	[Chance agreement]

bifurcation are not candidates for endarterectomy, for instance. Identifying these patients with duplex scanning and spectral analysis could therefore spare them an unnecessary invasive procedure. In a review of 109 patients with focal symptoms, Thiele et al. showed that 10% of the arteries were angiographically normal and that 7% were occluded. Although the number of normal and occluded arteries is lower than that found in other studies,[23,69] the use of duplex scanning in this patient population could have kept 17 of 100 patients from a needless contrast study. This number alone demonstrates that the test is cost-effective.[70]

Value in the Asymptomatic Patient

Whereas the evaluation of the symptomatic patient is reasonably well established, the finding of a bruit in the asymptomatic patient still provokes considerable controversy. The value of endarterectomy in this setting as a prophylaxis against stroke has been advocated by some authors[71,72] and refuted by others.[73,74] Although carotid endarterectomy is relatively safe when performed by experienced surgeons, it nevertheless carries a definite risk of stroke and death that must be weighed against that of withholding the surgery.[72,75] (See Chapter 25.)

The initial problem upon discovery of a bruit is to estimate its origin. If it is thought to be secondary to stenosis of the carotid artery, the possibility of arteriography is always raised. We have utilized duplex scanning in two separate settings in which some of these controversies occur today. A prospective study using duplex scanning and spectral analysis was performed to document the prevalence of carotid disease in 101 patients undergoing aortocoronary bypass surgery and to assess the value of preoperative, noninvasive screening.[76] Twenty-four studies (23%) were requested on the basis of a bruit or a history of neurologic symptoms, and 78 patients (77%) were not suspected of having carotid artery disease. In the requested group, 11 patients (46%) has stenoses that reduced luminal diameter by more than 50%, and two patients had a unilateral occlusion. Of the 78 patients with no signs or symptoms, five (6%) showed greater than 50% unilateral or bilateral narrowing of the internal carotid artery. No neurologic complications occurred in the requested group and only two neurologic events developed among those in whom there was no clinical evidence of carotid disease. Neither of these patients had high-grade stenoses. These findings are consistent with those reported by Barnes et al.[74] (Chapter 25) and Turnipseed et al.,[77] who could not relate the incidence of perioperative stroke to the presence of a severe lesion at the bifurcation. This does not mean that the detection of carotid disease is unimportant among these patients, but rather that they should be followed closely until they develop transient ischemic symptoms.

Another major point of interest and discussion is the management of patients with asymptomatic bruits. Although the presence of a bruit correlates with a higher risk of stroke, the side of the bruit is not a reliable indicator of the side of the stroke.[78] Furthermore, carotid bruits cannot be necessarily equated to high-grade carotid disease, nor will severe disease necessarily give rise to a bruit.[29,30] One hundred patients with 165 asymptomatic bruits were evaluated using duplex scanning and spectral analysis.[79] Twelve (7.5%) were normal, 83 (50%) had lesions reducing luminal diameter by less than 50%, 61 (37%) had lesions reducing luminal diameter by more than 50%, and 9 (5.5%) had an occlusion of the internal carotid artery. Using such an approach permits a more accurate estimation of the site and extent of involvement and obviates the need for arteriography in the majority of patients with this finding.

Intraoperative Assessment

Intraoperative contrast angiography remains the standard technique of detecting technical defects after an endarterectomy. Although this method is useful in the identification of technical errors, it provides only a single-plane view of the artery and does not assess the nature of the reestablished flow at the site of endarterectomy. The complications reported are similar to those associated with preoperative angiography and, although rare, have led some surgeons to abandon its routine application.[80]

These facts have justified the introduction of Doppler ultrasound for the intraoperative assessment of flow both before and after endarterectomy. A 20-MHz pulsed-Doppler probe and a FFT spectral analyzer were used at operation to study flow both before and after endarterectomy in 45 operated segments.[81] In all cases, intraoperative angiograms were available for comparison. Based on peak systolic velocity and spectral broadening, the flow disturbances were classified as mild, moderate, or severe (Table 16-6). The noninvasive studies prior to and following sur-

Table 16-6. Spectral Criteria for Classifying Internal Carotid Disease Using a 20-MHz Doppler

Flow Disturbance	Spectral Criteria
Mild	Systolic peak frequency up to 4 kHz; spectral broadening in decelerating phase of systole only
	or
	Any peak systolic frequency with no spectral broadening
Moderate	Systolic peak frequency up to 4 kHz; spectral broadening throughout most of systole
Severe	Systolic peak frequency above 4 kHz; spectral broadening throughout most of systole

gery were compared. Of 39 segments demonstrating significant pre-surgical flow disturbances, 34 showed improved spectral characteristics following the endarterectomy and four remained unchanged (Table 16-7). In one case the spectrum obtained at operation showed worsening flow characteristics, which were related to a technical error noted on the angiogram. The six remaining segments showed mild preoperative disturbances that persisted after the endarterectomy. Although much more detailed and longer-term follow-up studies are necessary to assess the relevance of these findings, this method may become a useful adjunct for detecting technical errors.

Postoperative Assessment

The estimated rate of symptomatic restenosis following endarterectomy has been reported to range from 1% to 5%.[82-84] Based on clinical suspicion, these results overlook the rate of recurrent stenosis in asymptomatic patients. Because arteriography cannot be performed routinely or

Table 16-7. Intraoperative Results before and after Endarterectomy[a]

Preendarterectomy	Postendarterectomy			Total
	Mild	**Moderate**	**Severe**	
Mild	6			6
Moderate	20	2		22
Severe	11	4	2	17
Total	37	6	2	45

[a] Using the criteria listed in Table 16-6.

repetitively following endarterectomy, noninvasive methods offer an appealing means of documenting recurrent stenosis in all patients undergoing carotid surgery.

Thirty-six patients were studied after carotid endarterectomy using duplex scanning with spectral analysis and angiography.[85] The mean follow-up interval was 28 months. Forty-four sides were available for comparison. When the arteriographic data from 44 operated arteries were compared to the results of the noninvasive study, duplex scanning combined with spectral analysis showed an overall accuracy of 80% (Table 16-8). The ability to predict a greater than 50% diameter reduction along with occlusions was 94%. The measure of agreement corrected for

Table 16-8. Accuracy of Duplex Scanning versus Angiography following Endarterectomy[a]

Angiography	Duplex					Total
	A	**B**	**C**	**D**	**E**	
Normal	0		1			1
1%–15%		3	2			5
16%–49%		1	16	4		21
50%–99%			1	14		15
100%					2	2
Total	0	4	20	18	2	44

[a] Kappa ± SE(K) = 0.675 ± 0.096.

chance between arteriography and duplex scanning as expressed by the Kappa statistic was 0.675 ± 0.096. These results compared favorably to those obtained preoperatively and justified the use of duplex scanning and spectral analysis in the routine follow-up of patients after endarterectomy. A total of 89 endarterectomized segments in 76 patients were noninvasively assessed, with a mean postoperative interval of 16 months.[86] Thirty-two sides demonstrated postoperative spectral changes consistent with a greater than 50% narrowing of the lumen. Serial follow-up on 22 sides revealed a persistent stenosis in 12, an occlusion in 1, and a regression of the lesion in 9. In this study the estimated rate of persisting severe narrowing was 19%. Nevertheless, only 4 of the 8 patients who presented recurrent focal symptoms on the side of the endarterectomy had a persisting stenosis greater than 50%.

When technical errors are excluded, recurrent stenosis is caused by fibromuscular hyperplasia and true atherosclerotic lesions.[83,84] Intimal myoproliferation is thought to be responsible for early recurrent stenoses. Usually seen in the first 24 months following endarterectomy, these smooth lesions appear to be the manifestation of the reparative process. Regression of fibromuscular hyperplasia has been observed[87,88] and could explain the apparent improvement of some high-grade lesions noted in our serial follow-up study. On the other hand, recurrent stenosis secondary to a typical atherosclerotic plaque is expected after a longer period of time, although the reasons for its recurrence remain unclear. In order to better understand the behavior of these two phenomena, further prospective studies combining intra- and postoperative data are required, and will constitute the basis for evaluating the role and value of carotid endarterectomy.

CONCLUSIONS

Noninvasive tests for the detection of carotid occlusive disease have focused primarily on the indirect assessment of the internal carotid artery by the analysis of arterial pressure and flow. These tests can only detect the presence of flow-reducing lesions and occlusions; they cannot differentiate between these two entities. Also, the assessment of bilateral disease is difficult using these techniques.

Direct noninvasive tests are ideal to evaluate atherosclerotic disease at the carotid bifurcation. The methods based on the auditory analysis of bruits are limited by the poor predictive value of the finding for the presence of internal carotid disease. Although the quantitative analysis of a bruit overcomes the inadequacy of auditory interpretation, the test is most suitable in combination with other techniques and most valuable in the follow-up of symptomatic patients with a bruit.

The introduction of ultrasonic methods has widened the diagnostic capabilities of noninvasive testing. The analysis of the envelope of the velocity waveform using zero-crossing detectors allows the highly accurate identification of normal and severly diseased arteries. Used alone, however, this technique is limited in its ability to detect occlusions and provides no information on the energy content of the velocity spectrum. Furthermore, because it is often difficult to identify with precision the sampling site, the method does have limitations. The development of imaging techniques has helped to overcome this difficulty. While B-mode scanning appears promising, reliance on the image alone may be misleading. By producing an acoustic shadow, calcification may in fact hide a lesion of interest. Also, the similar acoustic characteristics shared by soft plaques, thrombi, and blood make it difficult to identify accurately soft plaques and occlusions.

The addition of Doppler devices to ultrasonic imaging techniques provided instruments that produce an image of the artery from which the flow information is collected. The methods involving the combination of a pulsed Doppler and an imaging system are particularly useful in detecting flow from discrete points within the vessel, and they prevent errors associated with flow disturbances near the wall. Errors with these techniques are usually the result of misidentification of vessels and tend to decrease as the examiner gains experience. Although auditory interpretation of the Doppler signal has produced good results, the quantitative analysis of the spectra represents a considerable improvement in diagnostic accuracy. Correct vessel identification and more precise quantification of the degree of narrowing can be achieved with this technique. In a research setting it provides a useful means of assessing the natural history of carotid artery disease both before and after endarterectomy. Further improvements, such as the computer-based velocity waveform pattern-recognition technique, have shown great potential in the objective evaluation of carotid disease. Although a great deal of work remains to be done, such techniques should provide us with a better understanding and a more rational approach to the management of atherosclerotic disease at the carotid bifurcation.

REFERENCES

1. Hass WK, Field WS, North RR, et al: Joint study of extracranial arterial occlusion. II. Arteriography, techniques, sites and complications JAMA 203:159–166, 1968.
2. Mohr JP, Caplan LR, Melski JW, et al: The Harvard cooperative stroke registry; a prospective registry. Neurology 28:754–762, 1978.
3. Mani RL, Eisenberg RL: Complications of catheter cerebral angiography: analysis of 500 procedures. I. Criteria and incidence. Am. J Roentgenol 131:861–865, 1978.
4. Kartchner MM, McRae LP, Morrison FD: Noninvasive detection and evaluation of carotid occlusive disease. Arch Surg 106:528–535, 1973.
5. Kartchner MM, McRae LP: Noninvasive evaluation and management of the asymptomatic carotid bruit. Surgery 82:840–847, 1977.
6. Gee W, Oller DW, Wylie EJ: Noninvasive diagnosis of carotid occlusion by ocular plethysmography. Stroke 7:18–21, 1976.
7. Gee W: ocular pneumoplethysmography. In *Noninvasive Diagnostic Techniques in Vascular Disease,* second edition. Edited by EF Bernstein. St Louis, CV Mosby, 1982, pp 220–230.
8. Lye CR, Sumner DS, Strandness DE Jr: The accuracy of supraorbital examination in the diagnosis of hemodynamically significant carotid occlusive disease. Surgery 79: 42–45, 1976.
9. Barnes RW, Russell HE, Bone GE, et al: The Doppler cerebrovascular examination: improved results with refinements in technique. Stroke 8:468–471, 1977.
10. Duncan GW, Gruber JO, Dewey CF Jr, et al: Evaluation of carotid stenosis by phonoangiography. N Engl J Med 293:1124–1128, 1975.
11. Planiol TH, Pourcelot L: Diagnose des thromboses et stenoses carotidiennes: par effet Doppler. Rotterdam, Second World Congress on Ultrasonics in Medicine, 1973.
12. Gosling RG, King DH: Continuous wave ultrasound as an alternative and complement to X-rays in vascular examinations. In *Cardiovascular Application of Ultrasound.* Edited by RS Reneman. New York, Elsevier-North Holland, 1974.
13. Rutherford RB, Hiatt WR, Kreutzer EW: The use of velocity waveform analysis in the diagnosis of carotid artery occlusive disease. Surgery 82:695–702, 1977.
14. Hokanson DE, Mozersky DJ, Sumner DS, et al: Ultrasonic arteriography: a new approach to arterial visualization. Biomed. Engr 6:420, 1971.
15. Mercier LA, Greenleaf JF, Evans TC, et al: High resolution ultrasound arteriography: a comparison with carotid angiography. In *Noninvasive Diagnostic Techniques in Vascular Disease.* Edited by EF Bernstein. St Louis, CV Mosby, 1978.
16. Barber FE, Baker DW, Nation AWC, et al: Ultrasonic duplex echo-Doppler scanner. IEEE Trans Biomed Eng 21:109–113, 1974.
17. Phillips DJ, Blackshear WM Jr, Baker DW, et al: Ultrasound Duplex scanning in peripheral vascular disease. Radiol Nuc Med January–February: 6–10, 1978.
18. Blackshear WM Jr, Phillips DJ, Thiele BL, et al: Detection of carotid occlusive disease by ultrasonic imaging and pulsed Doppler spectrum analysis. Surgery 86:698–706, 1979.
19. May AG, VanDeBerg L, DeWeese JA, et al: Critical arterial stenosis. Surgery 54:250–259, 1963.
20. Thompson JE: *Surgery for Cerebrovascular Insufficiency.* Springfield, Illinois, CC Thomas, 1968.
21. Blaisdell WF, Clauss RH, Galbraith JG, et al: Joint study of extracranial carotid occlusion. IV. A review of surgical considerations. JAMA 209:1889–1895, 1969.

22. Moore WS, Hall AD: Importance of emboli from carotid bifurcation in the pathogenesis of cerebral ischemic attacks. Arch Surg 101:708–716, 1970.

23. Eisenberg RL, Nemzek WR, Moore WS, et al: Relationship of transient ischemic attacks and angiographically demonstrable lesions of the carotid artery. Stroke: 8:483–486, 1977.

24. Thiele BL, Young IV, Chikos PM, et al: Correlation of arteriographic findings with symptoms in patients with cerebrovascular disease. Neurology 30:1041–1046, 1980.

25. Blackshear WM Jr, Thiele BL, Harley JD, et al: A prospective evaluation of oculoplethysmography and carotid phonoangiography. Surg Gynecol Obstet 148:201–205, 1979.

26. Blackshear WM Jr: Comparative review of OPG–K-M, OPG–G, and pulsed Doppler ultrasound for carotid evaluation. Vasc Diagnosis Ther November:43–51, 1980.

27. Brokenbrough EC: Screening for the prevention of stroke: use of a Doppler flowmeter [product brochure]. Beaverton, Oregon, Parks Electronics, 1970.

28. Sumner DS: Non-invasive methods for preoperative assessment of carotid occlusive disease. Part 1. Statistical interpretation of test results. Vasc Diagnosis Ther June/July: 41–56, 1981.

29. Ziegler DK, Zileli T, Dick A, et al: Correlation of bruits over the carotid artery with angiographically demonstrated lesions. Neurology 21:860–865, 1971.

30. David TE, Humphries AW, Young TR, et al: A correlation of neck bruits and arteriosclerotic carotid arteries. Arch Surg 107:729–731, 1973.

31. Hammond JH, Eisenger RP: Carotid bruits in 1000 normal subjects. Arch Intern Med 109:563–565, 1962.

32. Keagy BA, Pharr WF, Thomas DD, et al: Comparison of oculoplethysmography/carotid phono-angiography with Duplex scan/spectral analysis in the detection of carotid artery stenosis. Stroke 13:43–45, 1982.

33. Kistler JP, Lees RS, Miller A, et al: Correlation of spectral phonoangiography and carotid angiography with gross pathology in carotid stenosis. N Engl J Med 305: 417–419, 1981.

34. Knox R, Breslau PJ, Strandness DE Jr: Quantitative carotid phonoangiography. Stroke 12:798–803, 1981.

35. Strandness DE Jr: *Peripheral Arterial Disease: A Physiological Approach.* Boston, Little, Brown, 1967.

36. Johnston KW, Taraschuk I: Validation of the role of pulsatility index in quantitation of the severity of peripheral arterial occlusive arterial disease. Am J Surg 131:295–297, 1976.

37. Stevens A, Roberts VC: On line signal processing of CW Doppler shifted ultrasound. Digest of XI International Conference on Medical and Biological Engineering, Ottawa, 1976, pp 160–161.

38. Nippa JH, Hokanson DE, Lee DR, et al: Phase rotation for separating forward and reverse blood velocity signals. IEEE Trans Sonics Ultrasonics 5:340–346, 1975.

39. Maruzzo BC, Johnston KW, Cobbold RSC: Real-time spectral analysis of directional Doppler flow signals. Digest of XI International Conference on Medical and Biological Engineering, Ottawa, 1976, pp 158–159.

40. Johnston KW, Maruzzo BC, Cobbold RSC: Inaccuracies of a zero-crossing detector for recording Doppler signals. Surg Forum 28:201–203, 1977.

41. Strandness DE Jr: Doppler ultrasonic techniques in vascular disease. In *Noninvasive Diagnostic Techniques in Vascular Disease,* second edition. Edited by EF Bernstein. St Louis, CV Mosby, 1982, pp 13–21.

42. Yao ST, Needham TN: Frequency analysis of Doppler-shift blood flow signals by a bandpass filter: preliminary report. Biomed Eng 5:438–442, 1970.

43. Light LH: A recording spectrograph for analyzing Doppler blood velocity signals (particularly from aortic flow) in real-time. J Physiol 207:42–44, 1971.

44. Coghlan BA, Taylor MG, King DH: On-line display of Doppler shift spectra by a zero line compression analyzer. In *Cardiovascular Applications of Ultrasound.* Edited by RS Reneman. New York, Elsevier-North Holland, 1974, pp 55–65.

45. Cooley JW, Tukey JW: An algorithm for the machine calculation of complex Fourier series. Math Comp 19:297–301, 1965.

46. Miyasaki M, Kato K: Measurement of cerebral blood flow by ultrasonic Doppler technique, theory. Jpn Circ J 29:375–382, 1965.

47. Gosling RG: Extraction of physiological information from spectrum analyzed Doppler shifted continuous wave ultrasound signals obtained noninvasively from the arterial system. In *IEEE Medical Electronics Monographs,* volumes 13–22. Edited by DW Hill, BW Watson. Stevenage, Hertfordshire, Peter Peregrinus, 1976, pp 33–125.

48. Baskett J, Beasly MG, Murphy GJ, et al: Screening for carotid junction disease by spectral analysis of Doppler signal. Cardiovasc Res 11:147–155, 1977.

49. Prichard DR, Martin TRP, Sherriff SB: Assessment of directional Doppler ultrasound techniques in the diagnosis of carotid artery disease. Neurol Neurosurg Psychiatry 42:563–568, 1979.

50. Spencer MP, Brockenbrough EC, Davis DL, et al: Cerebrovascular evaluation using Doppler continuous wave ultrasound. In *Ultrasound in Medicine,* volume 3B. Edited by D White, RE Brown. New York, Plenum Press, 1977, pp 1292–1310.

51. Weaver RG, Howard G, McKinney WM, et al: Comparison of Doppler ultrasonography with arteriography of the carotid artery bifurcation. Stroke 11(4):402–404, 1980.

52. White DM, Curry GR: A comparison of 424 carotid bifurcations examined by angiography and the Doppler Echoflow. *Ultrasound in Medicine,* volume 4. Edited by D White, RE Brown. New York, Plenum Press, 1978, pp 363–376.

53. Russell JB, Miles RD, Sumner DS: Pulsed Doppler ultrasonic arteriography with sound spectral analysis for evaluation of the carotid bifurcation. Bruit 6 (March):23–29, 1982.

54. Miles RD, Russell JB, Sumner DS: Computerized ultrasonic arteriography: a new technique for imaging the carotid bifurcation. IEEE Trans Biomed Eng 29:378–381, 1982.

55. Humber PR, Leopold GR, Wickbom IG, et al: Ultrasonic imaging of the carotid arterial system. Am J Surg 140:199–202, 1980.

56. Katz ML, Comerota JJ; Characterization of atherosclerotic plaque by real-time carotid imaging. Bruit 6 (March):17–22, 1982.

57. Knox RA, Phillips DJ, Breslau PJ, et al: Empirical findings relating sample volume size to diagnostic accuracy in pulsed Doppler cerebrovascular studies. JCU 10:227–232, 1982.

58. Fell G, Phillips DJ, Chikos PM, et al: Ultrasonic Duplex scanning for disease of the carotid artery. Circulation 64:1191–1195, 1981.

59. Breslau PJ, Knox RA, Phillips DJ, et al: The accuracy of ultrasonic Duplex scanning as compared with contrast arteriography in extracranial carotid artery disease. Vasc Diagnosis Ther 3 (6):17–22, 1982.

60. Langlois YE, Roederer GO, Chan AW, et al: Evaluating carotid artery disease: the concordance between pulsed Doppler/spectrum analysis and angiography. Ultrasound Med Biol 9:51–63, 1983.

61. Cohen J: A coefficient of agreement for nominal scales. Educ Psychol Measurement 20:37–46, 1960.

62. Wood CPL, Smith BT, Nunn CL, et al: Noninvasive detection of boundary layer separation in the normal artery bifurcation [abstract]. Stroke 13:11, 1982.

63. Phillips DJ, Greene FM, Langlois YE, et al: Flow velocity patterns in the carotid

bifurcations of young presumed normals. Ultrasound Med Biol 9:39–49, 1983.

64. Langlois YE, Roederer GO, Chan AW, et al: The use of common carotid waveform analysis in the diagnosis of carotid occlusive disease. Angiology (in press, 1983).

65. Roederer GO, Langlois YE, Chan AW, et al: Ultrasonic Duplex scanning of extracranial carotid arteries: improved accuracy using new features from the common carotid artery. J Cardiovasc Ultrasonography 1:373–380, 1982.

66. Greene FM Jr, Beach KW, Strandness DE Jr, et al: Computer based pattern recognition of carotid arterial disease using pulsed Doppler ultrasound. Ultrasound Med Biol 8:161–176, 1982.

67. Langlois YE, Greene FM, Roederer GO, et al: Computer-based method for classification of carotid arterial disease: methodology and results. Symposium on Noninvasive Diagnostic Techniques in Vascular Disease, San Diego, 1982.

68. Chikos PM, Fischer L, Hirsch JH, et al: Observer variability in evaluating extracranial carotid artery stenosis. Stroke (in press, 1983).

69. Marshall J: Angiography in the investigation of ischemic episodes in the territory of the internal carotid artery. Lancet 1(7702):719–722, 1971.

70. Chan AW, Beach KW, Langlois YE, et al: Evaluation of extracranial carotid artery disease by ultrasonic Duplex scanning. A clinical perspective. Australian New Zealand J Surg 52:562–569, 1982.

71. Javid H, Ostermiller WE, Hengesh JW, et al: Carotid endarterectomy for asymptomatic bruit. Arch Surg 102:389–391, 1971.

72. Thompson JE, Patman RD, Perrson AV: Management of asymptomatic carotid bruits. Am Surgeon 42(2):77–80, 1976.

73. Humphries W, Young JR, Santilli PH, et al: Unoperated asymptomatic significant internal carotid artery stenosis. A review of 182 instances. Surgery 80:695–698, 1976.

74. Barnes RW, Marszalek RH: Asymptomatic carotid disease in the cardiovascular surgical patient. Is prophylactic endarterectomy necessary? Stroke 12:497–500, 1981.

75. Thompson JE, Patman RD, Talkington CM: Asymptomatic carotid bruit: long-term outcome of patients having endarterectomy compared with unoperated controls. Ann Surg 188:308–316, 1978.

76. Breslau PJ, Fell G, Ivey TD, et al: Carotid arterial disease in patients undergoing coronary artery bypass operation. J Thorac Cardiovasc Surg 82:765–767, 1981.

77. Turnipseed WD, Berkoff HA, Belzer FO: Post-operative stroke in cardiac and peripheral vascular disease. Ann Surg 192:365–368, 1980.

78. Heyman A, Wilkinson WE, Heyden S, et al: Risk of stroke in asymptomatic persons with cervical bruits. N Engl J Med 302:838–841, 1980.

79. Fell G, Breslau PJ, Knox RA, et al: Importance of non-invasive ultrasonic doppler testing in the evaluation of patients with asymptomatic carotid bruits. Am Heart J 102:221–226, 1981.

80. Anderson CE, Collins GJ, Rich NM: Routine operative arteriography during carotid endarterectomy: a reassessment. Surgery 83:67–73, 1978.

81. Zierler RE, Bandyk DF, Berni GA, et al: Intraoperative pulsed Doppler assessment of carotid endarterectomy. Ultrasound Med Biol 19:65–71, 1983.

82. Stoney RJ, String ST: Recurrent carotid stenosis. Surgery 80:705–710, 1976.

83. French BN, Rewcastle NB: Recurrent stenosis at site of carotid endarterectomy. Stroke 8:597–605, 1977.

84. Cossman D, Callow AD, Stein A, et al: Early restenosis after carotid endarterectomy. Arch Surg 113:275–278, 1978.

85. Roederer GO, Langlois YE, Chan AW, et al: Post-endarterectomy carotid ultrasonic Duplex scanning: concordance with contrast angiography. Ultrasound Med Biol 9:73–78, 1983.

86. Zierler RE, Bandyk DF, Thiele BL, et al: Carotid artery stenosis following endarterectomy. Arch Surg 117:1408–1415, 1982.
87. Holder J, Binet EF, Flanigan S, et al: Arteriography after carotid endarterectomy. Am J Roentg 137:483–487, 1981.
88. Diaz FG, Patel S, Boulos R, et al: Early angiographic changes following carotid endarterectomy. Neurosurgery 10:151–161, 1982.

CHAPTER 17

K / M Oculoplethysmography and Carotid Phonoangiography

Valerie Crain and Lorin P. McRae

Stroke is the third most common cause of death in the United States, and therefore instrumentation and methodology to detect early changes in the extracranial circulation are urgently needed. Oculoplethysmography and carotid phonoangiography begin to fill that need. Both were developed to screen noninvasively the incipient stroke patient for obstructive disease in the carotid arterial system.[1-3]

TECHNIQUE

CAROTID PHONOANGIOGRAPHY

Carotid phonoangiography (CPA) is a method whereby the examiner holds a special hand-held microphone over the cervical carotid artery and records sounds from the carotid arteries in three positions: under the mandible lateral to the sternocleidomastoid muscle (the high position), approximately 2 cm below the high position (the middle position), and above the clavicle over the common carotid artery (the low position). The high and middle positions are considered to be at or about the carotid bifurcation, while the low position is clearly below the carotid bifurcation and is utilized to determine whether heart or arch vessels are the source of radiating murmur, turbulence, or bruit (Figure 17-1).

Auscultation is performed and oscilloscopic photographs of the maximum carotid sounds are obtained in each position. The subjective auscultatory evaluation is written on the back of the photograph. These photographs are evaluated and then stored for future comparisons.

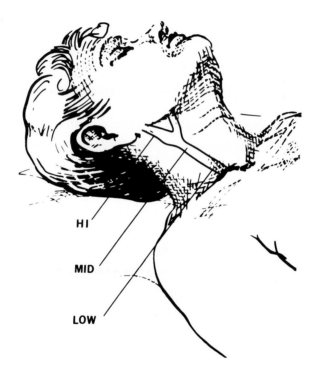

HI

MID

LOW

Figure 17-1. Microphone positions for carotid phonoangiography.

The patient is requested to hold his breath for approximately 3–4 seconds during recording. The patient and technician must be comfortable and relaxed or troublesome artifacts may be recorded.

Generally, to eliminate venous murmur and to reduce muscle-tension artifact, CPA is performed while the patient is in the supine position. If necessary, however, recordings may be performed with the patient in the sitting position. With an experienced technician and a cooperative patient, CPA testing takes only five minutes (Figure 17-2).

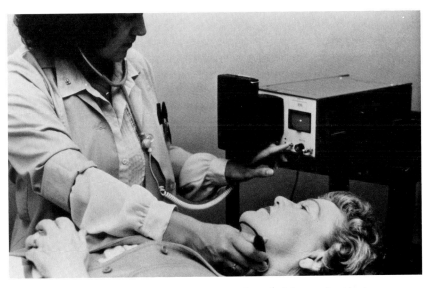

Figure 17-2. Carotid phonoangiograph, technician, and patient.

OCULOPLETHYSMOGRAPHY

Fluid oculoplethysmography (OPG) is performed with the patient sitting (Figure 17-3). Small corneal cups are placed on each anesthetized eye (0.5% proparacaine hydrochloride drops) and held in place with a mild suction of 40–60 mmHg. The cyclic ocular pulses are transmitted to pressure transducers through the closed, fluid-filled tubes, and then recorded graphically on light-sensitive paper for evaluation and subsequent storage. Light opacity earlobe sensors are placed on each earlobe to record their pulses, which represent the external carotid circulation.

The eye cups are usually applied twice on each patient, first directly with the right cup to the right eye and later with the cups reversed (right cup to left eye). This practice of reversing the cups helps to identify technically inadequate studies.

More recently, pneumatic (or air) OPG that uses similar pulse-timing principles has been introduced. With pneumatic OPG, the patient is tested most conveniently in the supine position (Figure 17-4). Both pneumatic and fluid OPG utilize a maximum of 60 mmHg suction to hold the cup to the eye, both require a testing time of 2–3 minutes with less than 60 seconds of cup contact on the eye, and both provide graphic recordings for interpretation and hard-copy documentation. This pulse-timing

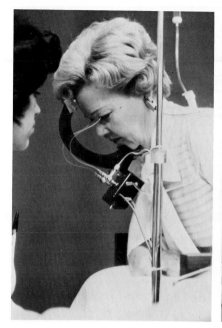

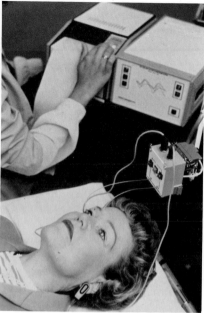

Figure 17-3. Fluid oculoplethysmography with patient in the sitting position.

Figure 17-4. Pneumatic oculoplethysmography with patient in the supine position.

pneumatic OPG is not the same as the oculopneumoplethysmograph (OPG-Gee) discussed in Chapter 18, which instead uses the pressure principle and requires much greater suction.

INTERPRETATION

OCULOPLETHYSMOGRAPHY

OPG is a functional test that measures hemodynamic changes in the eye. Proximal arterial stenosis reduces the rate at which blood flows into the eye, and a delay in the anacrotic or ascending portion of the ocular pulse is noted. Both ocular pulses are recorded simultaneously, and the difference between the volumetric filling of each eye is depicted by an additional electronically generated trace called the differential. This differential is used for interpretation of test results. The use of the differential measurement of pulse delays and pattern recognition (dual-sloping ocular pulse troughs in cases of bilateral stenosis, for instance), etc. are described in full detail in an interpretation manual.[4]

The most recent aid, applying the criteria established for OPG interpretation, is the Diff/Amp ratio. The Diff/Amp ratio is obtained by dividing the maximum differential deflection during midsystole by the ocular pulse amplitude (Figure 17-5). Table 17-1 correlates the Diff/Amp ratio with the degree of stenosis and notes the hemodynamic significance. If the differential deflection is 10%–20% of the ocular pulse amplitude (a ratio of 0.1 to 0.2), the study indicates 40%–60% stenosis. An increasing ratio of differential deflection to pulse amplitude correlates with increasing stenosis.[4]

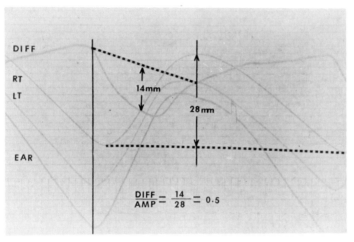

Figure 17-5. Calculations of the Diff/Amp ratio on pneumatic OPG trace. Ratio of 0.2 indicates severe stenosis of the internal carotid.

Table 17-1. Kartchner/McRae Diff/Amp Ratio Correlated to Percentage Distal Internal Carotid Diameter

Diff/Amp Ratio	Diameter Stenosis	Hemodynamic Significance
< 0.1	< 40%	Negative
0.1–0.2	40%–60%	Mild
> 0.2	> 60%	Severe

CAROTID PHONOANGIOGRAPHY

When interpreting CPA studies, one considers the course or location of the maximum bruit and its frequency (or pitch) and duration. Bruits that are longest and/or most dense in the low neck are transmitted from the heart and arch vessels and are not categorized as to the degree of stenosis. Bruits in the middle and high cervical positions originate at the carotid bifurcation (Figure 17-6). Figure 17-7 depicts the bruits occurring

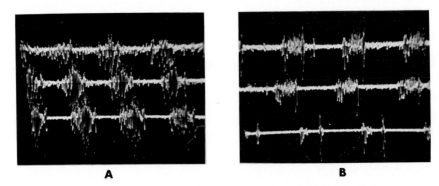

A   **B**

Figure 17-6. A Bruit originating below the carotid bifurcation. **B** Bruit originating at the carotid bifurcation.

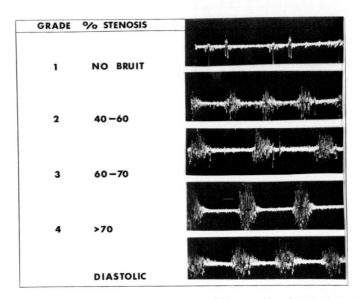

GRADE	% STENOSIS
1	NO BRUIT
2	40–60
3	60–70
4	>70
	DIASTOLIC

Figure 17-7. Representative bruits with corresponding grade and percentage stenosis.

at the carotid bifurcation and their corresponding percentage stenosis using the split-trace CPA. (Split-trace CPA enhances high-frequency bruits; it is a modification that can be installed on older units and is standard on all new units. OPG/CPA discussed herein is distributed by Narco Scientific, Bio Systems Division, Houston, Texas.) Bruits at the carotid bifurcation may originate from the external carotid or internal carotid arteries. Diastolic bruits have been found to originate from the internal carotid. Unique, high-pitched bruits terminating before the end of systole have been identified as external carotid bruits (Figure 17-8). Bruits of questionable origin are so reported; in these cases further non-invasive diagnostic evaluation is necessary.

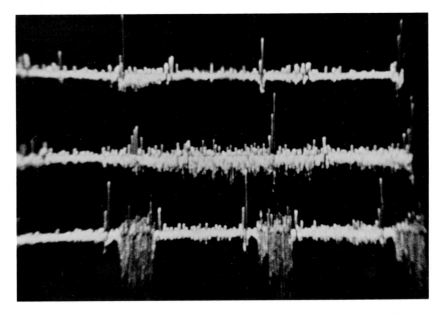

Figure 17-8. External carotid bruit, high-pitched and terminating before the end of systole.

INDICATIONS

The primary usefulness of the OPG and CPA studies is to screen patients with asymptomatic carotid bruits, vague symptoms, or other nonspecific clinical indications of increased risk of stroke. These studies are helpful in making decisions about carotid arteriography, but they are not intended to rule out arteriography in patients with lateralized transient ischemic attacks (see Chapter 15). OPG and CPA also help to screen patients prior to other major surgery, to follow patients, to determine progression of extracranial carotid disease, to document the benefits of surgery and establish a baseline following carotid endarterectomy, and to add complementary hemodynamic data to other noninvasive studies.

COMMON PROBLEMS, CONCERNS, AND QUESTIONS ABOUT OPG

INTERPRETATION

Variations in accuracy, sensitivity, and specificity may be the direct result of overreading or underreading the graphic recordings. The use of the objective Diff/Amp ratio interpretive method helps to reduce some difficulties of interpretation. A consistent use of both direct and reverse (or crossed) studies (see above) and a thorough understanding of this quality assurance technique increases interpretive accuracy.

Another problem of interpretation arises from the comparison of a hemodynamic physiologic test (OPG) to an anatomic standard (the arteriogram). Arteriograms may be overread, underestimated, or even inaccurate in identifying hemodynamic arterial stenoses leading to the eye. A cooperative effort between the vascular laboratory and the radiology department is necessary if the full potential of OPG is to be realized.

OCULAR PATHOLOGY

Glaucoma

The minimal suction utilized with the K/M fluid or pneumatic OPG has no effect on the patient with glaucoma, and these patients have been tested safely without complication. Conversely, glaucoma has had no observed effect on OPG results. Reductions in the amplitude of the ocular pulses have not been observed with glaucoma.

Eye Surgery and Injury

OPG testing is generally deferred for at least six weeks after eye surgery or injury unless the patient is cleared by his or her ophthalmologist. The patient who has undergone cataract surgery is most often in this category, and OPG has been performed safely six weeks postoperatively with no reported complication. Today, artificial intraocular lenses are surgically implanted in about one in three cataract patients to correct post-surgical aphakia, and OPG has been used successfully and safely on such patients six weeks after surgery. Unlike glaucoma, eye surgery or injury may restrict the expansion and contraction of the eye, reducing the amplitude of the ocular pulse in the affected eye, but will not cause ocular pulse delay.

Detached Retina

A patient who has had a detached retina is deferred from testing for a period of six months after the acute onset of symptoms. OPG has not been reported as the causative factor in any cases of detached retina, but testing is postponed nevertheless to eliminate the possibility of coincidentally increasing the symptoms. Again a reduction in ocular pulse amplitude from the affected eye may be anticipated.

Glass Eye

Because OPG compares simultaneously recorded bilateral ocular pulses, this comparison is impossible in a patient with a glass eye. Other non-invasive cerebrovascular studies may be suggested.

Eye Infections

In more than 25,000 patients tested in our laboratory over a ten-year period, we have not had a case of cross-contamination or eye infection. Infection control personnel were, however, concerned about the possibility of eye infection, and so we performed a six-month microbiological evaluation. Each week for six months we took cultures from each eye cup as well as from the outflow tubing of the fluid OPG. Eighty percent of the cultures contained no organisms. The remaining 20% cultured only those organisms that constitute the normal flora for the areas near the eye. It was concluded that the cleaning procedure was adequate and that the possibility of eye infection is not significant.

Unconscious and Uncooperative Patients

On occasion it becomes necessary to perform OPG on an anesthetized, comatose, or uncooperative patient. No problems have arisen in performing OPG on the comatose or the anesthetized recovery-room patient. Cup placement is easy, and there is little blink artifact with these patients. Suction cups generally fit best over the cornea, but they may be placed on any portion of the sclera. Amplitudes of the ocular pulses vary according to cup placement, but interpretation is not handicapped by these variations.

The most difficult patients to test are those who are combative and confused. Of five reported corneal abrasions from our laboratory, three have occurred in patients who could not cooperate. There is a significant difference between a sedated or comatose patient and a conscious but confused and combative patient. It is advisable to forego testing the uncooperative patient.

COMMON PROBLEMS, CONCERNS, AND QUESTIONS ABOUT CPA

PATIENT COOPERATION

It is important to reassure and to explain the CPA procedure to the patient before testing. This elicits the patient's cooperation and gives better test results. The patient is required to hold his breath for approximately 3–4 seconds during the photographic recording. If the patient is not under scrutiny, breathing artifacts can be mistaken for bruit. The patient is instructed that he will be asked to hold his breath, to relax, and not to tighten his neck muscles while holding his breath. Increased baseline artifact is recorded if muscle tension is present and recordings of good quality are difficult to obtain.

PULMONARY PATIENTS

Patients who demonstrate breathing difficulties—asthmatic and emphysemic patients, for example—may find it difficult to assume the supine position for the time required. A Fowler's or semi-Fowler's position may be used instead, but the technician must be aware of the possibility of venous murmur in this position. Patients who have long-standing breathing difficulties generally have more muscle tension in the neck. This tension makes it difficult to eliminate baseline artifact even with good relaxation. Also, patients with breathing problems may have difficulty

226

holding their breath for the 3–4 seconds needed to obtain CPA recordings. Several trials with good explanations usually allow the technician to obtain at least one set of heart sounds without breathing artifact. Together with the auscultatory findings, this evidence should be sufficient to determine the presence and extent of turbulence or bruit in each position.

If a patient is on a mechanical ventilator, sounds of the ventilator make it difficult to obtain quality CPA studies. In such a case the examiner should inquire whether the patient can tolerate disconnection of the ventilator for the few seconds needed for CPA recordings.

UNRESPONSIVE PATIENTS

Sometimes it is necessary to test patients who are unconscious, unresponsive, or semiconscious, and who cannot follow commands. If this situation arises, the examiner pushes the photo button during expiration, as there generally is a period between expiration and the next inspiration during which one heart complex can be recorded without noise or breathing artifact. Listening with the stethescope will probably prove more satisfactory than recordings in these cases.

NERVOUS TECHNICIAN

While it is important for the patient to be relaxed and comfortable for testing, it is also important that the technician control hand motion and be relaxed. Muscle tremor makes quality recordings very difficult.

NOISY ENVIRONMENT

To obtain minimum baseline and maximum carotid sounds, the testing environment should be quiet. Examination areas near elevators, noisy air conditioning, overhead paging, or busy highways may result in excessive baseline artifact. To determine the amount of environmental noise, the examiner turns the CPA volume to its maximum and places the microphone approximately two feet away from the CPA equipment on a soft surface such as a bed, pillow, or carpeting. If the baseline in the oscilloscope is more than ½ cm in height, the environment is not acceptable for CPA recordings. Elimination of the extraneous noises is imperative.

ANATOMIC AND PHYSIOLOGIC CONDITIONS

The CPA generally is adequate for picking up carotid sounds with sufficient amplitude to evaluate the bruit. Anatomic variations such as a large, fat neck or physiologic conditions such as poor cardiac output make it difficult to hear the carotid sounds. It may be helpful to have the patient hyperventilate approximately 3–4 times to increase the heart rate enough to obtain a quality recording.

MICROPHONE SEAL

An airtight seal of the microphone must be established to achieve quality recordings of carotid sounds. An airtight seal may be difficult to obtain on a patient who had a recent endarterectomy and whose neck is swollen. Even with extensive swelling and a suture line, one may obtain a good microphone seal by placing the microphone medially or laterally to the suture line. Patients with throat cancer, laryngectomies, or thyroid conditions may require altered microphone positioning, but quality recordings still can be obtained. Male patients should be shaved before recordings; if not, an acoustical gel should be applied to the microphone site. Even if the microphone does not seal and quality recordings cannot be obtained, the technician can hear the amplified sounds and suggest a diagnosis.

PNEUMATIC VERSUS FLUID OPG

The question of air-versus-fluid-OPG selection has existed since pneumatic OPG became available. It is our opinion that to date graphic recordings are necessary with either system for optimum interpretation. We do not advise reliance on presently available digital number systems.

The primary advantages of pneumatic OPG are its portability and ease of operation. Although the fluid OPG is portable, it is more difficult to transfer this unit in order to test patients outside the laboratory. And although both the fluid and pneumatic OPG must be calibrated initially, on a day-to-day basis the pneumatic OPG needs only to be turned on and it is ready for testing. Fluid OPG, on the other hand, requires 3 to 5 minutes to set up prior to daily testing and also requires disassembly at the end of the day. Supine testing using the pneumatic OPG has been considered an advantage; the patient can remain in a supine position for both the OPG and CPA tests.

The primary advantages of fluid OPG are its sensitivity, shorter cup application time, and more readable graphic recordings from difficult patients. In patients with significant bilateral stenosis, for instance, dual-sloping of the ocular pulse troughs is often observed by fluid OPG, but not by pneumatic OPG.

Shorter testing time is possible with the fluid OPG because of the availability of manual trace reset and ear gain controls. With pneumatic OPG, on the other hand, one must wait for automatic ear pulse adjustment. Without a reset button on the pneumatic OPG, any movement of patient or equipment causes the traces to move off scale, and additional time is spent waiting for the trace to return to midscreen.

Most of the controls for pneumatic OPG are located internally, so trouble-shooting adjustments, possible on the fluid OPG, are not available to the technician using the air OPG. This may be an advantage or disadvantage, depending on the user.

In summary, the volume of studies, the technical competence of the person performing the studies, the type of setting in which testing takes place (hospital, private office, mobile van), and the type of patient population are all significant factors in selecting between the pneumatic and fluid OPG. Patients have shown no preference themselves.

CONCLUSIONS

Oculoplethysmography offers hemodynamic information that complements anatomic testing procedures, such as B-mode ultrasound imaging, arteriography, and digital subtraction venous angiography, in evaluating carotid occlusive disease. The hemodynamic information from OPG supplements the pictures obtained by the anatomic methods and evaluates severity of disease and collateral circulation.

Used serially, carotid phonoangiography remains the least expensive and most effective method of detecting the formation of atherosclerotic plaques. When used together, OPG and CPA offer a safe, simple, inexpensive, and noninvasive means of screening patients for extracranial carotid occlusive disease.

REFERENCES

1. Kartchner MM, McRae LP: Auscultation for carotid bruits in cerebrovascular insufficiency. JAMA 210:494–497, 1969.

2. Kartchner MM, McRae LP, Morrison FD: Noninvasive detection and evaluation of carotid occlusive disease. Arch Surg 106:528–535, 1973.

3. Kartchner MM, McRae LP, Crain V, et al: Oculoplethysmography: an adjunct to arteriography in diagnosis of extracranial carotid occlusive disease. Am J Surg 132: 728–732, 1976.

4. McRae LP, Crain V, Kartchner MM: *Interpretation Manual: OPG/CPA Oculoplethysmography and Carotid Phonoangiography.* Tucson Medical Center, Ocular Pulse and Vascular Laboratory, 1978.

CHAPTER 18

PERIORBITAL DIAGNOSTIC TECHNIQUES

Earlene E. Slaymaker

Contrast arteriography prevails as the most widely accepted definitive study for the identification of carotid occlusive disease. Unfortunately, the discomfort, expense, and risks associated with this diagnostic technique limit its usefulness as a screening and follow-up procedure. As a result, numerous noninvasive testing techniques have been developed to assess cerebral circulation. This chapter discusses three of them, the periorbital cerebrovascular Doppler examination, supraorbital photoplethysmography, and ocular pneumoplethysmography.

THE CEREBROVASCULAR DOPPLER EXAMINATION

By monitoring the direction of blood flow in the frontal and supraorbital arteries, the periorbital cerebrovascular Doppler examination (PO CDE) permits the detection of hemodynamically significant obstruction of the internal carotid artery (i.e., $\geq$ 50% reduction in lumen diameter).

TECHNIQUE

The technique and accuracy of a complete PO CDE have been previously reported.[1] Figure 18-1 indicates the examination position.

In principle, the PO CDE identifies the periorbital arteries, determines the direction of blood flow in these vessels, and notes the responses to compression of the temporal, infraorbital, and facial arteries on each side of the head. Compression of these branches is necessary to identify prop-

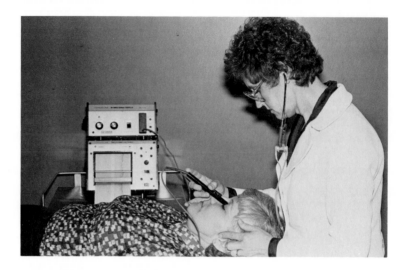

Figure 18-1. Typical position of patient and examiner during the periorbital cerebrovascular Doppler examination. Note how the hand holding the Doppler probe is stabilized.

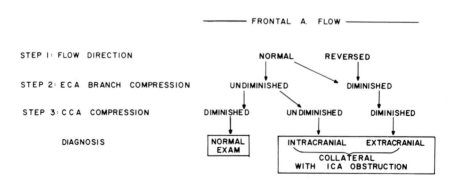

Figure 18-2. Algorithm summarizing possible responses to steps of the periorbital cerebrovascular doppler examination. *Abbreviations: ECA,* external carotid artery; *CCA,* common carotid artery; *ICA,* internal carotid artery. Reprinted with permission of the American Heart Association, Inc., from Barnes RW: Doppler cerebrovascular examination: improved results with refinements in technique. Stroke 8:468–471, 1977.

erly those branches that provide collateral supply to narrowed or occluded internal carotid arteries. Also, the common carotid artery, low in the neck, is compressed for only one to three heartbeats. With this maneuver, the examiner assesses the common carotid's contribution to intracranial circulation by observing the frontal artery's flow response (Figure 18-2).

Many centers regard carotid compression as potentially dangerous. In my experience, however, and with the precautions described, the method is safe and complications have been minor and rare, probably fewer than 1 in 10,000.

Using this technique, the overall accuracy of the PO CDE in detecting or excluding significant obstruction of the internal carotid artery is 94%–98%.[2-5]

DIAGNOSTIC CRITERIA

The PO CDE is considered abnormal if any or all of the following criteria are present:

1. Reversal of flow in the frontal and/or supraorbital arteries.
2. Diminution or reversal of flow with compression of branches of the external carotid arteries.
3. Failure of the signal to diminish with compression of the ipsilateral common carotid artery.
4. Diminution of the signal with compression of the contralateral common carotid artery.

False-negative examinations may result from any of four situations: combined internal and external stenosis with maintenance of normal pressure gradients between the two systems, intracranial collateral from the external carotid artery via the middle meningeal, failure to compress all branches of the external carotid artery, or failure to compress the common carotid artery.

False-positive examinations, on the other hand, may result from a number of technical errors that must be avoided if the examiner is to obtain the maximal level of accuracy. Common sources of errors are the erroneous identification of the vessel being examined (nasal-frontal, palpebral-supraorbital); inadvertent movement and application of excessive probe pressure, especially during compression maneuvers; incorrect positioning of the Doppler probe, resulting in erroneous assessment of flow direction (probe placed above orbital rim; this error is more common with the supraorbital than with the frontal artery); and inadequate stabilization and compression of the common carotid artery.

SUPRAORBITAL PHOTOPLETHYSMOGRAPHY

By photoelectric means, supraorbital photoplethysmography (SO PPG) detects hemodynamically significant obstruction of the extracranial internal carotid artery on the basis of altered ophthalmic artery flow dynamics in response to compression of all branches of the external carotid and the common carotid arteries.

TECHNIQUE

The SO PPG technique and results have been previously reported.[6] Infrared photocell transducers are positioned over the supraorbital region of the patient's forehead (Figure 18-3). Analogue recordings are obtained of the simultaneous pulsations during sequential bilateral compression maneuvers of the external carotid artery branches and each common carotid artery (Figure 18-4).

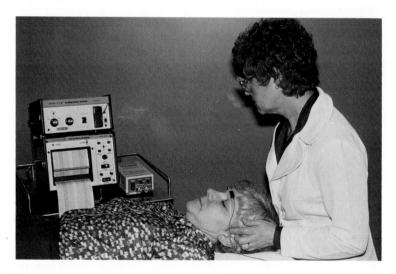

Figure 18-3. Correct locations for photocell transducers and compression of the temporal artery for the supraorbital photoplethysmographic examination.

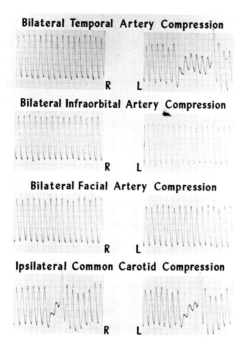

Figure 18-4. Analogue recordings obtained with compression maneuvers during the supra-orbital photoplethysmographic examination. These results are abnormal, indicating stenosis of the left internal carotid artery with the left temporal artery serving as the primary collateral.

DIAGNOSTIC CRITERIA

The SO PPG is abnormal if any of the following criteria is present:

1. $\geq$ 33% reduction in pulse amplitude with compression of the temporal artery.
2. Reduction in amplitude with simultaneous compression of either the temporal and facial arteries or the temporal and infraorbital arteries.
3. $\geq$ 15% reduction in pulse amplitude with compression of the facial or infraorbital artery.
4. Failure of the pulse amplitude to decrease with compression of the ipsilateral common carotid artery.

SO PPG is a relatively sensitive test with a low incidence of false-negative studies. On the other hand, the test is less specific and the percentage of false-positive studies is high. Barnes, Duke, and Lynch reported a false positive rate of 11%, 19%, and 21.1%, respectively.[3,5,7] The majority of the false-positive results were caused by anomalies of supraorbital perfusion. Like the Doppler, the SO PPG is highly accurate—94%–100%[3,5,6]—in detecting significant stenoses of the internal carotid artery.

OCULAR PNEUMOPLETHYSMOGRAPHY

Ocular pneumoplethysmography (OPG-Gee) simultaneously measures systolic blood pressure in both ophthalmic arteries. In addition, hemispheric collateral blood pressure is estimated by measuring the ophthalmic arterial pressure during compression of the ipsilateral common carotid artery.

TECHNIQUE

OPG-Gee has been described by Gee (Figure 18-5).[8] With the patient in the supine position, several drops of 0.5% proparacaine hydrochloride without epinephrine are instilled into both eyes. Eye cups, previously

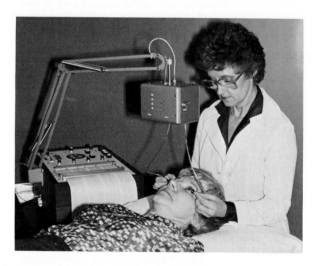

Figure 18-5. Typical position of patient and examiner during application of the eye cups for the ocular pneumoplethysmographic examination.

cleansed with a 70% alcohol swab, are applied to the anesthetized sclera of each eye, lateral to the cornea. A vacuum, either 300 mmHg or 500 mmHg, is applied to both ocular globes. As the vacuum is increased, the intraocular pressure increases gradually. The vacuum is released slowly and reappearance of the arterial pulsations of both eyes are recorded simultaneously. The systolic ophthalmic arterial pressures are calculated from the analogue recordings. These measurements are compared with each other and with the brachial systolic pressure (Figure 18-6).

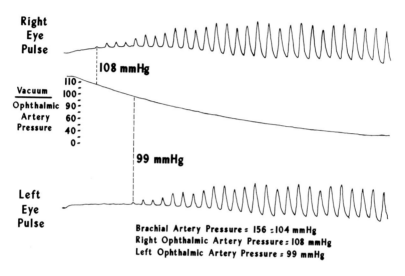

Figure 18-6. A tracing of simultaneously recorded ophthalmic arterial pressures. Note that the appearance of the systolic pulsation of the left eye occurs at a pressure significantly lower ($\geq$ 5 mmHg) than that of the right eye.

DIAGNOSTIC CRITERIA

Development of an instrument capable of a maximum vacuum of 500 mmHg necessitated modification of the diagnostic criteria applicable to studies obtained with a maximum vacuum of 300 mmHg. Gee modified the simple ratio used to compare ophthalmic systolic pressure (OSP) and brachial systolic pressure (BSP). The test is abnormal if the difference between ophthalmic arterial pressures is $\geq$ 5 mmHg, or if the OSP/BSP correlate lies below the line represented by the formula OSP = 39 + 0.42 BSP.

As reported by Lynch et al., OPG-Gee has an 8.1%–15.4% false-negative rate and a low false-positive rate, 4.9%–6.7%.[7,12] False-negative studies may result from combined internal and subclavian artery stenosis, excess collateralization, stenoses of 50%–70%, or subcritical stenoses. False-positive studies may result from improper placement of the eye cups and eye blink artifact, both of which problems are correctable by the examiner. If not corrected, the tracing may indicate a pressure-significant stenosis, and identification of the first true eye pulse may be difficult. The accuracy of OPG-Gee equals that of the most favorable cerebrovascular Doppler studies, 85%–97% for significant stenoses.[7,9-12]

RESULTS

A number of investigators have made valuable contributions to the field of noninvasive diagnostic techniques. Results have been inconsistent, however, with accuracy being influenced by technique, examiner experience, and the definition of hemodynamically significant disease.

In my experience, the complete cerebrovascular Doppler examination provides a means of quickly, accurately, and noninvasively detecting hemodynamically significant carotid artery lesions. Our data demonstrate that most of the false-negative studies occur in the subgroup of vessels with 50%–70% stenoses.[11,7] The physiologic significance of angiographically demonstrated stenoses of 50%–70% is variable, as noted in recently published data on coronary artery disease.[13]

At our institution, SO PPG has always been combined with the PO CDE. Our reports have demonstrated it to be a relatively sensitive test with a low incidence of false-negative results.[3,5-7] The primary disadvantage of the SO PPG is its high rate of false-positive examinations,[3,5-7] many of which are due to abnormal supraorbital circulation resulting from traumatic lacerations of the forehead near the eyebrow.

It has been our practice to employ a combination of studies in the evaluation of cerebrovascular disease. OPG-Gee, the most recent addition, provides a method, different than the PO CDE, by which the physiologic alterations resulting from significant carotid obstruction can be monitored. Like the PO CDE, most false-negative studies occur in vessels with 50%–70% stenoses.[12,7]

DISCUSSION

Any noninvasive examination should fulfill certain criteria in terms of simplicity, portability, expense, accuracy, and reproducibility. The directional Doppler used in the PO CDE is relatively inexpensive and easily transported from one area to another. There are no contraindications to its use, test performance time is approximately 10–15 minutes, and interpretation of the results is subjective. It does require extensive technician training and a high level of competence.

The equipment used to perform SO PPG is also relatively inexpensive and easily transported. The test is simple to perform and technician training is minimal. A study can be completed in 5–10 minutes, providing a hard-copy record for objective interpretation. It is a very sensitive test for the identification of stenotic vessels. Its use is, however, limited by scars on the forehead and by arrhythmias, which cause an irregular and unsatisfactory baseline.

The OPG-Gee is considerably more expensive and not as transportable as the Doppler and SO PPG equipment. Technically, though, it is an easy test to perform, and it produces a hard-copy record for review and interpretation. As mentioned in Chapter 17, there are absolute and relative contraindications to its use, including acute or chronic conjunctivitis, untreated or unstable glaucoma, history of spontaneous retinal detachment, recent eye surgery or trauma, and allergy to local anesthetic.

CONCLUSIONS

Most noninvasive diagnostic techniques for carotid artery disease are insensitive to stenoses of, or less than, 50%, which are not likely to be physiologically significant. A limitation of these techniques is the fact that they do not discriminate between operable stenosis and inoperable occlusion of the internal carotid artery.

Noninvasive diagnostic techniques do, however, play an important role in the evaluation and management of patients with suspected carotid occlusive disease. The clinical information derived from the periorbital cerebrovascular Doppler examination, supraorbital photoplethysmography, and ocular pneumoplethysmography is useful in managing patients in the following categories:

1. Asymptomatic carotid bruit.
2. Ambiguous cerebral symptoms.
3. Vertebrobasilar symptoms (concomitant carotid disease).
4. High risk (strong family history of arteriosclerosis obliterans, hypertension, hyperlipidemia).
5. Serial follow-up (natural history, influence of medical or surgical therapy).

Noninvasive techniques also provide an adjunctive means of screening patients with symptoms of cerebral ischemia, although contrast arteriography is recommended for patients with hemispheric transient ischemic attacks and for those who have completed a stroke and have had significant recovery. The clinical use of any noninvasive diagnostic screening technique does, of course, require careful consideration of its role and limitations.

REFERENCES

1. Barnes RW, Wilson MR: *Doppler Ultrasonic Evaluation of Cerebrovascular Disease.* Iowa City, University of Iowa Press, 1975.
2. Barnes RW, Russell HE, Bone GE, et al: Doppler cerebrovascular examination: improved results with refinements in technique. Stroke 8:468–471, 1977.
3. Barnes RW, Garrett WV, Slaymaker EE, et al: Doppler ultrasound and supraorbital photoplethysmography for noninvasive screening of carotid occlusive disease. Am J Surg 134:183–186, 1977.
4. Barnes RW, Reinertson JE, Slaymaker EE, et al: Predictive value of noninvasive screening tests in identifying symptomatic candidates for carotid endarterectomy. In *Noninvasive Cardiovascular Diagnosis: Current Concepts.* Edited by EB Diethrich. Baltimore, University Park Press, 1978, pp 19–28.
5. Duke LJ, Slaymaker EE, Lamberth WC, et al: Results of ophthalmosonometry and supraorbital photoplethysmography in evaluating carotid arterial stenoses. Circulation 60:2, I-127–I-131, 1979.
6. Barnes RW, Clayton JM, Bone GE, et al: Supraorbital photoplethysmography. Simple, accurate screening for carotid occlusive disease. J Surg Res 22:319–327, 1977.
7. Lynch TG, Wright CB, Miller EV: Oculopneumoplethysmography, Doppler examination, and supraorbital photoplethysmography: a comparison of hemodynamic techniques in assessing cerebrovascular occlusive disease. Cerebrovascular noninvasive testing. Ann Surg 194:731–736, 1981.
8. Gee W, Smith CA, Hinsen CE, et al: Ocular pneumoplethysmography in carotid artery disease. Med Instrum 8:244–248, 1974.
9. Machleder HI, Barker WF: Noninvasive methods for evaluation of extracranial cerebrovascular disease. Arch Surg 112:944–946, 1977.

10. McDonald PT, Rich NM, Collins GJ, et al: Doppler cerebrovascular examination, oculoplethysmography, and ocular pneumoplethysmography: use in detection of carotid disease. A prospective clinical study. Arch Surg 113:1341–1349, 1978.
11. McDonald KM, Gee W, Kaupp HA: Screening for significant carotid stenosis by ocular pneumoplethysmography. Am J Surg 137: 244–249, 1979.
12. Lynch TG, Wright CB, Miller EV, et al: Evaluation of cerebrovascular Doppler examination and oculopneumoplethysmography in a clinical perspective. Stroke 12:325–330, 1981.
13. Wright CB, Doty DB, Eastham CL, et al: Measurement of coronary reactive hyperemia with a Doppler probe. J Thorac Cardiovasc Surg 80:888–897, 1980.

CHAPTER 19

DIRECT DOPPLER
AUSCULTATION
OF THE CAROTID ARTERIES

Lee Nix

In the past, noninvasive screening for carotid arterial disease has primarily involved indirect or periorbital techniques that detect changes in pressure or flow in branches of the ophthalmic artery. These indirect methods cannot detect nonobstructing or ulcerating plaques, nor can they distinguish operable internal carotid stenosis from inoperable occlusion. Because of these limitations, several noninvasive methods of directly evaluating the cervical carotid have been developed, namely the ultrasonic B-scan and Doppler imaging systems. These techniques are useful, but expensive and complicated. Moreover, rapid changes in technology have delayed and limited their widespread use. There is an alternative, however. Commonly available bidirectional, continuous-wave Doppler devices provide a rapid, accurate, and inexpensive means of investigating the carotid artery in the neck.

TECHNIQUE

A bidirectional continuous-wave Doppler detector for the auditory assessment of the common, internal, and external carotid segments has been used to screen patients with suspected cerebrovascular disease. This instrument permits the operator to listen to flow both toward and away from the probe. In the flow-away-from-probe mode, the detector screens out the venous signals and allows the supraclavicular common carotid to be examined through the bifurcation and into the extracranial portions of the internal and external carotid artery up to the jaw.

The patient is examined in the supine position with the head on a pillow to relax the neck muscles (Figure 19-1). After applying a coupling gel to the skin, the examiner begins above the clavicle in the common carotid, holding the bidirectional Doppler probe at a 45-degree angle. The probe is advanced in a cephalad direction along the common carotid until the bifurcation is reached. The internal and external carotid, recognizable by their characteristic signals, are distinguished by changes in the signal and traced to the jawline.

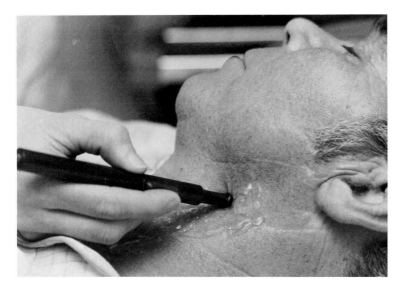

Figure 19-1. Position of patient and probe for direct Doppler examination of the carotid artery bifurcation. Reprinted with permission of the American Medical Association from Barnes RW, Nix L, Rittgers SE: Audible interpretation of carotid Doppler signals. Arch Surg 116:1185–1189, 1981.

Signals from the different carotid segments are distinguished by sound. Normal common carotid arterial signals are smooth and pulsatile with a strong systolic component and a moderate diastolic component. Normal internal carotid arterial signals are recognizable because of their prominent diastolic component, which is continuous as a result of the brain's very low cerebrovascular resistance. The normal external carotid arterial signals are smooth and markedly pulsatile, with high velocity in systole and relatively low velocity in diastole as a result of the higher peripheral resistance of the face and scalp. These characteristic signals help the examiner to identify the bifurcation and the location of stenotic lesions.

A stenotic area is recognized by the sharp increase in velocity (pitch) at the stenosis. Just distal to the stenosis, where the arterial lumen becomes more normal, is an area of disturbed flow. Just at the stenosis the signal (pitch) increases sharply because the blood velocity increases to pass through the narrow lesion. This signal is recognized by its high-pitched hiss or rasping sound. Distal to the stenotic lesion, disturbed, lower-pitched sounds are heard as the high-velocity flow enters a segment of increased volume.

Occlusion of the internal carotid causes changes other than an absent signal. The ipsilateral common carotid may assume characteristics of the external carotid—notably low diastolic components—or the external carotid, which provides abundant collateral circulation to the brain, may develop some diastolic components that somewhat resemble those of the internal carotid.

RESULTS

Of 775 consecutive patients examined during a three-year period, 101 required arteriograms. Films of 199 carotid systems were available for comparison. The direct carotid examinations were performed by nurse technologists in the vascular laboratory prior to arteriographic studies.

The interpretations of the carotid Doppler signals by the vascular technologist were tabulated and analyzed without knowledge of the contrast arteriograms. The Doppler velocity signals were classified as normal (no detected stenosis), abnormal (stenosis associated with a significantly increased or disturbed velocity), and absent (occlusion of the named carotid segment). The degree of stenosis on the contrast arteriogram was determined according to the percentage reduction in diameter and was classified as < 50% stenosis, which included ulcerated plaques, ≥ 50% stenosis, or occlusion. Based on these arteriographic findings, the results of the carotid Doppler examinations were expressed in terms of their sensitivity, specificity, and negative and positive predictive values.

The results of the carotid Doppler examinations and contrast arteriograms are presented in Table 19-1. The overall sensitivity of the carotid Doppler examinations in detecting severe stenosis or occlusion of the carotid artery was 92%. The Doppler studies correctly differentiated these two conditions in 84% of the diseased vessels. In carotid arteries with stenosis greater than or equal to 50%, the sensitivity of the Doppler examinations was 90%, and these studies suggested stenosis in all but two of the 36 abnormal examinations. In two patent carotids with greater than 90% stenosis, a signal could not be elicited, presumably because of the low blood flow through the severely stenotic segment. The four false-negative studies were probably the result of the examiner's mistaking the flow signals of the external carotid artery for those of the internal carotid. Such errors may arise from the external carotid's compensatory increase in diastolic component when providing abundant collateral flow to the internal carotid.

Table 19-1. The Results of Carotid Arteriography Correlated with Those of the Direct Doppler Examination

Carotid Arteriogram	Number of Vessels	Carotid Doppler Signal		
		Normal	Abnormal	Absent
Normal	46	42	4	0
<50% Stenotic	90	63	27	0
≥50% Stenotic	40	4	34	2
Occluded	23	1	3	19

The sensitivity of the Doppler examinations in detecting occluded vessels was 96%, and all but three of the Doppler abnormalities consisted of absent flow signals that correctly suggested occlusion of the carotid segment. Three examinations suggested disturbed (rather than occluded) flow of the internal carotid, perhaps because the examiner misinterpreted abnormal flow signals from a branch of the external carotid artery that, possibly, served as a collateral for the occluded internal carotid. It is also possible that a severely stenotic segment of the internal carotid occluded prior to arteriography. The one false-negative Doppler examination probably resulted from the examiner's misinterpreting the external carotid artery as the high-flow internal carotid artery because of a compensatory increase in diastolic collateral flow.

The Doppler flow signal was abnormal in 30% of the nonobstructive stenoses, but these studies were not considered falsely positive because the arteriograms revealed carotid disease sufficient to disturb flow. The specificity in identifying normal carotid arteries was 91%. These four false-positive results may have been caused by excessive pressure of the Doppler probe, which could compress the underlying carotid artery and disturb its flow.

The negative predictive value of a normal carotid Doppler examination in excluding significant carotid occlusive disease was 95%. The positive predictive value of an abnormal carotid Doppler signal suggesting disturbed flow was 94%, and 90% of these findings were confirmed when subsequent carotid arteriography revealed stenosis. The positive predictive value of an absent flow signal was 100%, and 90% of these were associated with angiographically proven occlusion of the carotid and the remainder with greater than 90% stenosis on arteriogram.

DISCUSSION

The results of auditory interpretation of direct carotid Doppler interrogation surpass our previous results with indirect methods and approach those of ultrasonic imaging.

The use of direct Doppler auscultation to evaluate the velocities of carotid flow is recognized as an integral, helpful part of B-scan and Doppler ultrasonic imaging systems. B-scan systems use Doppler assessment of flow to detect changes caused by soft plaques and to prove patency in the presence of severe atherosclerotic plaque or occlusion by fresh thrombosis. Ultrasonic imaging systems use direct Doppler auscultation to determine flow velocities in the presence of calcified plaques, which often obscure the carotid image.

There are also limitations to examining the carotid artery directly with continuous-wave Doppler: (1) it relies on the examiner's subjective evaluation (there usually is no hard-copy confirmation), (2) its successful use depends on the experience of the examiner, (3) it cannot detect thin plaques, which cause no audible disturbances of flow, and (4) it is susceptible to anatomic variations, which may be confusing without an image to guide the examiner.

The direct, continuous-wave Doppler examination is valuable in the important discrimination between stenosis and occlusion of the internal carotid artery. It is more sensitive than indirect techniques, and it requires only the equipment frequently used in other noninvasive tests. If hard-copy results are desired, the signals may be recorded and the spectrum analyzed. Direct Doppler examinations of the carotid can be performed by an experienced vascular technologist; the examiner's experience with and knowledge of the flow characteristics of the internal carotid provide an invaluable adjunct to imaging systems.

The accuracy (with or without an ultrasonic imaging system) of the direct carotid Doppler examination makes it the most rapid, accurate, and inexpensive method of evaluating extracranial carotid occlusive disease.

BIBLIOGRAPHY

1. Barnes RW: Noninvasive evaluation of the carotid bruit. Annu Rev Med 31:201–218, 1980.
2. Barnes RW, Wilson MR: *Doppler Ultrasonic Evaluation of Cerebrovascular Disease.* Iowa City, University of Iowa Press, 1975.
3. Baskett JJ, Beasley MG, Murphy GJ, et al: Screening for carotid junction disease by spectral analysis of Doppler signals. Cardiovascular Res 11:147, 1977.
4. Lewis R, Beasley G, Hyams E, et al: Imaging the carotid bifurcation using continuous-wave Doppler-shift ultrasound and spectral analysis. Stroke: 9:465, 1978.
5. Prendes JL, McKinney WM, Buonanno FS, et al: Anatomic variations of the carotid bifurcation affecting Doppler scan interpretation. J Clin Ultrasound 8:147–150, 1980.

CHAPTER 20

EARLY DETECTION OF STROKE-RELATED LESIONS BY REAL-TIME DOPPLER SPECTRAL ANALYSIS

Stanley E. Rittgers, William W. Putney, and Robert W. Barnes

S everal studies have demonstrated that plaques too small to cause hemodynamic changes frequently cause transient ischemic symptoms and completed strokes.[1] Therefore, one must detect not only the severe, flow-reducing stenoses, but also the lesser, flow-disturbing plaques in order to identify those individuals at risk for strokes. Directly monitoring and recording Doppler velocity signals over the extracranial carotid arteries and visually processing this information with real-time spectral analysis helps to assess flow disturbances and to diagnose many of these arterial lesions.

INSTRUMENTATION

Direct carotid Doppler spectral analysis is performed with an 8-MHz bidirectional, continuous-wave ultrasound probe. The audio and tape outputs of the Doppler-shifted signals are switched so that only flow away from the probe is recorded.

The frequency content of the carotid artery Doppler signal is analyzed with a real-time sound spectral analyzer (Figure 20-1).[2] This device provides a continuous display of Doppler frequency shifts in preselected ranges shown on the vertical axis. Time is displayed in either a continuous or a freeze-frame mode on the horizontal axis while the amplitude of the Doppler signal at each frequency is displayed as modulated intensity in 16 shades of gray.

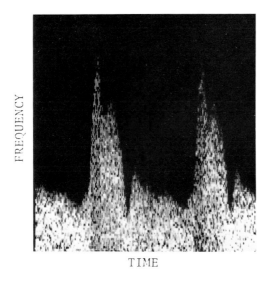

Figure 20-1. Real-time spectral analyzer showing Doppler-shift frequency vertically, time horizontally, and frequency amplitude as brightness intensity.

TECHNIQUE

The position of the probe is adjusted until an optimal common carotid flow signal is elicited (Figure 20-2). The probe is then moved slowly along the course of the common carotid artery until the carotid bifurcation is reached, at which point the pitch of the Doppler signal changes slightly. Next the probe is advanced along the course of the internal carotid artery, which is recognized by the distinctive high-flow velocity that continues during diastole. The examiner repositions the probe over the carotid bifurcation and angles it slightly more toward the lower border

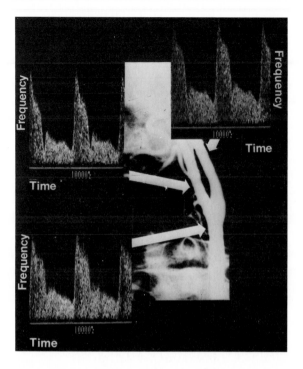

Figure 20-2. Doppler spectral waveforms from normal common (*lower left*), external (*upper left*), and internal (*upper right*) carotid arteries.

of the mandible. A flow signal from the external carotid artery is elicited and distinguished by its multiphasic character and lower diastolic velocity.

The normal internal carotid arterial waveform is characterized by its low distal resistance, allowing high flow during both systole and diastole. The velocity of the internal carotid artery is typically higher than that of the common carotid artery because of the large proportion of total flow passing through this smaller vessel. A brightness concentration appears at higher frequencies near the waveform outline and a darkened "window" is seen during systole indicating uniformly high velocity and no flow disturbances.

Velocity in the external carotid artery is less peaked and, because of higher peripheral vascular resistance, there is proportionately less diastolic flow. A more rapid systolic deceleration phase and a more prominent notch distinguish the external carotid artery from the other branches.

At a mild stenosis of the internal carotid artery, peak frequency may be maintained or slightly elevated (Figure 20-3). Surface irregularities and separation zones near the stenosis do cause some disturbance of flow; there is a slight loss of flow concentration at high velocities with some filling in of the systolic window.

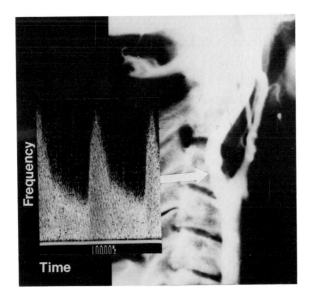

Figure 20-3. Doppler spectral waveform in a case of mild stenosis of the internal carotid artery.

A stenosis that reduces luminal diameter by 50% produces peak systolic frequencies above those normally observed (Figure 20-4). The Doppler signal is characterized by a high pitch accompanied by a bubbling sound from flow eddies distal to the stenosis. The waveform contains low-velocity flow near the baseline with no intensity concentration along the upper-frequency envelope. The outline is faint and the systolic peak appears irregular and jagged because of the turbulent flow. When the probe is moved distal to the site of maximum stenosis, peak frequency drops rather abruptly because the flow channel widens and average flow velocity decreases.

In the case of a stenosis greater than 90%, the Doppler waveform is similar to, but more exaggerated than, that produced in cases of moderate stenosis (Figure 20-5). Peak systolic frequency often is extremely

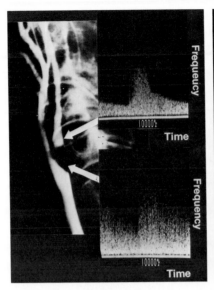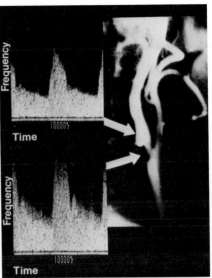

Figure 20-4. Doppler spectral waveforms at (*top*) and distal to (*bottom*) a moderate stenosis of the internal carotid artery.

Figure 20-5. Doppler spectral waveforms at (*top*) and distal to (*bottom*) a severe stenosis of the internal carotid artery.

elevated with a distinct hissing sound. The waveform is distinguished by a very weak upper outline and by an irregular, turbulent systolic peak. Simultaneously, there are high intensities near the baseline, caused by stagnated, eddylike flow outside the main jet. When the probe is moved distally, the peak frequency decreases and there is a considerable shift of blood-cell concentration toward the baseline.

When the internal carotid artery is completely occluded, the common carotid arterial waveform reveals low peak velocity during systole and virtually no flow during diastole (Figure 20-6). The external carotid arterial waveform often appears elevated throughout the cardiac cycle due to the development of a collateral pathway via this channel. The distinctive features of the external carotid artery generally remain, however, although flow may be somewhat disturbed because of stenotic lesions in this branch or because of the turbulence caused by the additional flow carried through this small-caliber vessel. An extremely abnormal velocity waveform may be detected in the internal carotid stump, representing whirlpoollike motion.

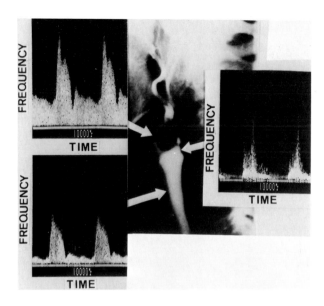

Figure 20-6. Doppler spectral waveforms from common (*lower left*), external (*upper left*), and proximal internal (*upper right*) carotid arteries with totally occluded distal internal carotid artery.

DIAGNOSTIC CRITERIA AND RESULTS

A summary of the criteria used to categorize the degree of blood flow disturbance is presented in Table 20-1.

From September 1978 to March 1980, direct carotid Doppler spectral analysis was performed on 124 internal carotid arteries of 72 patients who underwent arteriography for the conditions indicated in Figure 20-7. Biplanar contrast arteriograms of both extracranial and intracranial cerebrovascular arteries were obtained on all patients. The internal carotid arterial segments were classified as normal, <50% stenotic, ≥50% stenotic, or occluded.

The results of real-time spectral analysis of carotid Doppler flow signals are shown in Table 20-2. An abnormal or absent Doppler spectrum was present in all but one of the vessels with severe stenosis or occlusion, yielding an overall sensitivity of 98% in identifying hemodynamically significant disease. The sensitivity in detecting occlusions was 95%, and an absent Doppler signal correctly identified the occlusion in 77% of the vessels. Flow abnormalities were present in all of the stenoses greater than or equal to 50%, and a spectral flow disturbance was identified in 42 of the 60 arteries with stenosis less than 50%, for a sensitivity of 70% in the detection of mild disease. Therefore, the overall sensitivity in detecting carotid disease of any severity was 83%. The specificity in identifying normal carotid arteries was 53%; in five of the seven normal carotid arteries in which a flow disturbance was elicited, however, the spectral abnormality was mild.

Table 20-1. Doppler Spectral Waveform: Diagnostic Criteria

Classification	Waveform Characteristics
Normal	Intensity concentration near upper envelope, regular waveform
Mild	Small increase in intensity at low frequencies, regular waveform
Moderate	Uniform intensity across frequency range, elevated peak frequency
Severe	Marked intensity near baseline, indistinct upper envelope, extreme peak frequency
Occluded	Absence of signal

The positive predictive value of an absent Doppler signal in identifying internal carotid occlusion was 94%, while the value of a disturbed Doppler spectrum in predicting internal carotid stenosis of any severity was 86%. Therefore, the positive predictive value of either an abnormal or an absent Doppler spectrum in identifying carotid disease of any severity was 91%. The negative predictive value of a normal Doppler spectrum being associated with truly normal internal carotid arteries was 30%, but the negative predictive value of a normal Doppler spectrum in identifying insignificant carotid disease was 96%. Although the specificity of carotid artery spectral analysis was relatively poor, most of the falsely positive errors were associated with interpretation of mild spectral disturbances. We believe that specificity can be improved through use of more quantitative measurements of flow disturbances. Also, it is important to realize that these results were obtained by audio and visual pattern recognition of Doppler signals, without the aid of an imaging system. Coupling Doppler spectral analysis to such a system would further improve the results.

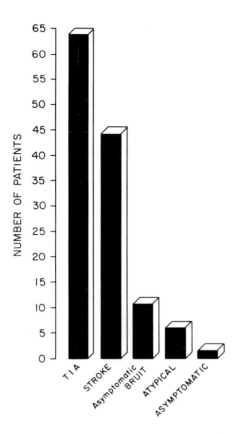

Figure 20-7. Presenting symptoms of patients in study group. Four females and 124 males from 27 to 84 years of age (mean age, 59) were evaluated both noninvasively and invasively.

Table 20-2. The Results of Real-Time Spectral Analysis of Doppler Flow Signals

Severity of Disease on Arteriogram	Number of Arteries	Flow Disturbance Classification				
		None	Mild	Moderate	Severe	Absent
Normal	15	8	5	1	1	0
<50% stenoses	60	18	29	12	1	0
≥50% stenosis	27	0	5	6	15	1
Occlusion	22	1	0	1	3	17

CONCLUSIONS

The data from this study confirm the value of direct carotid Doppler spectral analysis in the diagnosis of carotid artery disease. This technique is sensitive to both severe stenoses and total occlusions and can differentiate between the two. It also detects most non-hemodynamically significant lesions. Consequently, direct carotid Doppler spectral analysis may be used to screen asymptomatic and atypically symptomatic patients, and to follow patients with carotid disease over the long term. Because of its excellent sensitivity, this test may also be used to improve the criteria for ordering angiography in symptomatic patients. Since the present system can be readily coupled to any continuous-wave or pulsed Doppler ultrasonic system, real-time spectral analysis now offers a significant advance to the use of conventional Doppler equipment.

Recently, instrumentation has been developed to quantify further the spectral waveform information (AngioScan II, Unigon Industries, Inc., Mt. Vernon, New York). A Z-80 based microprocessor system with compiler BASIC software has been interfaced with a real-time frequency analyzer, and programs have been written to extract and store selected parameters from each waveform and to correlate the results with known angiographic information. The parameters chosen were the mode frequency (frequency with maximum amplitude), the peak frequency (frequency with amplitude 18 db down from the mode amplitude), and the upper and lower bandwidth frequencies (frequencies with amplitudes 12 db down from the mode amplitude). Additionally, a systolic window was defined as the ratio of the area under the lower bandwidth curve to the area under the upper bandwidth curve taken over 100 msec, beginning at peak systole.

The results of a sample of 58 arteries show that both the ratio of peak frequency in the proximal internal carotid artery to that in the distal (+1 cm) internal carotid artery and the systolic window at the distal internal carotid artery correlate with the degree of stenosis. The diagnostic accuracy of each of these parameters was determined using receiver-operator characteristic curves. Index values for the peak frequency ratio and the systolic window—1.1 and 38%, respectively—were found to be most effective in differentiating normal from diseased vessels. Combining these criteria and considering a positive value of either parameter to indicate a positive study resulted in a specificity of 89% and sensitivities of 40%, 50%, 89%, 100%, and 100% to stenoses of 1%–20%, 21%–40%, 41%–60%, 61%–80%, and 81%–99% diameter reduction, respectively.

256

REFERENCES

1. Pessin MS, Duncan GW, Mohr JP, et al: Clinical and angiographic features of carotid transient ischemic attacks. N Engl J Med 296:358–363, 1977.
2. Rittgers SE, Putney WW, Barnes RW: Real-time spectrum analysis and display of directional Doppler ultrasound blood velocity signals. IEEE Trans Biomed Eng 27:723–728, 1980.

CHAPTER 21

Three-Dimensional Ultrasonic Arteriography

Richard D. Miles

Most noninvasive techniques now available for the detection of carotid disease are sensitive only to hemodynamically significant lesions, but many strokes and prestroke symptoms are caused by emboli arising from lesions that cause only minor hemodynamic changes. This limitation prompted us to develop computerized ultrasonic arteriography, a new technique for noninvasively imaging the carotid bifurcation for the diagnosis of occlusive disease. The basic theories behind our computerized imaging system are discussed in this chapter; the instrument's application and the results of clinical trials are explained in the following chapter.

BACKGROUND

Pulsed-Doppler ultrasonic arteriography was introduced[1] to overcome the limited usefulness of other noninvasive techniques in cases involving lesions that are not hemodynamically significant. This technique employs transducer-position information and Doppler flow signals to form a projection image of the carotid lumen on an oscilloscope screen (Figure 21-1). By analyzing these standard oscilloscope images and by listening to changes in the Doppler flow sound, 86% of the lesions reducing luminal diameter by more than 40% were detectable.[2] In addition, the diameter

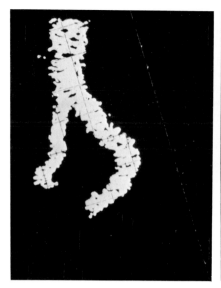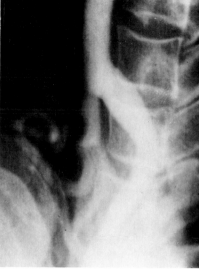

Figure 21-1. *Left:* Image of a normal carotid bifurcation produced by a standard Hokanson pulsed-Doppler ultrasonic arteriograph. *Right:* X-ray of the same vessel confirmed the diagnosis.

of stenoses, measured from ultrasonic and x-ray images, agreed within ±20% in 81% of the cases.

In spite of its diagnostic usefulness, though, ultrasonic arteriography has its limitations: 14% of the stenoses are missed and 19% of those that are detected are incorrectly interpreted. Many of these errors are errors of projection involving lesions that are invisible or only partially visible in a single projection. If the vessel diagrammed in Figure 21-2 were imaged from the top by standard ultrasonic arteriography or by x-ray angiography, for example, it would appear normal. This is called a projection error.

To reduce projection errors we need other views, so we took a Hokanson pulsed-Doppler ultrasonic arteriograph and added a microcomputer with a keyboard, floppy disk drive, video monitor, and keypad (Figure 21-3). This instrument, which we call a Computascan, produces multiplanar images of the carotid bifurcation. During a patient examination, orthogonal plane and depth views develop simultaneously on the video screen while transverse cross sections are drawn at selected sites along the vessel.[3] These multiple views identify lesions that are not visible in a single view alone. The instrument reduces projection errors by allowing

**Plane View
Appears Normal**

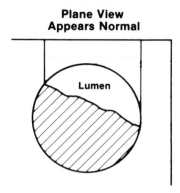

Lumen

Figure 21-2. Cross-sectional diagram of a stenosed artery. Projection errors can occur in standard ultrasonic arteriography and x-ray angiography when a three-dimensional artery is projected onto a two-dimensional plane.

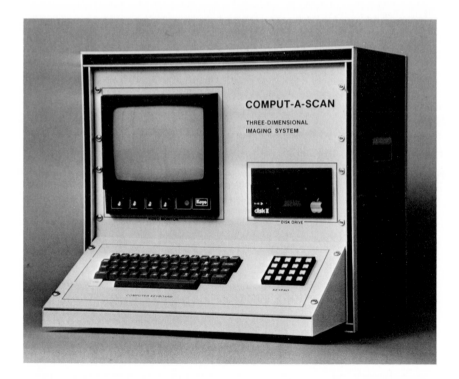

Figure 21-3. Instrument that interfaces with a Hokanson pulsed-Doppler arteriograph for the production of multiplanar images.

one to look at the vessels from different directions simultaneously. In Figure 21-4A, for example, the plane view appears normal, but the stenosis is visible in the depth and cross-sectional views. In other cases disease is evident in all three views (Figure 21-4B).

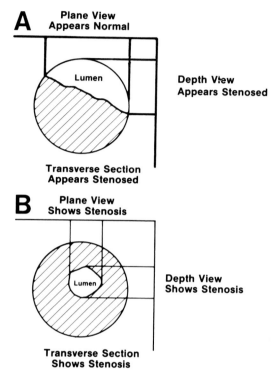

Figure 21-4. Computascan reduces projection errors by simultaneously producing cross-sectional, lateral, and anterior-posterior views of the carotid bifurcation. **A** Asymmetric stenosis leads to projection errors. **B** Symmetric stenosis appears in all views.

DOPPLER PHYSICS

PRINCIPLES

To better understand this instrument, let us briefly review the Doppler principle (see also Chapter 23). A stationary observer perceives a constant tone emanating from an approaching vehicle to be at a pitch higher than what is broadcast; the same tone seems lower than what is broadcast when the vehicle passes and moves away. In both cases the tone perceived is shifted up or down by a Doppler frequency Δf, which is proportional to the velocity of the vehicle. This principle applies to both audible sound and (inaudible) ultrasonic sound waves.

When ultrasound is beamed into tissue and reflected by moving red blood cells, the reflected ultrasonic waves are shifted up or down in frequency by a value Δf, which is proportional to several variables, as follows:

$$\Delta f = \frac{2v f_0 \cos\Theta}{c}$$

In this equation v is the velocity of the red blood cells, c is the velocity of ultrasound in tissue, Θ is the angle between the ultrasound beam and the velocity vector, f_0 is the transmitted frequency, and f is the Doppler-shifted frequency. The values of f_0 and c are considered constant; the only variables are the relative beam angle Θ and the velocity v of the blood cells.

APPLICATIONS

With continuous-wave ultrasound, one crystal in the transducer continuously transmits the ultrasonic signal while an adjacent crystal continuously receives the reflected ultrasonic waves. Electronic circuitry separates forward from reverse flow.[4] Continuous-wave ultrasound can also be used in vessel-imaging systems.[2] Because it cannot determine the depth of the vessel, however, pulsed-Doppler ultrasound is necessary.

The pulsed-Doppler transducer transmits a burst of ultrasound into the tissue from a single crystal. The same crystal also detects the reflected ultrasonic waves and converts them back into electricity.

The distance between the transducer and the red blood cells is determined by the time Δt it takes for the echo to return. This interval lasts only microseconds, and electronic circuitry is required to measure it accurately.

The distance the ultrasound travels equals the velocity of the ultrasound (c) multiplied by the time it takes to make the round trip (Δt). Hence round trip distance = c × Δt. By sampling the reflected ultrasound for a brief instant, it is possible to measure blood flow in a small volume within the vessel.[5] The depth of this sample volume is determined by the length of the time interval Δt, which can be manually or automatically adjusted to place the sample volume at the proper depth.

Figure 21-5 clarifies this sampling process. In the Hokanson pulsed-Doppler arteriograph, there are six sample (or range) gates that detect flow at six points across the vessel lumen. When the moving hand in the figure is straight up, the ultrasonic burst is transmitted. The hand rotates in clockwise fasion, and after Δt the ultrasound has traveled out to the vessel and back again. The hand touches the Gate 1 position, causing the gate to sample briefly the reflected ultrasound present at that time, and continues to rotate. It touches Gate 2, which also samples the reflection, and the process continues through Gate 6. Once the hand is straight up again, another burst of ultrasound is transmitted to start the cycle again. By changing the time Δt between the transmission and sample Gate 1, the depth of the sample can be varied from 4 to 40 mm.

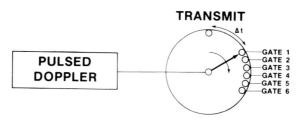

Figure 21-5. Time (Δt) between transmission and gate contact determines sample depth.

PRACTICE

During an examination with the standard Hokanson arteriograph, the examiner moves the six sample gates up and down by push-button control until they are located within the vessel lumen. When a gate detects flow, a dot appears on an oscilloscope screen. As the examination progresses, the dots accumulate to form an outline of the vessel lumen. The finished image is a lateral projection of the vessel. The instrument acts essentially as a continuous-wave Doppler, since it does not use flow detection by the individual sample gates to produce these lateral views.

The Computascan gathers additional information, using, in addition to transducer position, the sample depth and flow data from each gate to produce the multiplanar images. The main components of the Computascan interface are dual-channel analog-to-digital converters, which digitize the transducer's position on the skin; a depth converter, which allows the computer to vary, either automatically or manually, the depth of the sample gates; and a circuit that latches the flow signals from the six gates (Figure 21-6). These signals are continuously loaded into the microcomputer to be used by the program to draw images on the video screen. The transducer is moved manually back and forth across the neck to produce these images.

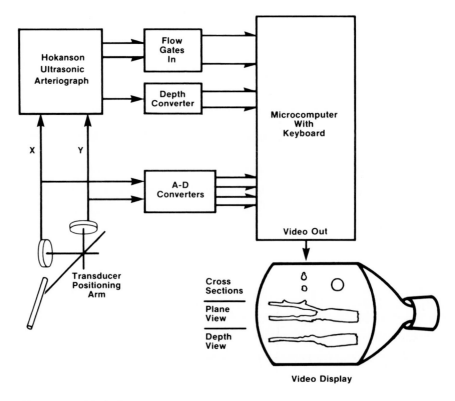

Figure 21-6. Block diagram of Computascan interface to a Hokanson pulsed-Doppler arteriograph.

THE EXAMINATION

To start the examination, the examiner inserts a floppy disk into the disk drive and turns on the computer. A series of questions are asked of the examiner—the patient's name, the date of the examination, and the side being examined. The examiner then places the transducer on the neck above the common carotid artery and begins the scan.

The video screen the examiner watches is represented in Figure 21-7, which shows a lateral and an anterior-posterior view. The internal carotid artery appears in both views, but the external carotid is shown only in the lateral view to prevent superimposing the two branches in the anterior-posterior view. The horizontal white line represents the skin line (zero depth). The distance between the line and the image of the vessel indicates the depth of the vessel beneath the skin. The patient's name and the date and site of examination are displayed at the bottom of the screen along with the mode the examiner selected. In this case a key was pressed to produce "both" the lateral and anterior-posterior views. On the right side of the screen, the display shows the depth at which the sample volumes are located, and six bars that flash from short to long indicate when flow is detected by the particular gate. The examiner moves the gates up and down until they are located within the center of the lumen, as indicated by all six bars flashing the position of the transducer relative to the vessel.

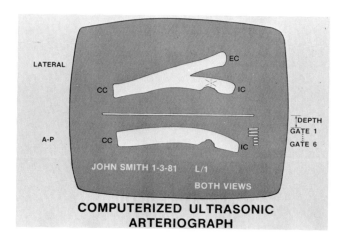

Figure 21-7. Video screen on which computer displays vessel images.

In this example, both the lateral and anterior-posterior views reveal narrowing of the vessel lumen. At the location of the transducer, the three upper sample gates would be detecting the flow and the bottom three gates would not because they are located in the obstructed part of the lumen.

To produce a cross-sectional view, the examiner presses the cross-section key at any time during the examination (Figure 21-8). The computer displays the selection at the bottom and draws a temporary vertical line through the vessel in the lateral view. As the transducer is moved along that vertical line, dots appear directly above it to indicate the size

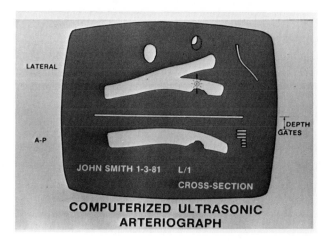

Figure 21-8. Cross sections can be produced at any location by the computer.

of the lumen. Cross sections are especially valuable in regions of stenosis, since the actual size of the lumen can be determined. If a band of calcium prevents penetration of ultrasound, the calcified region is assumed to be patent if cross sections distal to the calcium are of normal size.

Once the examination is complete, another key is used to trace the position of the mandible for anatomic reference. A photograph of a normal bifurcation taken from the Computascan printout is shown in Figure 21-9.

CONCLUSIONS

Three-dimensional views of the carotid artery and its main branches can now be obtained with the Computascan, a device that increases the accuracy and usefulness of the Hokanson ultrasonic arteriograph.

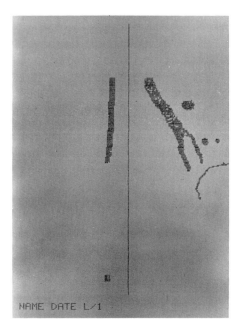

Figure 21-9. Printout from a computerized examination of a normal bifurcation.

REFERENCES

1. Hokanson DE, Mozersky D, Sumner DS, et al: Ultrasonic arteriography: a new approach to arterial visualization. Biomed Eng 6:420, 1971.
2. Reid JM, Spencer MP: Ultrasonic Doppler techniques for imaging blood vessels. Science 176:1235–1236, 1972.
3. Miles RD, Russell JB, Sumner DS: Computerized ultrasonic arteriography: a new technique for imaging the carotid bifurcation. IEEE Trans Biomed Eng 5:378–381, 1982.
4. McLeod FD: A directional Doppler flowmeter. Digest of the VII International Conference on Medicine and Biomedical Engineering, Stockholm, 1967, pp 13–14.
5. Baker DW: Pulsed ultrasonic Doppler blood-flow sensing. IEEE Trans Sonics Ultrasonics 17:170–185, 1970.

CHAPTER 22

PULSED-DOPPLER
ULTRASONIC
ARTERIOGRAPHY

James B. Russell

As the previous chapter indicates, pulsed-Doppler ultrasonic arteriography is a relatively new procedure that permits noninvasive imaging of the arterial lumen and provides audio information regarding the velocity patterns of blood flow. It has been shown to be quite accurate for the detection of extracranial carotid arterial lesions, especially those that narrow the diameter of the arterial lumen by at least 45%. Our laboratory has been using an ultrasonic arteriograph (D. E. Hokanson, Inc., Issaquah, Washington) since February 1977 to study more than 1,800 patients suspected of having carotid occlusive disease. This chapter reviews our experience with this noninvasive procedure.

INSTRUMENTATION

The ultrasonic arteriograph utilizes a 5-MHz pulsed Doppler that is connected to a position-sensing arm. A single piezoelectric crystal transmits and receives the ultrasonic signal, which is then processed by six range gates or flow channels that allow the pulsed Doppler to examine flow at small regions within the arterial lumen. Using a hand-held control, the examiner moves the sampling area up or down, to a maximum depth of 4 cm below the skin's surface. Six LEDs indicate when arterial flow is detected. Furthermore, by adjusting the sample volume, flow signals from adjacent arteries or veins can be excluded. An image of the arterial lumen is produced on a storage oscilloscope by blending together dots that correspond to the x and y locations of arterial flow. The frequencies present in the Doppler audio signal correspond to the velocities of the red blood cells as they pass through the ultrasonic beam. Channel three is used to examine blood flow in the center of the arterial lumen, where the velocities are greatest, and its audio signal is subjected to spectral analysis. Therefore, channel three has a wider frequency response (200 Hz to 5.6 kHz) than the other five channels (200 Hz to 2.2 kHz).

In 1979, Richard Miles, working in our laboratory, successfully interfaced a microcomputer to the ultrasonic arteriograph. The computerized version produces a plan view similar to the standard system and, in addition, simultaneously generates depth and cross-sectional views. Chapter 21 describes this new imaging system.

Recent electronic advances have permitted the manufacture of real-time spectral analyzers simple and convenient enough for the vascular laboratory. In May 1980, we began analyzing the spectra of the Doppler audio signal in conjunction with ultrasonic imaging. The spectral analyzer (Unigon Industries, Inc., Mt. Vernon, New York) uses the Fast Fourier Transform (FFT) method of analysis and displays the spectrum on a video monitor with frequency on the y-axis, time on the x-axis, and amplitude as shades of gray. The display can be frozen at any time and the spectrum photographed.

TECHNIQUE

The examiner begins by reassuring the patient that the study is safe and painless and by explaining its nature. Patient cooperation is essential because movement distorts the image of the lumen. The patient is examined in the supine position with the head slightly tilted to extend the neck. The examiner positions the Doppler transducer so that it approaches the flow stream at an angle of 45–60 degrees and adjusts the position-sensing box to obtain an oblique projection of the carotid bifurcation. This configuration usually separates the images of the external and internal carotid arteries adequately and avoids superimposing the two vessels. Depending on the patient's anatomy, however, other projections and angles of approach may be required to obtain a clear picture of the arterial lumen.

The examiner locates the flow signal and adjusts the depth of the ultra-sonic beam to position all six range gates within the arterial lumen. By moving the transducer along the surface of the neck, the examiner pro-duces a "flow map" while listening to and interpreting the audio signal. Periodic depth adjustments are made to keep the ultrasonic beam within the arterial lumen. Upon completion of the image, the intensity of the scope is increased and a line is drawn on the screen to denote the loca-tion of the mandible. This provides an anatomic reference for the image.

Spectral analysis of the Doppler audio signal is performed while the image is being produced, which helps the examiner to identify the ves-sels. After finishing the image, the examiner uses the audio output of channel three to study carefully the spectra of the common carotid, bi-furcation, and internal and external carotid arteries. By using the image, the depth-control switches, and the flow-indicating LEDs, the examiner positions this single channel in the center of the arterial lumen. A photo-graph of a spectrum from the internal carotid artery is taken approxi-mately 1 cm distal to the bifurcation or, if there is a region of suspected stenosis, at the area of highest frequency. Figure 22-1 diagrammatically illustrates the examination process.

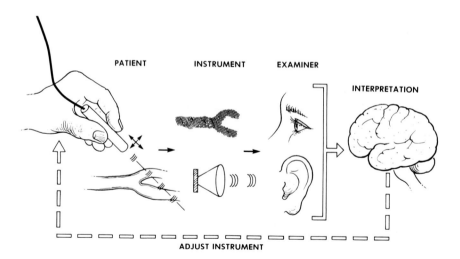

Figure 22-1. Diagrammatic representation of the examination process. The examiner receives audio and visual information that is used to adjust the instrument and to form a diagnostic impression.

270

INTERPRETATION

A typical, normal computerized image (Figure 22-2) shows the plan (or lateral) view of the common, internal, and external carotid arteries in the upper portion of the photograph. Cross sections of each vessel are shown above the plan view. The horizontal line represents the surface of the skin, and the depth view is produced below this. Because the internal and external carotid arteries are often oriented in the same plane, only the common carotid and internal carotid arteries are shown in the depth view to avoid superimposing the two vessels. Normal images show a smooth outline of the arterial lumen and are approximately the same size throughout the course of the artery. Normal audio signals help to confirm the absence of disease.

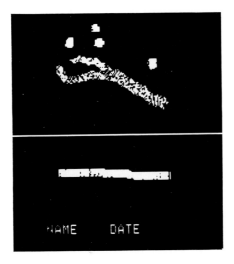

Figure 22-2. A normal computerized image. Lateral view and cross sections are placed above the horizontal line; depth (anterior-posterior) view appears below. The external carotid artery is not shown in the depth view. Reprinted with permission from Russell JB, Miles RD, Sumner DS: Computerized ultrasonic arteriography: a noninvasive technique for producing multiplanar images of the carotid bifurcation. Bruit 4 (September):27–29, 1980.

Normal spectra (Figure 22-3) are characterized by a peak systolic frequency of 2–3 kHz, a well-defined envelope of sound energy with most of it concentrated around the edge of the waveform, producing the "window" effect, and the absence of spectral broadening. Because this system

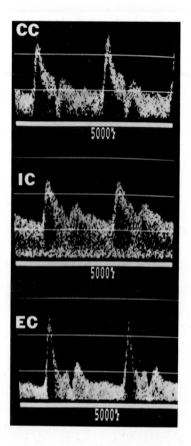

Figure 22-3. Normal spectra from the common carotid (*CC*), internal carotid (*IC*), and external carotid (*EC*) arteries obtained with the pulsed Doppler. The "window" and smooth profile typify normal spectra. Reprinted with permission from Russell JB, Miles RD, Sumner DS: Pulsed-Doppler ultrasonic arteriography with sound spectral analysis for evaluation of the carotid bifurcation. Bruit 6 (March):23–29, 1982.

employs a pulsed Doppler, the spectra vary somewhat from those obtained with a continuous-wave Doppler (Figure 22-4). With a pulsed Doppler, the window is much more pronounced since this instrument can sample from the central flow stream, where most of the red blood cells are traveling at nearly the maximum velocity. The presence of a window throughout systole has been a useful criterion for identifying normal arteries. However, care must be taken in positioning the sample volume because flow near the wall does not have the same pattern as flow in the center of the lumen.

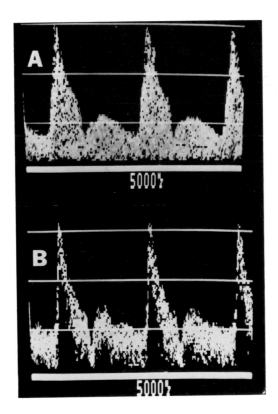

Figure 22-4. Normal spectra from the common carotid artery: (**A**) using a 5-MHz continuous-wave Doppler and (**B**) using a 5-MHz pulsed Doppler with the sample volume positioned in the central flow stream. Reprinted with permission from Russell JB, Miles RD, Sumner DS: Pulsed-Doppler ultrasonic arteriography with sound spectral analysis for evaluation of the carotid bifurcation. Bruit 6 (March):23–29, 1982.

Because of the limited resolution of the Doppler, the ultrasonic image may not show minor lesions (<20% diameter stenosis). These lesions are usually accompanied by minor disturbances of flow that in some cases may be detected audibly by the examiner and illustrated by the spectrum (Figure 22-5). Spectral patterns of minor lesions have nearly normal frequency characteristics with some disturbance of the pattern at peak systole and with spectral broadening during midsystole. Stenoses that reduce diameter by 20%–40% are usually demonstrated by changes in both image and audio frequency. In some cases, the narrowing may be

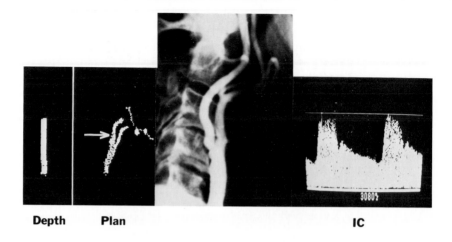

Depth   **Plan**   **IC**

Figure 22-5. Ultrasonic image and spectrum from the internal carotid artery. The image does not show the minor lesion, but the broad spectrum suggests flow disturbances and implies a minor stenosis. Reprinted with permission from Russell JB, Miles RD, Sumner DS: Pulsed-Doppler ultrasonic arteriography with sound spectral analysis for evaluation of the carotid bifurcation. Bruit 6 (March):23–29, 1982.

more apparent in one view than another (Figure 22-6). With more severe lesions, both techniques usually detect the disease. The image often shows distinct areas of narrowing, and in cases of very severe disease (>80% diameter stenosis) some regions may appear blank. (The strength of the reflected ultrasonic signal depends on the number of red blood cells scattering the sound energy. As flow is reduced, the number of moving RBCs decreases and the signal strength may fall below the threshold required for imaging.) Spectral patterns with elevated systolic and diastolic frequencies and with spectral broadening characterize more severe (>40% diameter reduction) lesions (Figure 22-7).

If internal carotid arterial flow signals are not detected, a diagnosis of occlusion is made (Figure 22-8). Usually, the pattern of audio signals from the external carotid artery has a low diastolic component, characteristic of the high distal impedance. Frequently, this pattern is also heard in the common carotid artery. When only a single vessel is detected distally, it is very important that the examiner search for the internal carotid at several depths and in other projection planes. This practice helps to prevent errors associated with tortuous or superimposed vessels.

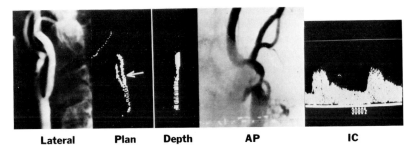

Lateral   **Plan**   **Depth**   **AP**   **IC**

Figure 22-6. A 50% internal carotid arterial stenosis most pronounced in the anterior-posterior angiographic view and in the ultrasonic depth view. The broad spectrum also suggests a carotid lesion. Reprinted with permission from Russell JB, Miles RD, Sumner DS: Pulsed-Doppler ultrasonic arteriography with sound spectral analysis for evaluation of the carotid bifurcation. Bruit 6 (March):23–29, 1982.

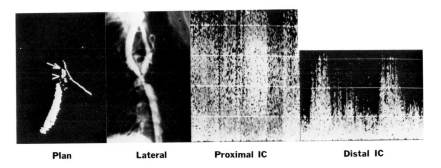

Plan   **Lateral**   **Proximal IC**   **Distal IC**

Figure 22-7. A severe internal carotid arterial lesion demonstrated on the ultrasonic image by the broken lumen. The spectrum from the proximal internal carotid artery (*first arrow*) reveals high-frequency components and is quite broad. The distal spectrum (*second arrow*) shows that flow is being reestablished but is still very disturbed. Reprinted with permission from Russell JB, Miles RD, Sumner DS: Pulsed-Doppler ultrasonic arteriography with sound spectral analysis for evaluation of the carotid bifurcation. Bruit 6 (March):23–29, 1982.

LIMITATIONS

The major limitations of ultrasonic arteriography are the subjective nature of the test and the need for an experienced examiner to perform the procedure. Several months of experience are usually required before an individual can correctly assess normal and abnormal flow signals and produce accurate images. Spectral analysis helps by providing hard-copy

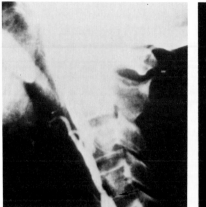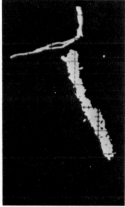

Figure 22-8. An internal carotid occlusion (*arrow:* bifurcation). On the ultrasonic image, the external carotid artery takes a more anterior course toward the mandible.

documentation of flow information, but it remains the responsibility of the examiner to position the transducer correctly in order to obtain unambiguous spectra.

Calcification of the arterial wall and anatomic variations also limit the ability of the ultrasonic arteriograph to diagnose disease clearly. In about 7% of patients, calcium deposits in the arteries block the passage of ultrasound and create blank regions on the image (Figure 22-9). Although

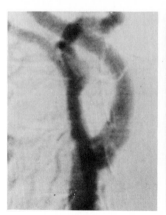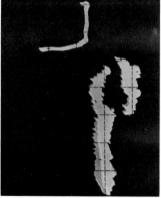

Figure 22-9. The ultrasonic arteriogram reveals a calcified region at the origin of the internal carotid artery. The flow signals distal to the blank area were normal, implying calcification rather than stenosis.

an analysis of the distal flow signal helps to determine the status of the artery in the blank or opaque zone, minor stenoses cannot be ruled out. Tortuous arteries and superimposed vessels may cause the examiner to miss the internal carotid artery or they may reflect a confusing signal and create an abnormal image (Figure 22-10). Most of these problems can be circumvented by repeating the examination from a different angle.

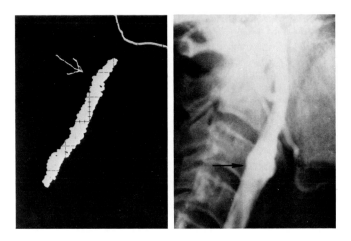

Figure 22-10. The internal and external carotid arteries are superimposed on the x-ray (*arrow:* bifurcation). On the ultrasonic image, only one vessel was detected distally. Flow signals were consistent with those of the external carotid artery, and a diagnosis of internal occlusion was made. This error could have been avoided if the examiner had searched for the internal carotid artery at a greater depth.

ACCURACY

A comparison of ultrasonic scans with standard contrast angiograms showed that the two examinations were significantly correlated ($P <$ 0.001), with an r value of 0.75. The linear regression line was UA % stenosis = (0.71 $\pm$ 0.04) x-ray % stenosis + (6.3 $\pm$ 2.0). Because the resolution of the ultrasonic arteriograph and measurement accuracy of the x-ray image are about 1 mm, and assuming a 5-mm lumen, any value within $\pm$20% of perfect correlation was felt to represent a fairly high degree of correspondence. We found that 81% of the ultrasonic scans and x-ray images agreed within $\pm$20%. Table 22-1 presents our results in

Table 22-1. Accuracy of Ultrasonic Arteriography[a, b]

Measure	>0%[c]	≥40%[c]
Sensitivity	77%	87%
Specificity	81%	91%
Positive predictive value	86%	82%
Negative predictive value	71%	93%

[a] Data from Sumner DS, Russell JB, Ramsey DE, et al: Noninvasive diagnosis of extracranial carotid arterial disease. Arch Surg 114: 1222–1229, 1979.

[b] N = 209 arteries.

[c] Diameter stenosis considered positive on ultrasonic arteriogram and x-ray.

detecting carotid arterial disease with the ultrasonic arteriograph in terms of sensitivity and specificity. (Not surprisingly, ultrasonic arteriography is most accurate for detecting more severe lesions.) These results were obtained prior to the addition of the spectral analyzer and before the computer interface.

Reports from other laboratories reveal great variability in the sensitivity and specificity at the 40%–50% criterion (Table 22-2). Although the median sensitivity at this level is 88%, the reported sensitivities range from 48% to 93%. There have been fewer reports on the accuracy of ultrasonic arteriography in detecting *any* disease, but, as Table 22-2 indicates, these results have shown more agreement.

Our initial results with the computerized ultrasonic arteriograph reveal improved sensitivity in detecting disease at both the >0% and

Table 22-2. Reported Accuracy of Pulsed-Doppler Imaging[a]

Measure	40%–50%[b]	>0[c]
Sensitivity[d]	88% (48%–93%)	75% (70%–77%)
Specificity[d]	85% (55%–92%)	81% (77%–88%)

[a] Data from Sumner DS: Noninvasive methods for preoperative assessment of carotid occlusive disease. Vasc Diagnosis Ther 2(4):41–56, 1981.

[b] Diameter stenosis considered positive on ultrasonic arteriogram and x-ray: six reports.

[c] Diameter stenosis considered positive on ultrasonic arteriogram and x-ray: three reports.

[d] Median (range).

$\geq 40\%$ criteria. Currently, new imaging programs are being implemented and results are being studied. Additional analyses will be required to determine the ultimate benefit of the new system.

As Chapter 20 indicates, spectral analysis has also shown promise for improving the sensitivity of the technique, particularly at the $\geq 40\%$ level. Recent work indicates that the sensitivity increased to 97% for the detection of lesions that reduce luminal diameter by at least 40%. Specificity, however, decreased to 65%. In our hands, spectral analysis has not improved results for the detection of mild disease ($> 0\%$), although this failure may be at least partly attributable to incorrect placement of the Doppler sample volume.

DISCUSSION

Ultrasonic arteriography is an accurate means of diagnosing carotid occlusive disease. It quite accurately detects stenoses that reduce luminal diameter by at least 40%. Unlike indirect methods, ultrasonic arteriography does not depend on reduced pressure or flow to detect abnormalities and is therefore capable of diagnosing minor lesions that may have clinical significance. Results in this area are quite respectable, and further refinements of both equipment and technique may improve its diagnostic accuracy.

It must be emphasized that ultrasonic arteriography requires a high level of technical expertise to be used accurately and that considerable experience may be required for a technician to obtain maximal results. It is our experience that most mistakes are attributable to errors of interpretation and procedure rather than to limitations of the equipment. We feel that it is essential for the technician and physician to review arteriograms jointly and to compare noninvasive and invasive results. Nevertheless, in the hands of a trained technician, pulsed-Doppler ultrasonic arteriography is a valuable diagnostic tool for the noninvasive vascular laboratory.

REFERENCES

1. Barnes RW, Bone GE, Reinerston J, et al: Noninvasive ultrasonic carotid angiography: prospective validation by contrast arteriography. Surgery 80:328–335, 1976.

2. Barnes RW, Nix ML, Rittgers SE: Audible interpretation of carotid Doppler signals. Arch Surg 116:1185–1189, 1981.

3. Blackshear WM, Phillips DJ, Chikos PM, et al: Carotid artery velocity patterns in normal and stenotic vessels. Stroke 11:67–71, 1980.

4. Blackshear WM, Phillips DJ, Thiele BL, et al: Detection of carotid occlusive disease by ultrasonic imaging and pulsed Doppler spectrum analysis. Surgery 86:698–706, 1979.

5. Hobson RW, Berry SM, Katocs AS, et al: Comparison of pulsed-Doppler and real-time B-mode echo arteriography for noninvasive imaging of the extracranial carotid arteries. Surgery 87:286–293, 1980.

6. Hokanson DE, Mozersky DJ, Sumner DS, et al: Ultrasonic arteriography: a new approach to arterial visualization. Biomed Eng 6:420, 1971.

7. Lewis RR, Beasley MG, Hyams DE, et al: Imaging the carotid bifurcation using continuous-wave Doppler-shift ultrasound and spectral analysis. Stroke 9:465–471, 1978.

8. Miles RD, Carlson DL, Russell JB, et al: Microcomputer aided three-dimensional ultrasonic imaging. Proc Annu Conf Eng Biol 32:135, 1979.

9. Mozersky DJ, Hokanson DE, Baker DW, et al: Ultrasonic arteriography. Arch Surg 103: 663–667, 1971.

10. O'Donnell TF, Pauker SG, Callow AD, et al: The relative value of carotid noninvasive testing as determined by receiver operator characteristic curves. Surgery 87:9–19, 1980.

11. Rittgers SE, Putney WW, Barnes RW: Real-time spectrum analysis and display of directional Doppler ultrasound blood velocity signals. IEEE Trans Biomed Eng 27:723–728, 1980.

12. Russell JB, Miles RD, Sumner DS: Computerized ultrasonic arteriography: a noninvasive technique for producing multiplanar images of the carotid bifurcation. Bruit 4 (September):27–29, 1980.

13. Russell JB, Miles RD, Sumner DS: Pulsed-Doppler ultrasonic arteriography with sound spectral analysis for evaluation of the carotid bifurcation. Bruit 6 (March):23–29, 1982.

14. Sumner DS: Noninvasive methods for preoperative assessment of carotid occlusive disease. Vasc Diagnosis Ther 2(4):41–56, 1981.

15. Sumner DS, Russell JB, Ramsey DE, et al: Noninvasive diagnosis of extracranial carotid arterial disease. Arch Surg 114:1222, 1979.

16. Wolf EA: Discussion of Sumner et al: Noninvasive diagnosis of extracranial carotid arterial disease. Arch Surg 114:1229, 1979.

CHAPTER 23

REAL-TIME B-MODE ULTRASONIC CAROTID IMAGING WITH GATED DOPPLER

Lorin P. McRae and Mark M. Kartchner

The use of high-resolution, real-time B-mode ultrasonic imaging in the evaluation of the cervical carotid arteries is an exciting and promising advance in the effort to reduce the disability and death caused by avoidable strokes. This technology has great potential (although there have been some extravagant and unwarranted claims), and the relatively expensive equipment is justified in the medium- to high-volume vascular laboratory. To achieve effective cost and risk benefits, though, it is important to recognize the capabilities and limitations of the technique, as well as the economic and motivational factors involved in considering its use.

Real-time ultrasonic imaging is not new in medicine. The challenge, rather, has been (and is) to achieve high resolution, broad gray scale, and minimum artifact in order to examine adequately the internal structure of arteries with atherosclerosis, stenosis, and ulcerations. Commercially available units have advanced to the point that they are very attractive as diagnostic instruments, but we hope for continued improvement toward the ideal unit. In the meantime, each potential user must evaluate the performance of the available ultrasonic imaging units and make decisions based on cost, performance, usage, and benefit factors, as they apply to a laboratory's particular situation.

BASIC CONCEPTS OF ULTRASONIC IMAGING AND DOPPLER

Chapter 16 contains a brief outline of Doppler physics. For a detailed account of Doppler physics, see Chapter 21. The following section reviews the physical phenomena of ultrasound, especially their role in clinical applications.

PHYSICAL PHENOMENA

Sound is the movement of waves of pressure through air, tissue, or other matter, similar to the movement of waves or ripples over the surface of water (Figure 23-1). A *cycle* is the positive and negative (up and down) variation from a designated point on one wave to the corresponding point on the next wave. *Frequency* is the number of waves or cycles passing a point of observation per unit of time. *Ultrasound* refers to high-frequency soundwaves above our hearing range, generally considered to be above 20,000 cycles per second (*hertz* or *Hz*). *Wavelength* is the spatial or linear

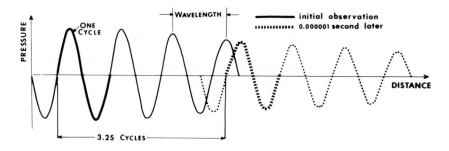

Figure 23-1. A four-cycle burst of a 3.25-MHz (3,250,000 cycles per second) sound wave as observed at two time intervals one millionth of a second apart.

distance between two corresponding points on the waveform, or the linear length of a single cycle. In a given medium, the product of the frequency and wavelength is a constant (the *propagation velocity* of the medium), so the higher the frequency, the shorter the wavelength.

When sound energy encounters junctions between two media (from skin to muscle to arterial wall to intima to blood, and so forth), some of it is reflected back toward the source (Figure 23-2A). The reflection is

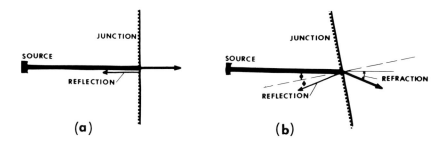

Figure 23-2. Reflection of sound at the junction of two media: **(a)** perpendicular incidence reflecting directly back to the source; **(b)** nonperpendicular incidence giving angled reflection and causing refraction of sound penetrating the junction.

directly back to the source only if the junction between the two media is exactly perpendicular to the direction in which the ultrasonic wave is moving. If the sound path is not perpendicular to the media junction, most of the reflected sound energy returns at an angle twice the deviation from perpendicular away from the source (Figure 23-2B). Furthermore, sound energy is refracted away from a straight course when it penetrates an oblique media junction. The extent and direction of the refraction depends on the propagation velocities of the two media and on the angle of incidence.

In order for a distinct medium or tissue to produce discernable reflections, it must have a length along the soundpath greater than the wavelength of the ultrasound. *Axial resolution* refers to the ability of an ultrasonic imaging system to distinguish between distinct, separate structures or tissues along the direction (axis) of ultrasonic beam propagation.

In addition to being reflected, ultrasonic waves are scattered or diffused by irregular surfaces and refracted or transmitted forward in a new direction at nonperpendicular interfaces. Eventually, all of the sound energy is absorbed by conversion to heat. Therapeutic ultrasound uses the conversion of ultrasonic energy to heat to elevate the temperature of deep tissue without noticeably heating the skin. In diagnostic ultrasonic imaging and Doppler evaluations, though, absorption of the ultrasonic energy is an undesirable but unavoidable side effect. Although the risk factors associated with this side effect appear negligible in light of the very low levels of ultrasonic energy used in diagnostic equipment, the long-term risks are unknown. It is advisable not to use more ultrasonic energy (time or intensity) than necessary in areas of sensitive nerves or tissue, such as the eye.

TECHNICAL CONSIDERATIONS

The technical factors involved in the use of an ultrasonic imaging system are a function of these physical phenomena. In order to achieve sufficient axial resolution, for instance, the ultrasonic frequency must be increased to reduce the wavelength. The higher the frequency, however, the greater the rate of energy absorbtion. This fact limits the extent of effective penetration that can be achieved with reflected energy sufficient enough to be detected and displayed as an echo or image. Ultrasonic energy is absorbed not only during its transmission to the tissue interface, but also during its reflection back to the receiving transducer. Also, a given irregularity of tissue interface scatters very short-wavelength ultrasound more than lower-frequency ultrasound. This scattering causes more diffusion of the high-frequency energy and greater potential for artifact.

Even good-quality ultrasonic units that use 3 MHz (3,000,000 Hz) or lower ultrasound for adult abdominal or heart imaging generally do not provide enough resolution to image the carotid arteries. As ultrasonic frequency is increased to provide axial resolution of less than 0.5 mm, a major problem is achieving penetration adequate enough to visualize arteries in heavier patients. That problem aside, tissue composition varies enough among individuals that a unit providing very good penetration to 4–5 cm in one patient may give only fair or poor visualization at 3 cm in another patient. Thus, to compare carotid imaging units, the potential user is wise to evaluate and compare the performance of the various units on two patients, one with good and one with poor penetration.

Lateral or *angular resolution* is related to the width of the ultrasonic beam at the depth of the tissue interface being displayed (Figure 23-3). The ultrasonic image does not reliably distinguish between structures whose lateral separation is less than the width of the beam at a given depth. Mechanical configuration of the ultrasound transducer crystal or reflecting mirrors and electronic techniques are used to focus the beam at a certain depth within the tissue. Ideally, a real-time B-mode imaging system would transmit an extremely thin beam at all depths to produce the theoretical razor-thin slice through the tissue. No system achieves this, however, and there is a tendency to pull tissue structure from outside the supposed plane of image and to display these artifacts as apparent tissue structure within the artery under examination. As an extreme example, the walls of adjacent veins are occasionally displayed as though they were located within the arterial lumen. A more common error connected with poor lateral resolution is a tendency to overestimate

284

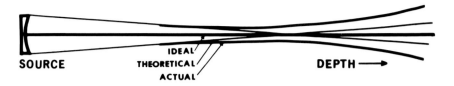

Figure 23-3. Width of ultrasonic beam varies with depth.

the severity of stenosis when reflective echoes from the outer edges of the ultrasonic beam appear as plaque in an area where blood is actually flowing (Figure 23-4). This limitation of lateral resolution is further illustrated when Doppler flow signals are obtained from what appears to be atherosclerotic plaque.

Some units use a gated pulsed-Doppler (see Chapters 16, 21, 22) to supplement the B-mode scan. With gated pulsed-Doppler, most of the aforementioned basics of ultrasound still apply, but its transmitted ultrasonic beam is held stationary in a single line rather than scanning back and forth in a plane, and the reflected signals sensed by the receiving crystal are electronically processed in terms of a shift in frequency rather than as intensity or brightness, as in B-mode. The Doppler shift is to a higher frequency when reflections originate from tissue or particles moving toward the sound source, and to a lower frequency for particles moving away from the sound source, as Chapter 21 explains in detail. The magnitude of the change in frequency is proportional to the vector component of velocity along the axis of the ultrasonic beam. Therefore,

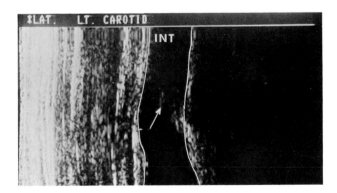

Figure 23-4. Apparent stenosis of an internal carotid artery in which there is no appreciable narrowing. A thin calcific plaque on the posterior wall reflects the edge of the ultrasonic beam and projects as though occupying a major portion of the arterial lumen.

Doppler responses depend on the angle between the directional flow of particles and the axis of the ultrasonic beam. By using short-duration pulses of ultrasound and by gating (activating) the receiver at specific time intervals, only energy reflected from a specified depth is processed. To minimize the depth range of response (axial length of the Doppler sample volume), the duration of the pulses must be minimized, which in turn reduces the quality of the Doppler response. On the other hand, increasing the duration of pulses to improve the quality of response also increases the uncertainty about the exact location of the blood flow that is creating the Doppler flow signal.

Depth of penetration becomes a matter of concern with Doppler ultrasound because only a small portion of transmitted ultrasonic energy is reflected back to the receiving transducer by the small moving particles. The rest is scattered. To compensate for the inefficient return of the Doppler signal, an ultrasonic signal of higher intensity usually is transmitted. The alternative is to use lower frequency for better penetration. The higher-energy approach increases the heating effect from energy absorption, while reduced frequency enlarges the sample volume because of reduced axial and lateral resolution. In either case, adequate Doppler signal samples do not come from a single point, but rather from a space larger than the smallest structure that can be visualized with the imaging echoes. Unless the examiner has specific information to the contrary for a given piece of equipment, the caution to avoid excessive ultrasound in sensitive areas is even more applicable to Doppler than to B-mode imaging.

CLINICAL EXPERIENCE

During the first 12 months of using ultrasonic carotid imaging (UCI), we performed 939 bilateral carotid image evaluations. Initially, the average technician time for performing the test was nearly one hour, with an additional half hour devoted to viewing the tapes and dictating reports. Those times have now been reduced to an average of 15–20 minutes for test performance and 10–15 minutes for interpretation.

RESULTS

Table 23-1 relates the severity of carotid disease found with UCI to patient age. Each patient is rated as to the most significant finding on either side of the neck. *Mild* indicates definite atherosclerotic plaque, but

Table 23-1. Severity of Carotid Pathology Found by Real-Time B-Mode Ultrasonic Carotid Imaging with Gated Doppler according to Age of 939 Patients

Age Group	Severity of Carotid Pathology						
	Negative	Mild	Questionable Ulceration	Moderate	Ulcerative Crater	Significant Stenosis	Total Occlusion
≤39	86	9	—	—	—	—	—
40–49	43	21	3	1	—	1	1
50–59	52	58	6	3	4	6	6
60–69	58	107	14	31	20	11	23
70–79	34	114	19	51	31	15	30
≥80	7	30	6	19	6	9	4

without irregularities that suggest ulceration and without significant stenotic intrusion into the arterial lumen. *Questionable ulceration* is characterized by irregularities or roughness of the plaque surface that suggests the possibility of underlying ulceration. No well-defined craters are seen. *Moderate* denotes either extensive atherosclerosis or localized stenosis that reduces the diameter of the arterial lumen by more than 50%, but which leaves a residual diameter of more than 2.5 mm, implying no significant alterations of flow or pressure. An *ulcerative crater* has at least one distinct depression in the ultrasonic image of the plaque or arterial lumen, strongly suggesting ulceration. A residual lumen less than 2.5 mm in diameter is considered a *significant stenosis. Total occlusion* means that no Doppler blood flow was detected in the distal internal carotid artery.

Patients under the age of 40 have a high incidence of negative UCI studies. Only 9% have mild atherosclerosis. In contrast, patients more than 80 years of age who are referred for noninvasive cerebrovascular evaluations have a low incidence of negative studies. Only 9% were free of atherosclerosis in the cervical carotid arteries. Among patients more than 50 years of age without lateralized neurologic symptoms, the mere presence of atherosclerosis appears to have little significance. A high-quality ultrasound image study that reveals no evidence of cervical carotid atherosclerosis or abnormality in patients with lateralized symptoms of transient ischemic attack should direct the physician's attention to other potential causes of the symptoms. If atherosclerosis is visualized, however, the failure to locate an ulcerative crater or significant stenoses certainly does not rule out emboli-producing carotid ulcerations.

UCI versus Arteriography

Arteriograms are available for comparison on 74 of the UCI patients. With the UCI equipment and techniques used, ultrasonic imaging probably does better than arteriography in demonstrating the presence and characteristics of mild or moderate atherosclerotic plaque in the cervical carotid arteries. However, in patients with hemodynamically significant stenosis (i.e., an effective lumen of 2.5 mm diameter or less), ultrasonic imaging is not as accurate in defining the severity of the stenosis. Among the 74 patients undergoing arteriography, six had luminal diameters smaller than 2.5 mm that were reported by UCI to be from 3 mm to 5 mm (oculoplethysmography correctly identified the five with a lumen of 2.0 mm or less). Nonreflecting soft atheroma or thrombus was the apparent cause of four of the six false-negative UCI findings. One error resulted from incorrect identification of the internal and external carotid arteries and the other was the result of a nonvisualized, more severe stenosis just distal to the one reported by UCI. There were also two false-positive UCI studies in evaluating hemodynamically significant stenosis. One was technical, a 3.5 mm lumen visualized as 2.0 mm because too much attention was paid to displaying the plaque as opposed to the lumen. The other false positive was an interpretive error caused by echo artifact from the bifurcation and by the external carotid appearing as soft internal carotid plaque. Following arteriography, the error became quite apparent on more careful examination of the taped UCI study.

The reliability with which either arteriography or UCI detects and evaluates carotid ulcerative disease is controversial. No definite ulcerations were reported by arteriography in carotid arteries found to be free of atherosclerosis by UCI. For four of 16 arteries with craters reported by UCI, there was no arteriographic confirmation of ulceration. The radiologist reported at least some arteriographic indication of carotid ulceration in approximately half of the remaining nonoccluded carotid arteries in which some atherosclerosis was reported by UCI without well-defined craters. A high-resolution ultrasonic imaging system can demonstrate some craters potentially associated with ulcerative disease, and the probability of clinically significant ulceration is proportional to the extent and roughness of the atherosclerosis visualized.

Besides the obvious advantage of being noninvasive, UCI with gated Doppler has several unique advantages over arteriography. These advantages also would apply to comparisons with computer-enhanced intravenous injection arteriography (see Chapter 7).

In three patients, UCI with gated Doppler demonstrated blood flow in patent internal and external carotid arteries in the presence of total occlusion of the common carotid artery. Also, the extent of atherosclerosis at the bifurcation could be well demonstrated. Arteriography, on the other hand, demonstrated total occlusion of the common carotid with no evidence of the patent internal and external carotid arteries.

The arteriograms of another patient were interpreted as showing occlusion at the origin of the internal carotid artery. Because of real-time UCI and Doppler demonstrations of proximal internal carotid artery patency with atypical blood flow, the patency was confirmed by reviewing the delayed arteriographic films.

UCI is often more revealing of the true extent of atherosclerosis than arteriography when there is a fairly normal-size lumen through an enlarged carotid bulb whose outside diameter is much larger than the more distal internal carotid artery. Arteriography demonstrates only the configuration of the present lumen and may not reasonably estimate the original lumen (Figure 23-5). As previously noted, however, arteriography provides a more reliable indication of both the true dimensions of the patent lumen and the hemodynamic significance of the stenosis. The clinical value of UCI's ability to demonstrate the extent of non-flow-reducing atherosclerotic disease is still to be determined.

In specific cases real-time B-mode UCI has demonstrated (1) strong vibrations of loose tissue or plaque within the carotid arterial lumen, (2) intimal dissection with minimal narrowing of the arterial lumen, (3) extrinsic compression causing indentations in the carotid arterial lumen, (4) fibromuscular hyperplasia near the internal carotid origin, and (5) aneurysmal dilation with excessive pulsatility.

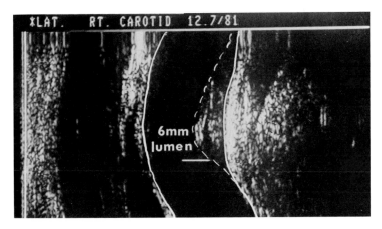

Figure 23-5. A large smooth atherosclerotic plaque with a residual lumen of 6 mm diameter is more impressive by ultrasound imaging than by arteriography.

It is not unusual for UCI to demonstrate soft atheroma covering older, more calcific plaque. In some cases of marked change in bruit or other noninvasive indications of rapidly progressing carotid occlusive disease, UCI shows calcific plaque apparently portruding farther into the arterial lumen because of nonreflecting hemorrhage beneath the original plaque. With ever-increasing improvements in the range of gray scale and the quality of resolution, we can anticipate significant new insight into the atherogenesis of carotid occlusive disease as UCI is used more for the long-term follow-up of and research into carotid occlusive disease and its relationship to strokes.

SELECTING EQUIPMENT

High-quality resolution with sufficient gray scale to differentiate between blood, soft plaque, and bright calcific plaque is a primary consideration in equipment selection. Also, high-quality resolution should provide good penetration to at least 4 cm and preferably more. One should not accept a demonstration showing only the common carotid artery, since this is relatively simple and straightforward compared to satisfactory visualization of the internal and external carotid arteries. Insist that any demonstration emphasize the visualization of the carotid bifurcation.

Do not be distracted from the search for quality resolution by claims emphasizing Doppler. If flow-related information and Doppler evaluation are the primary objective, one should invest in the less expensive Doppler imaging systems or even the well-proven, much less expensive indirect noninvasive techniques. Reasonable-quality gated Doppler, however, is essential for differentiating total occlusion from severe stenosis, and even in some cases for detecting total occlusion when very little atherosclerotic disease is visualized. In the stenotic arteries without occlusion, moving the gated Doppler across the lumen helps to differentiate artifact from echoes of real intraluminal material and helps to identify nonreflecting fresh atheroma or thrombus by the absence of blood flow in the vicinity of visualized plaque. Doppler further assists in the differentiation between the internal and external carotid arteries and helps to prevent following the jugular vein as an extension of the internal carotid artery, especially when the artery is excessively tortuous.

If a demonstration of the equipment can be arranged where selected patients can be examined, a patient with a fairly recent total occlusion of the internal carotid artery, one with a known severe stenosis, and one with a relatively large thick neck will provide a good challenge for most units.

A video recorder is recommended to provide a permanent record for the physician's review. We also recommend that a control tape be made after purchase of the equipment. Recordings should be taken from two or three control subjects who will be available for subsequent comparative recordings. These recordings should display the results with the various controls at several representative settings. Each time the equipment is adjusted or when there is a question of performance, a limited study can be performed on the control subjects and direct comparisons made. This practice enables one to establish a much more objective performance target than is otherwise possible.

TESTING

TECHNIQUE

We find a reclining dental-type chair with adjustable elevation and head-rest to be the most convenient for patient testing (Figure 23-6). Testing also can be performed with reasonable facility with the patient on a stretcher, examining table, or even seated in an ordinary chair.

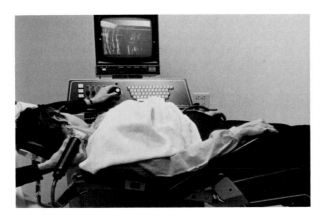

Figure 23-6. Testing procedure demonstrating use of adjustable reclining chair and ultrasonic imaging unit.

A quick cross-sectional or transverse projection starting at the base of the neck and moving up to just behind the angle of the jaw generally provides a good impression of the level and configuration of the bifurcation, as well as the general location and extent of disease. Doppler signals are obtained from the common, internal, and external carotid arteries during this transverse scan to confirm the patency and identity of the arteries.

The cervical carotid arteries are examined next with longitudinal views from anterior oblique, lateral, and posterior oblique projections. Upon noting atherosclerosis, the technician should rock slowly back and forth across the plaque to show the maximum extent of the disease. However, equal effort should be spent in attempting to show the residual lumen to its best advantage. It is often possible to show a plaque as creating nearly total occlusion even though the actual stenosis is minimal. This error can occur when the examiner approaches the arterial wall, concentrating on the plaque rather than on the lumen. Serious overinterpretation may result if the technician concentrates excessively on pathology without a balanced effort to show the maximum patent lumen at all levels (Figure 23-7).

Even though high-contrast settings often produce more attractive images, adequate gray scale must be maintained at all times to avoid overlooking soft atheroma (Figure 23-8). Also, gated pulsed-Doppler can be used to advantage on a real-time B-mode background to differentiate artifactual echoes from soft plaque. It is important to remember that Doppler signals may not be obtained from areas of ultrasonic shadowing even though blood flow is present. It is not always possible to get ade-

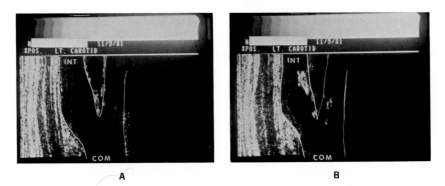

A   B

Figure 23-7. Slight rocking of the ultrasonic probe, concentrating on the lumen (**A**) and on the pathology (**B**) of the same carotid bifurcation with mild, nonstenotic atherosclerosis.

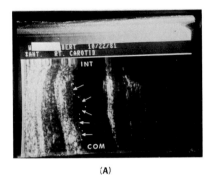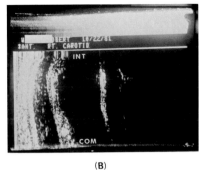

(A)   (B)

Figure 23-8. Very soft atherosclerotic plaque faintly seen but reasonably well delineated with broad gray scale (**A**) is obliterated by an excessive contrast adjustment with inadequate gray scale (**B**).

quate Doppler signals when moving the Doppler curser across an artery with extensive bright calcific plaque. One should in turn scan across the artery with the gated Doppler just proximal and just distal to hard plaques.

The technician can enhance the quality of the recorded test and minimize both technician and interpretive time by making a preliminary determination as to whether hemodynamically significant stenosis or emboli-producing ulcerations are the primary concern. Excessive use of the Doppler wastes time and detracts from a study when the patient is referred for focal lateralized symptoms; hemodynamic tests give no indication of flow reduction in the patient, and atherosclerosis with minimal arterial narrowing is observed. A priori judgment in such a case should direct the technician's attention to careful visualization of the plaque with concentration on any irregularities observed. Conversely, a question of total occlusion versus severe stenosis requires a much greater portion of the testing time for Doppler evaluation. Also, more Doppler time should be used to search for nonreflecting thrombus or soft atheroma in patients with positive noninvasive hemodynamic tests for whom the UCI image shows apparent lumen greater than 2.5 mm.

A continuous oral commentary from the technician is extremely important to the physician who reviews the UCI video tapes. The commentary should identify the location on the neck and the direction of any movement of the probe. When rocking over a plaque or stenotic lumen, or when searching for the branches of the carotid bifurcation, the technician should clarify each movement of the probe—medial, lateral, angle, and the like. Also, it is helpful for the commentary to note abnormalities observed by the technician.

INTERPRETATION

The same general factors should be kept in mind while interpreting the results as when performing the test. Additional caution should be exercised in attempting to identify craters as possible ulcerations. Dark spots or apparent ultrasonic shadows can be created by refraction or diverse angling of the ultrasonic waves. This is most easily demonstrated on a transverse projection with the side walls of the artery producing refractive as opposed to reflective shadows (Figure 23-9). A slight variation of this phenomenon often occurs at the distal and proximal ends of atherosclerotic plaques, tempting some to interpret these dark spots as ulcerative craters. In attempting to identify craters representing potential

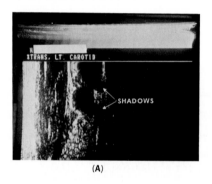 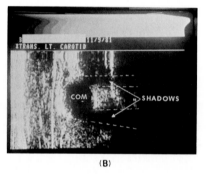

(A)   (B)

Figure 23-9. Ultrasonic shadows in the transverse projection from (**A**) refraction at the side walls of a common carotid artery of a young patient and (**B**) from both refraction and reflection in the presence of calcific plaque.

ulcerations as sources of emboli, one should be wary of dark areas that may arise from angled reflection and refraction at oblique surfaces (Figure 23-10A). An additional phenomenon, which can be readily misinterpreted as an ulcerative crater, is occasionally seen when there is hemorrhage or blood clot within an atherosclerotic plaque. The thin intima covering the distal end of a blood clot probably will not be visualized (Figure 23-10B). Generally, caution should be exercised in reporting nonreflective spaces at the extreme distal end of atherosclerotic plaques as ulcerative craters. If present, true ulcerative craters are more often visualized in the mid or proximal portion of the plaque.

In reporting UCI findings it is more meaningful to provide the dimensions of the residual patent lumen than the percentage stenosis. The limited UCI field of view seldom shows the effective outflow arterial diameter for comparison with the lumen through the stenosis. The extent of local dilatation about the carotid bifurcation varies so much among patients that a percentage of this exaggerated diameter has little meaning without an absolute dimension for reference.

Very bright echoes, as from calcific plaque, may result in an underestimation of the actual lumen size. On the other hand, with very soft, dull echoes, the actual lumen is often smaller than indicated. Also, with rapidly developing atherosclerosis or thrombotic stenosis, soft deposits within the arterial lumen often do not show on the B-mode image at all, falsely indicating an arterial lumen considerably larger than the effective blood flow visualized by arteriography. This is an inherent limitation of real-time B-mode UCI, but noninvasive hemodynamic studies can compensate for it.

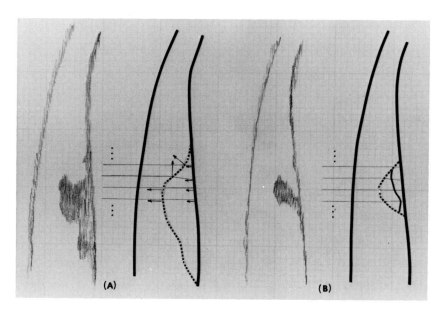

Figure 23-10. Illustration of the possibility of false crater images (**A**) created by angled reflections and refraction at the distal end of a plaque and (**B**) as a result of nonvisualization of intima over blood clot within an atherosclerotic plaque.

The Relative Role of UCI in the Noninvasive Cerebrovascular Laboratory

A common argument for expensive UCI equipment is that there is a need to detect those patients with less than 50% strenosis. Because 80% of the patients over 50 years of age show some degree of atherosclerosis in their cervical carotid arteries, it is not clear why there is an urgency to detect all patients with early extracranial carotid atherosclerosis. The primary objective of the noninvasive cerebrovascular laboratory should remain stroke prevention, not plaque detection.

For asymptomatic patients and patients with nonlateralizing neurologic symptoms, oculoplethysmography (OPG) and carotid phonoangiography (CPA) provide a very effective means of detecting those with significant risk of stroke.[1,2] As an effective hemodynamic noninvasive test for extracranial carotid occlusive disease, OPG also provides good screening for those patients scheduled for other major surgery who are at risk of perioperative strokes.[3-5] The reports of such screening with UCI and Doppler have not shown similar benefit, apparently because they are unable to evaluate adequately the functional significance of stenoses.[6,7] OPG/CPA, being much more time-efficient and less expensive than UCI, provides a convenient means of sequentially screening patients to determine those with active atherogenesis.[8] Very active atherogenesis producing changes noticeable by CPA may not be detected by UCI when the resulting atheroma or thrombus is not sufficiently organized to produce visible echoes. Also, the lumen often is not visualized well enough to determine progression in the presence of lumen tortuosity or shadows caused by extensive calcific plaque. Finally, UCI is not comfortably used on a fresh incision after carotid endarterectomy, but OPG reliably identifies patients with acute thrombotic occlusion.

UCI is considerably more effective than OPG/CPA for the patient with lateralized hemispheric neurologic symptoms suggestive of emboli. High-quality UCI presently stands alone among the many noninvasive tests for extracranial carotid occlusive disease in its ability to search for and reveal carotid ulcerations and atherosclerotic plaques that do not affect blood flow. Thus UCI, a structural test, and OPG/CPA, a functional test, do not duplicate and compete with each other, but rather are highly complementary tests.

In addition to testing patients with symptomatic, suspected ulcerative disease, real-time B-mode UCI with gated pulsed-Doppler complements OPG/CPA and Doppler studies in a number of other ways:

1. UCI with gated Doppler has been much more effective than Doppler alone in differentiating between ophthalmic artery stenosis, severe internal carotid stenosis, and total occlusion in the patient with marked ocular pulse delay and absence of a bruit representing tight stenosis.
2. UCI helps to clarify the extent of bilateral extracranial carotid occlusive disease in some patients for whom OPG/CPA is indeterminant.
3. UCI with Doppler helps to differentiate between progressing contralateral stenosis and development of ipsilateral collateral circulation in the presence of known occlusion of an internal carotid artery when the ocular pulses equalize.
4. UCI adds an element of confidence in following patients with asymptomatic carotid bruits but without significant reduction of internal carotid flow.
5. UCI helps to clarify unusual phenomena, such as variable pulse-to-pulse delays, clinically inappropriate positive or negative OPG results, chronic asymptomatic postoperative tests, and the like.

Real-time B-mode ultrasonic carotid imaging with gated Doppler has added an exciting and rewarding new dimension to our noninvasive vascular laboratory. Many noninvasive tests merely compete with one another, adding confidence to the results when in agreement, but forcing one to choose his champion when there is disagreement. UCI stands apart from the others, providing information about the patient's carotid disease not otherwise available and holding great promise for the future in our continued efforts to prevent stroke.

REFERENCES

1. Kartchner MM, McRae LP: Noninvasive evaluation and management of the asymptomatic carotid bruit. Surgery 82:840–847, 1977.
2. Kartchner MM, McRae LP: Guidelines for noninvasive evaluation of asymptomatic carotid bruit. Clin Neurosurg 28:418–428, 1981.
3. Kartchner MM, McRae LP: Carotid occlusive disease as a risk factor in major cardiovascular surgery. Arch Surg 117:1086–1088, 1982.
4. Diethrich EB, Reiling M, Ibrahim F, et al: Stroke screening prior to coronary artery bypass. Bull Tex Heart Inst 4:262–276, 1977.
5. Kartchner MM, McRae LP: The clinical use of oculoplethysmography and carotid phonoangiography. In *Diagnosis and Treatment of Carotid Artery Disease*. Edited by WH Baker. Mt Kisco, Futura, 1979, pp 55–81.

6. Breslau PJ, Fell G, Miller DW, et al: Incidence of carotid arterial disease in patients undergoing coronary artery bypass surgery. Sixth Joint Meeting on Stroke and Cerebral Circulation, Los Angeles, 1981.

7. Barnes RW, Liebman PR, Marszalek PB: The natural history of symptomatic carotid disease in patients undergoing cardiovascular surgery. Surgery 90:1075–1083, 1981.

8. Kartchner MM, McRae LP: Noninvasive assessment of the progression of the extra-cranial carotid occlusive disease. In *Noninvasive Cardiovascular Diagnosis: Current Concepts.* Edited by EB Diethrich. Baltimore, University Park Press, 1978, pp 213–218.

CHAPTER 24

THE PREDICTIVE
VALUE OF
CEREBROVASCULAR STUDIES

Falls B. Hershey, Arthur I. Auer, H. Bradley Binnington,
Joseph J. Hurley, and Dennistoun K. Brown

The main purpose of noninvasive cerebrovascular studies is to find correctable lesions in the carotid arteries and to help prevent strokes. We hope to detect carotid stenosis and its location, and to estimate its severity in order to help plan the treatment. When the referring physician inquires, ''How bad is the stenosis?'' he also would like to know how accurate we are. *Accuracy* is easy to calculate, of course:

$$\frac{\text{number of correct diagnoses}}{\text{total number of tests}} = \text{accuracy}$$

We also can calculate the *sensitivity* of cerebrovascular studies—their ability to detect desease:

$$\frac{\text{number of true positive tests}}{\text{number of all positive diagnoses (i.e., true } \oplus + \text{ false } \ominus \text{ tests)}} = \text{sensitivity}$$

And by calculating the *specificity* of these studies, we gain yet another measure of their worth, in this case their ability to exclude disease and to detect normality:

$$\frac{\text{number of true negative tests}}{\text{number of negative diagnoses (true } \ominus + \text{ false } \oplus \text{ tests)}} = \text{specificity}$$

The best, most practical reply to such an inquiry does not involve accuracy, sensitivity, or specificity, but rather the predictive value of the test—i.e., how often its prediction is correct. The positive predictive value, sometimes defined as the true positive fraction, is the percentage of correct predictions, the number of true positives divided by all positive diagnoses. A similar calculation expresses the negative predictive value.

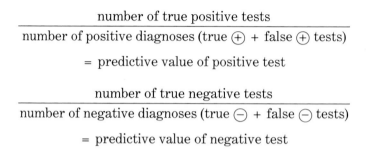

$$\frac{\text{number of true positive tests}}{\text{number of positive diagnoses (true } \oplus + \text{ false } \oplus \text{ tests)}}$$

$$= \text{predictive value of positive test}$$

$$\frac{\text{number of true negative tests}}{\text{number of negative diagnoses (true } \ominus + \text{ false } \ominus \text{ tests)}}$$

$$= \text{predictive value of negative test}$$

The referring physician understands these predictive values more readily than sensitivity and specificity.

The primary message of this chapter is that a combination of conflicting test results may be interpreted more accurately by use of the Bayes theorem. Interpretation is easy when all tests agree, but when the results conflict it is difficult to know which tests to trust. Each test has its strengths and weaknesses for different degrees of stenosis. The Bayes theorem permits us to calculate the likelihood of disease when faced with various combinations of positive and negative noninvasive tests. Formerly, our interpretation was a hopeful, possibly enlightened hunch about the conflicting results. Now, with the Bayes theorem, the guiding principle is always to avoid unnecessary arteriograms and not to overread the tests.

ANALYZING EARLY DATA

We began in 1977 with carotid phonoangiography[1] and oculoplethysmography,[2] both of which are the subjects of Chapter 17. Later we introduced the periorbital cerebrovascular Doppler examination (PO CDE), which, as Chapter 18 explains, involves directional Doppler interrogation of the supraorbital and frontal arteries to detect the reversal of the flow from the orbit that may occur in severe stenosis or total occlusion. We began also to listen to the effects of compression of the various sources of collateral circulation via these branches of the external carotid artery. Hard-copy documentation became possible when we added supraorbital photoplethysmography (SO PPG), enabling us to obtain tracings of the collateral compression effects (Chapter 18). On the whole we did well, and by September 1979 there were only three patients who had unnecessary arteriograms, solely on the basis of laboratory errors. There were more than three errors, of course, but the other errors caused no serious harm because the arteriograms were already necessitated by TIAs or other indications, or because a severe stenosis had been diagnosed correctly on the other side of the neck. As Tables 24-1 and 24-2 indicate, our

Table 24-1. Accuracy, Sensitivity, Specificity, and Predictive Values of Noninvasive Diagnosis of Critical Carotid Stenosis: The Early Experience at St. John's Mercy Medical Center[a]

Measure	Calculation	Value (%)
Accuracy	number correct/total	88
Sensitivity	true positive/total positive	78
Specificity	true negative/total negative	92
Positive predictive value	true positive diagnoses/total positive diagnoses	77
Negative predictive value	true negative diagnoses/total negative diagnoses	89

[a] From July 1, 1977, to December 31, 1979, 1,595 patients were examined, 249 arteriograms were performed, and 396 arteries were scored. There were 371 correct and 49 incorrect diagnoses. Critical stenosis ≥ 50%.

Table 24-2. Accuracy, Sensitivity, and Specificity of Noninvasive Cerebrovascular Examinations from January 1, 1980, to June 30, 1980[a]

Study	Accuracy (%)	Sensitivity (%)	Specificity (%)
Carotid phonoangiography	82.1	54.1	97.1
Oculoplethysmography	84.6	66.7	91.4
Directional Doppler			
Reversal	82.2	51.3	100.0
Compression	84.1	71.1	91.3
Photoplethysmography	78.4	47.9	84.4
Combined interpretation	86.9	86.5	87.1

[a] Fifty-five arteriograms were performed, and 107 carotid arteries were suitable for scoring.

early results were not as sensitive or specific as the best reports in the literature, but neither were they the worst.

Figure 24-1 compares the blood flow laboratory's final interpretations with the arteriographic measurements. Internal carotid arteries were classified as normal, mild, moderate, severe, or either nearly or completely occluded. A positive test was 50% stenosis of the internal carotid artery measured after the manner of Kartchner and McRae (see Chapter 17), namely the ratio of the narrowest part of the stenosis to the diameter of the uniform cylindrical internal carotid artery in its middle portion.[2] Most errors occurred in cases of moderate stenoses (column C). Our interpretations of normal and severe cases were very accurate, as are those from other laboratories. If the threshold for positive tests were moved to the right to include only columns D and E—i.e., the severely stenotic and nearly or completely occluded arteries—accuracy would improve markedly, but this manipulation would not improve reality. The problem remains, and all of us are searching for better methods of detecting the moderate stenoses that do not cause the hemodynamic changes or audible murmurs on which we now rely (see Chapters 19, 20, and 22).

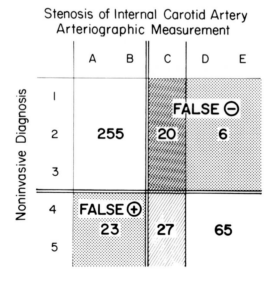

Figure 24-1. Matrix comparing arteriographic diagnosis (*abscissa*) of internal carotid artery stenosis and the final combined interpretation of the noninvasive tests (*ordinate*). *Key to arteriographic ratings: A* and *1,* normal; *B* and *2,* mild; *C* and *3,* moderate (50%–75% stenosis; *D* and *4,* severe; *E* and *5,* nearly or completely occluded. Threshold for true positive is *C* and/or *3* (i.e., 50% stenosis).

Which tests are the most reliable, then, and for which degree of stenosis? Figure 24-2 compares the accuracy of OPG/CPA, PO CDE, and SO PPG, and that of the combined final interpretation for each level of arteriographic stenosis. (Later data will separate the OPG and CPA interpretations.) It is evident that these methods often overlook moderate (50%) stenosis. Further, our SO PPG examination was not very satisfactory even for severe stenoses. The PO CDE produced a number of false positives, even in cases of normal and mild stenosis, but this was the result of inexperience and in the next six months the PO CDE score improved markedly. The results of OPG/CPA and our final diagnoses were highly accurate in cases of normal, mild, and severe stenosis.

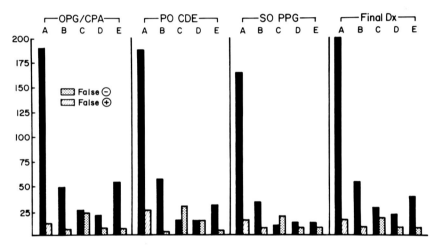

Figure 24-2. Comparison of the accuracies of various noninvasive examinations in cases of "critical" stenosis of the carotid artery. *Final diagnosis:* interpretation of all noninvasive results. *Ordinate:* number of cases. *Each pair of columns:* number of correct and incorrect diagnoses. True negative <50% stenosis; true positive ≥50% stenosis. See legend to Figure 24-1 for key to arteriographic ratings of stenosis.

ANALYZING LATER DATA

Accuracy improved somewhat during the next six months. As Table 24-2 indicates, though, none of the tests were as sensitive as the combined interpretation. CPA was very helpful when it was positive, but the OPG with a negative CPA was only 67% sensitive. PO CDE examinations were helpful. The compression tests were more sensitive than in the previous two years and were positive in some cases that did not demonstrate reversal in the frontal arteries. Reversal was noted in only 51% of the critical 50% stenoses, but happily there were no falsely positive reversals during this series. SO PPG showed poor sensitivity and specificity, appeared to offer nothing additional, and therefore was abandoned. The sensitivity of our combined interpretation improved from the 78% of our first series to 86.5%. A glance at the predictive values of these tests (Table 24-3) is very revealing. When the CPA was positive, it was very helpful, as was OPG. Both had improved since the previous report. Experience also increased the predictive values of the PO CDE, but of course the 100% predictive value for reversal will drop slightly when we inevitably have a false positive.

Table 24-3. Predictive Values of Noninvasive Cerebrovascular Studies from January 1, 1980, to June 30, 1980[a]

Study	Positive Predictive Value (%)	Negative Predictive Value (%)
Carotid phonoangiography	90.9	79.8
Oculoplethysmography	85.7	84.2
Periorbital directional Doppler		
Reversal	100.0	78.2
Compression	81.8	85.1
Supraorbital photoplethysmography	37.7	89.1
Combined interpretation	78.0	87.1

[a] Fifty-five arteriograms were performed, and 107 internal carotid arteries were suitable for scoring.

USING THE BAYES THEOREM

Bayes theorem calculations can help to determine the likelihood of stenosis $\geq 50\%$ when the battery of tests is a mixture of positive and negative results.[3,4] We must know the specificities and sensitivities of the individual tests, and we must know the "mix," i.e., the percentage of disease in the population examined. For our purposes, disease was defined as stenosis $\geq 50\%$, and we assumed that the patients referred to the laboratory were the same types as those in our first series.

According to the following formula, the positive or negative results of the various tests can be expressed as the "likelihood" that the patient has or does not have a critical stenosis. Using a positive result from the first test L_x, for instance,

$$L_x^+ = \frac{(L_{x-1})\,(S_n)}{(L_{x-1})\,(S_n) + (1 - L_{x-1})\,(1 - S_p)}$$

where L_{x-1} = pretest likelihood of critical stenosis of the internal carotid artery, L_x = posttest likelihood of critical stenosis, S_n = sensitivity of test X, and S_p = specificity of a given test, we can calculate the pretest likelihood of disease and then use this value in the formula to calculate the posttest likelihood of disease for each subsequent test.[4]

The pretest likelihood for our total group was 0.06. The likelihood of disease in the case of a positive CPA diagnosis was 0.41, and this value became the pretest likelihood of disease for the OPG. In the case of a positive OPG, the likelihood of disease was 0.86, while that for a negative OPG with positive CPA was 0.27.

Figure 24-3 presents a flow chart of the results of our five steps of Bayes theorem calculations. The sequence of such calculations does not affect the results; any sequence will yield the same value for likelihood in the final interpretation. No calculations are needed when all the tests are positive or negative because the interpretation is clear.

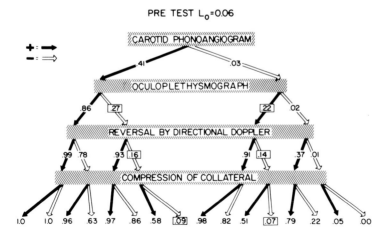

Figure 24-3. Flow chart of Bayes theorem calculations of likelihood of critical ($\geq 50\%$ stenosis) of the internal carotid artery for patients with various combinations of positive and negative tests. See text for details.

These Bayes theorem calculations revealed that the last step, the SO PPG examination, offered no additional accuracy, and so it is no longer performed in our laboratory. Our good luck with the PO CDE reversal is somewhat unusual and probably cannot be sustained. For the present calculation, though, reversal of the directional Doppler by itself is sufficient to prove critical stenosis of the internal carotid artery. One must remember, however, that there are many false negatives for this test, and so nonreversal does not score heavily against critical stenosis. Note the influence of a positive compression test even when there is no reversal.

The Bayes theorem formulas can be set up and calculated for all possible combinations of positive and negative tests. The table of likelihoods calculated in this fashion for each patient can be helpful for future interpretations and can be revised at intervals.

Recalling Figures 24-1 and 24-2, however, we still need more accurate tests for moderate stenosis. The direct Doppler examination of the carotid bifurcation is promising in this respect (see Chapter 19). Even with our ordinary continuous-wave Dopplers, the direct Doppler examination reveals turbulence and increased velocity in cases of mild and moderate stenosis (Table 24-4). This is also true for spectral analysis (AngioScan, Unigon Industries, Inc., Mt. Vernon, New York) of the continuous-wave

Table 24-4. Sensitivity, Specificity, and Predictive Values of Direct Doppler/AngioScan Diagnosis of Critical Stenosis of the Internal Carotid Artery[a]

Measure	Value (%)
Sensitivity	94.70
Specificity	88.65
Positive predictive value	78.00
Negative predictive value	97.00

[a] A comparison of the results of the direct Doppler/ AngioScan examination with those of arteriography revealed that 102 of 105 negative results and 54 of 69 positive results were confirmed arteriographically.

Doppler (Figure 24-4) (see Chapter 20). The falsely positive results of the AngioScan are attributable to both inexperience and misinterpretation of stenoses of the external and internal carotid arteries. False negatives occur when the external carotid carries collateral flow to the brain and has considerable diastolic flow that mimics the internal carotid artery. The scanning by the ultrasonic arteriograph (D.E. Hokanson, Inc., Issaquah, Washington), as noted in Chapter 22, may be helpful in this distinction, and in the diagnosis of total occlusion of the internal carotid artery.

Arteriographic Stenosis

		N	B	C	D	E total	
(102)	N	62	25	0	0	0	(3)
	A	5	10	2	1	0	
	B	1	8	6	2	1	
(15)	C	1	2	7	23	1	(54)
	D	3	0	0	7	7	

Angioscan Results

Figure 24-4. Matrix comparing arteriographic (*abscissa*) and AngioScan (*ordinate*) diagnosis of internal carotid artery stenosis.

CONCLUSIONS

The predictive value of a positive or negative interpretation is the most satisfactory expression of the accuracy of noninvasive cerebrovascular examinations for the referring physician.

When a series of laboratory tests gives conflicting values, the likelihood of disease for a particular combination of positive and negative tests may be calculated by use of the Bayes theorem.

Direct Doppler examination, coupled with spectral analysis, offers more accurate diagnosis of moderate stenoses ($\leq 50\%$) of the internal carotid arteries.

REFERENCES

1. Kartchner MM, McRae LP: Auscultation for carotid bruits in cerebrovascular insufficiency. JAMA 210:494–497, 1969.
2. Kartchner MM, McRae LP, Morrison ED: Noninvasive detection and evaluation of carotid occlusive disease. Arch Surg 106:528–535, 1973.
3. Needham TN, Levien L, Nicolaides A: Improving predictive value by combining complementary tests: an application to the diagnosis of carotid disease. Bruit 5 (June):14–16, 1981.
4. Nicolaides AN, Needham TN: Carotid phonoangiography combined with Doppler ultrasound examination. In *Investigation of Vascular Disorders*. Edited by AN Nicolaides, JST Yao. London, Churchill Livingstone, 1981, pp 221–218.

CHAPTER **25**

PREOPERATIVE SCREENING
FOR ASYMPTOMATIC
CAROTID OBSTRUCTION

Robert W. Barnes and Phyllis B. Marszalek

The role of prophylactic carotid endarterectomy for asymptomatic carotid occlusive disease is controversial. There are three categories of patients with asymptomatic carotid disease, those with (1) isolated carotid bruit, (2) asymptomatic carotid disease contralateral to a symptomatic lesion, and (3) asymptomatic carotid disease in the preoperative patient. Asymptomatic carotid disease is usually detected by the presence of an audible bruit from the carotid artery or by incidental discovery on a cerebrovascular arteriogram. During the past decade noninvasive diagnostic techniques have played an increasingly important role in detecting asymptomatic carotid occlusive disease. This chapter reviews the results of a prospective screening study designed to detect asymptomatic carotid disease in patients undergoing coronary artery bypass or major peripheral arterial reconstruction.

Supported by an NIH grant No. 5-21075. An earlier report of this series appeared in Stroke 12:497–500, 1981, and a modified version appears in Diethrich EB (ed): *Noninvasive Assessment of the Cardiovascular System: Diagnostic Principles and Techniques.* Littleton, MA, John Wright/PSG, 1982, pp 53–60.

PATIENTS AND METHODS

PATIENTS

Between March 1979 and December 1980, 452 patients undergoing coronary artery bypass or peripheral arterial reconstruction at the Medical College of Virginia or the Richmond Veterans Administration Medical Center were prospectively screened for asymptomatic carotid occlusive disease. There were 384 men and 68 women who ranged in age from 33 to 90 years, with a mean age of 58 years. The indications for operation were coronary artery disease in 325 patients and peripheral arterial occlusive disease in 127 patients. Hypertension was evident in 189, previous myocardial infarction in 181, and diabetes mellitus in 79 individuals. Patients with a prior history of transient ischemic attack or previous carotid endarterectomy were excluded from this study.

DIAGNOSTIC METHODS AND FINDINGS

All patients were evaluated by one experienced noninvasive vascular technologist. The presence of a cervical bruit recorded by the admitting physician was documented. All patients underwent a periorbital Doppler cerebrovascular examination,[1] as well as direct interrogation of the carotid artery and bifurcation with a bidirectional Doppler ultrasonic velocity detector (Model D9, Medasonics, Inc., Mountain View, California).[2] Normally, the periorbital examination revealed antegrade ophthalmic arterial flow that was not affected by compressing the branches of the external carotid artery. In the presence of significant obstruction of the extracranial internal carotid artery, periorbital ophthalmic arterial flow was often reversed and attenuated by compressing the branch of the external carotid artery that supplied collateral circulation to the orbit. The normal direct carotid arterial velocity signal was smooth and pulsatile, with high flow velocity in the internal carotid artery and lower multiphasic flow velocity in the external carotid artery. The common carotid signal had auditory characteristics intermediate between the flow characteristics of its two branches. Carotid stenosis was characterized by increased flow velocity at the site of stenosis and by an abnormal turbulent flow signal distal to the stenosis. Occlusion of the carotid artery was manifested by the absence of a detectable flow signal at the expected location.

DATA ANALYSIS

The variables of interest in this study included the presence of audible cervical bruit and the presence of asymptomatic carotid obstruction manifested by an abnormal periorbital and/or direct carotid arterial flow velocity signal. All patients were assessed for perioperative neurologic deficits, including transient ischemic attack or stroke, occuring within 30 days of operation. All perioperative deaths and their causes were recorded. In addition, patients were followed during the late postoperative period for both neurologic deficits and late deaths.

RESULTS

ASYMPTOMATIC CAROTID BRUIT

Among the 452 patients, cervical bruits were heard in 63 arteries of 44 patients (9.7%). Bruits were significantly more prevalent among patients with peripheral vascular disease (18.1%) than in patients with coronary artery disease (6.5%, $P < 0.005$). Of the 63 arteries with bruit, only 25 (39.7%) were associated with significant carotid obstruction, as manifested by an abnormal noninvasive screening study.

CAROTID OBSTRUCTION

Significant carotid obstruction was present by noninvasive techniques in 87 arteries of 64 patients (14.2%). The prevalence of carotid obstruction was somewhat higher in patients with peripheral vascular disease (18.1%) than in patients with coronary artery disease (12.6%). A cervical bruit was present in only 25 (28.7%) of the 87 arteries with significant obstruction.

PERIOPERATIVE NEUROLOGIC DEFICIT

A neurologic deficit occured in six patients within 30 days of operation. In five of these six patients, neither a cervical bruit nor carotid obstruction was present. In one patient a stroke developed two weeks after a peripheral vascular procedure on the side of a carotid bruit, but the vessel was not significantly obstructed according to noninvasive Doppler testing. No patient with hemodynamically significant carotid occlusive disease suffered a perioperative neurologic deficit.

PERIOPERATIVE DEATHS

There were seven deaths (1.5%) within 30 days of operation. Six of the seven deaths occured in patients with hemodynamically significant carotid occlusive disease. The remaining patient who died had a carotid bruit. Thus, all patients who died during the perioperative period had some evidence of carotid disease. The incidence of death among patients with significant carotid obstruction (9.3%) was substantially higher than that among patients without significant carotid occlusive disease (0.3%, $P < 0.005$).

LATE NEUROLOGIC DEFICITS

Although the patients with significant carotid obstruction suffered no perioperative neurologic deficits, three of them did experience late episodes of transient ischemic attack. No patient has suffered neurologic deficit.

DISCUSSION

Asymptomatic carotid artery disease is usually detected by the presence of a cervical bruit. Unfortunately, cervical bruits are a nonspecific guide to hemodynamically significant obstruction of the extracranial internal carotid artery.[3] Many cervical bruits arise from the subclavian artery, the common carotid artery, or the great vessels within the thorax. Such lesions are considered less likely to cause stroke than lesions causing bruits at the carotid bifurcation, but bruits at the carotid bifurcation do not necessarily denote significant obstruction of the internal carotid artery. Some bruits may arise from the external carotid artery, and many carotid bruits are not associated with flow-reducing lesions as manifested by abnormal noninvasive diagnostic screening. Furthermore, many patients with severe stenosis of the carotid artery or occlusion of the internal carotid artery may not have a cervical bruit. So it is more appropriate to identify patients with extracranial carotid atherosclerosis as individuals with asymptomatic carotid disease, rather than as individuals with asymptomatic carotid bruit.

The prognosis of patients with asymptomatic carotid bruit is incompletely understood. Thompson et al. suggested that such patients suffer a 17% incidence of future stroke and that 27% develop subsequent transient ischemic attacks.[4] Several other authors have reported a subsequent stroke rate of 14%–19% following identification of an asymptomatic carotid bruit.[5-7] Unfortunately, the incidence of stroke without antecedent transient ischemic attack is not clearly defined. Kartchner and McRae reported a stroke rate of 11.9% in patients with asymptomatic carotid bruit who had an abnormal ocular plethysmographic examination, compared to 1.9% in patients with a normal noninvasive study.[8]

The reported risk of prophylactic carotid endarterectomy for asymptomatic carotid bruit includes a stroke rate of about 1.5% and a mortality rate of about 0.5%.[4,9,10] In four separate studies of nonoperative follow-up of angiographically proven asymptomatic carotid artery disease contralateral to symptomatic lesions, the subsequent stroke rate without antecedent transient ischemic attacks was less than 1%.[11-14] The incidence of perioperative stroke among patients undergoing concomitant vascular surgery was 0.8% in 1,032 patients.[15-17] Although carotid bruits were noted in 16% of patients, no patient with a bruit suffered a perioperative stroke. These results compare favorably with reported series of combined prophylactic carotid endarterectomy and cardiovascular operations in which the stroke rate was 1.8%.[18-22] These data raised questions about the validity of performing prophylactic carotid endarterectomy, particularly in patients undergoing major cardiovascular operations.

The present study fails to support the correlation of perioperative stroke and detectable asymptomatic carotid occlusive disease. Indeed, no patient with an abnormal carotid screening study suffered a perioperative stroke. All neurologic deficits were in patients who had no significant carotid obstruction, and only one of the six deficits occurred in a patient with an asymptomatic carotid bruit. Nevertheless, the incidence of perioperative myocardial infarction and death among patients with detectable carotid disease was significantly higher than that among patients who had no carotid obstruction. Furthermore, during the late follow-up period there was a significant incidence of late neurologic deficits among patients with detectable obstruction of the carotid artery. Fortunately, all deficits have presented as transient ischemic attacks, and no patient has suffered a permanent neurologic deficit during the follow-up period.

Our results are similar to those reported by Turnipseed et al., who could not document a correlation between carotid occlusive disease detectable by noninvasive technique and perioperative stroke.[23] Breslau and coworkers have reported a similar lack of correlation of detectable carotid disease and perioperative stroke in patients undergoing coronary artery bypass.[24]

One may question the appropriate role of noninvasive screening techniques in patients with asymptomatic carotid occlusive disease. We feel that noninvasive detection of hemodynamically significant carotid obstruction does identify patients who may be at future risk of transient ischemic attacks. Such patients should be closely followed and appropriately educated about the symptoms of transient cerebral ischemia, which should alert them to seek immediate medical attention. Once symptoms of transient ischemia develop, prompt arteriography and appropriate surgical or medical management should be undertaken. The detection of asymptomatic carotid occlusive disease should not, however, lead to prophylactic carotid endarterectomy prior to necessary major cardiovascular procedures. Noninvasive techniques also may be valuable in identifying the integrity of the collateral cerebral circulation via the circle of Willis.[25] In patients with significant carotid obstruction and inadequate collateral circulation, prophylactic carotid endarterectomy might be considered, but longitudinal follow-up of such patients must define the natural history of their asymptomatic disease to determine whether or not the risk of nonoperative management exceeds the risk of prophylactic endarterectomy.

CONCLUSIONS

This study suggests that asymptomatic carotid occlusive disease is common among patients undergoing coronary artery bypass or major peripheral arterial reconstruction, but it also indicates that asymptomatic carotid bruit does not correlate well with significant obstruction of the extracranial internal carotid artery. Conversely, the majority of patients with hemodynamically significant carotid stenosis do not have an audible cervical bruit. Our prospective study failed to document any correlation between detectable carotid obstruction and perioperative neurologic deficits, although it did reveal a significant correlation between detectable carotid disease and perioperative myocardial infarction and death. Furthermore, patients with significant carotid obstruction had an increased incidence of transient ischemic attack during the follow-up period. This study suggests that noninvasive diagnostic techniques are useful in identifying patients who may be at risk of future transient ischemic attack. It failed to support the common practice of prophylactic carotid endarterectomy prior to major cardiovascular operation, however.

REFERENCES

1. Barnes RW, Russell HE, Bone GE, et al: Doppler cerebrovascular examination; improved results with refinements in technique. Stroke 8:468–471, 1977.

2. Rittgers SE, Barnes RW: *Doppler Ultrasonic Evaluation of Carotid Velocity Signals: An Audio Instruction.* Richmond, The Medical College of Virginia Commonwealth University, 1980, p 37.

3. Barnes RW: Noninvasive evaluation of the carotid bruit. Annu Rev Med 31:201–218, 1980.

4. Thompson JE, Patman RD, Talkington CM: Asymptomatic carotid bruit: long-term outcome of patients having endarterectomy compared with unoperated controls. Ann Surg 188:308–316, 1978.

5. Coopermen M, Martin EW, Evans WE: Significance of asymptomatic carotid bruits. Arch Surg 113:1339–1340, 1978.

6. Dorazio RA, Ezzet F, Nesbitt NJ: Long-term follow up of asymptomatic carotid bruits. Am J Surg 140:212–213, 1980.

7. Heyman A, Wilkinson WE, Heyden S, et al: Risk of stroke in asymptomatic persons with cervical arterial bruits: a population study in Evans County, Georgia. N Engl J Med 302:838–841, 1980.

8. Kartchner MM, McRae LP: Noninvasive evaluation and management of the "asymptomatic" carotid bruit. Surgery 82:840–847, 1977.

9. Javid H, Ostermiller WE, Hengesh JW, et al: Carotid endarterectomy for asymptomatic patients. Arch Surg 102:389–391, 1971.

10. Moore WS, Boren C, Malone JM, et al: Asymptomatic carotid stenosis: immediate and long-term results after prophylactic endarterectomy. Am J Surg 138:228–233, 1979.

11. Humphries AW, Young JR, Santilli PH, et al: Unoperated, asymptomatic significant internal carotid artery stenosis: a review of 182 instances. Surgery 80:695–698, 1976.

12. Johnson N, Burnham SJ, Flanigan DP, et al: Carotid endarterectomy: a follow-up study of the contralateral non-operated carotid artery. Ann Surg 188:748–752, 1978.

13. Levin SM, Sondheimer FK, Levin JM: The contralateral diseased but asymptomatic carotid artery: to operate or not? An update. Am J Surg 140:203–250, 1980.

14. Padore PC, De Weese JA, May AG, et al: Asymptomatic contralateral carotid endarterectomy. Surgery 88:748–752, 1980.

15. Treiman RL, Foran RF, Shore EH, et al: Carotid bruit. Significance in patients undergoing an abdominal aortic operation. Arch Surg 106:803–805, 1973.

16. Carney WI Jr, Steward WB, De Pinto DJ, et al: Carotid bruit as a risk factor in aorto-iliac reconstruction. Surgery 81:567–570, 1977.

17. Evans WE, Cooperman M: The significance of asymptomatic unilateral carotid bruits in preoperative patients. Surgery 83:521–522, 1978.

18. Bernhard VM, Johnson WD, Peterson JJ: Carotid artery stenosis: association with surgery for coronary artery disease. Arch Surg 105:837–840, 1972.

19. Lefrak EA, Guinn GA: Prophylactic carotid artery surgery in patients requiring a second operation. Southern Med J 67:185–189, 1974.

20. Hertzer NR, Loop FD, Taylor PC, et al: Staged and combined surgical approach to simultaneous carotid and coronary vascular disease. Surgery 84:803–811, 1978.
21. Ennix CL Jr, Lawrie GM, Morris GC Jr, et al: Improved results of carotid endarterectomy in patients with symptomatic coronary disease: an analysis of 1,546 consecutive carotid operations. Stroke 10:122–125, 1979.
22. Crawford ES, Palamara AE, Kasparian AS: Carotid and noncoronary operations: simultaneous, staged, and delayed. Surgery 87:1–8, 1980.
23. Turnipseed WD, Berkoff HA, Belzer FO: Postoperative stroke in cardiac and peripheral vascular disease. Ann Surg 192:365–368, 1980.
24. Breslau PJ, Fell G, Miller DW, et al: Incidence of carotid arterial disease in patients undergoing coronary artery bypass surgery. Stroke 12:9, 1981.
25. Bone GE, Slaymaker EE, Barnes RW: Noninvasive assessment of collateral blood flow of the cerebral hemisphere by Doppler ultrasound. Surg Gynecol Obstet 145:873–876, 1977.

Part IV

ASSOCIATED TECHNOLOGICAL CONSIDERATIONS

CHAPTER 26

PROGRESS IN DOPPLER INSTRUMENTATION

Stanley E. Rittgers

The Doppler effect (named for Christian Doppler about 1843) is simply the observation that a series of energy waves that strike a moving object at one frequency are reflected back at a different frequency (Figure 26-1). The change in frequency is directly proportional to the velocity of the moving object. Examples of this phenomenon include radar (radio waves), astronomical measurement of star velocity (light), and the common change in pitch heard from a passing train whistle (sound), from which the effect was first observed.

BASIC PRINCIPLES

As they apply to current and developing systems, the principles of Doppler physics are outlined below. For detailed coverage of Doppler physics, see Chapter 21, and for an account of the physical phenomena associated with clinical applications, see Chapter 23.

Supported by a grant from the Veterans Administration.

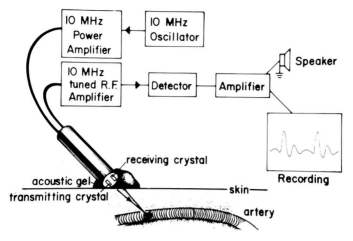

Figure 26-1. Doppler ultrasonic velocity detector.

DOPPLER SHIFT VERSUS ANGLE

Velocity consists of both speed and direction, and so it is important to keep in mind that the Doppler frequency shift varies according to the angle between the probe and the artery (Figure 26-2). When ultrasonic waves strike the blood cells in a direct line (small angle between probe and artery), there is a large frequency shift (Doppler effect). As angles increase, frequency shifts decrease until a minimal waveform is obtained with a 90% orientation. Further rotation of the probe reverses this sequence of frequency changes, with the sense of direction now opposite because blood cells are moving away from the probe.

DEPTH OF PENETRATION VERSUS FREQUENCY

Depth of penetration of sound through tissue is inversely related to the frequency of the Doppler instrument (Figure 26-3). Sound energy is gradually lost as it travels through any tissue medium, and it is especially attenuated when it strikes interfaces between two different tissues, such as muscle and bone. High-frequency sound waves decay with depth faster than low-frequency waves. As a general rule, there is about a 7% loss in signal amplitude per centimeter of tissue depth for every megahertz of transducer frequency. This means, for example, that a 1-MHz

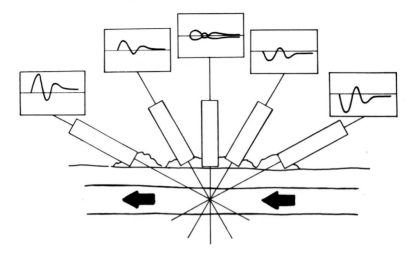

Figure 26-2. Doppler frequency shift versus probe angle.

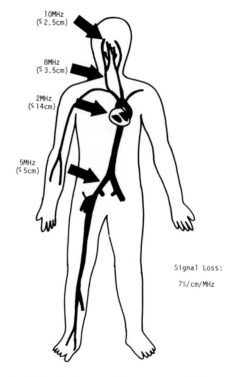

Figure 26-3. Depth of penetration versus probe frequency.

probe would retain about 93% $(1-0.07)**1$ of its original amplitude at a depth of 1 cm, and about 48% $(1-0.07)**10$ at a depth of 10 cm. A 10-MHz probe, on the other hand, would have about 48% $(1-0.07)**10$ of its original amplitude at 1 cm and about 0.06% $([1-0.07]**10)**10$ at 10 cm. This rapid decline in usable signal strength dramatically illustrates why there are large variations in Doppler outputs and why care must be taken in choosing the proper transducer for a given application.

Why not just use the lowest frequency transducer to examine all regions of the body? First, the Doppler frequency shift is proportional to the probe frequency, and thus a high transmitting frequency produces a large Doppler frequency shift, which is more detailed and easier to interpret. Second, the width of the beam being transmitted is usually larger with a low-frequency probe, and so only wide areas may be interrogated with this device. A compromise, then, is generally reached in which the probe having the best frequency resolution and sufficient depth penetration is chosen for each application.

OUTPUT DEVICES

The output of a Doppler device may be auditory, visual, or both. Most commonly, stereo headsets or speakers are used to separate the forward-flow and reverse-flow channels. Simply listening to the Doppler shift signal provides information about signal quality, source, and physiologic condition. It is a sufficient format for many examinations. Visual displays complement sound and provide a record of the waveform. Such displays may be either a strip-chart recording from a zero-crossing detector or real-time spectral analysis displayed on a television monitor. The strip chart provides bidirectional information in a compressed, single-line waveform. The tracing is not mean velocity, but actually weights high frequencies more heavily than low frequencies. Frequency spectral analysis provides a full display of all frequency components in the waveform and may be used to obtain true mean and peak frequencies.[1]

PRESENT SYSTEMS

POCKET DOPPLERS

Currently available Doppler units come in many forms for a variety of purposes. A number of pocket, battery-operated Dopplers are available for general screening. Their chief advantage is their size and portability, and they have become widely popular for bedside and clinical monitoring. Low-frequency devices operating at 2–3 MHz have good depth penetration and are thus excellent for obstetrics and deep-vessel detection. Mid-range devices of 5–7 MHz combine depth and frequency resolution. They are essential for the femoral arteries and veins in the thigh, but are also well suited for most major vessels of the extremities. High-frequency devices from 8–10 MHz have shallow depth penetration but excellent frequency range and narrow beams. These are the "pencil probes" most often used for examining the more superficial arteries and veins of the face, neck, and extremities.

STANDARD DOPPLERS

The standard sized Doppler units are general purpose instruments that, although they often have optional battery power, find greatest use in vascular and research laboratories. These instruments come with transmitting frequencies of from 2 MHz to 10 MHz, but many now offer interchangeability of probes with the same basic unit. Also, bidirectional capability is standard, with output provided as either a true separation of forward and reverse flow or a quadrature output. Integral speakers, strip-chart recorders, and panel meters are available.

CONTINUOUS-WAVE VERSUS PULSED DOPPLER

Up to this point my discussion of the ultrasonic Doppler has focused on only continuous-wave operation. A modification of this technique, with unique implications, is the pulsed Doppler (Figure 26-4). A continuous-wave Doppler consists of two transducer crystals, one continuously sending and the other continuously receiving sound waves. Because these waves travel outward to all depths (with varying attenuation) and are then reflected back, the received signal represents virtually all sources of Doppler frequency shifts in the beam path. This includes all flow in a given vessel as well as any flow in other vessels (arteries or veins) in the beam path. The pulsed Doppler, on the other hand, consists of only one transducer crystal that alternately transmits and receives sound waves. Because the pulse burst is very brief and is sent at precise intervals, the blood volume sampled is small and the source of the returning signals is readily identified. Therefore, the pulsed Doppler affords the capability of precisely locating a desired vessel and of even selecting one region of flow within that vessel. This greatly reduces artifacts from adjoining vessels and provides recordings from specific regions of interest.

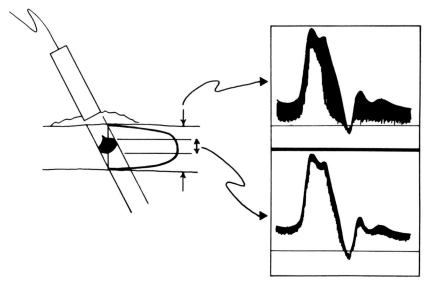

Figure 26-4. Continuous-wave versus pulsed Doppler operation.

DOPPLER IMAGERS

Ultrasonic Doppler detectors have been incorporated into vascular imaging systems. These instruments are based on either continuous-wave or pulsed Dopplers and generate an image by recording the presence or absence of flow at each location that the probe passes. The image is a physiologic representation of the flow channel rather than the morphologic image of arterial structures provided by ultrasonic echo devices. Continuous-wave Doppler imagers provide a plane view only, while pulsed Doppler imagers can also provide a cross-sectional view by virtue of their range-gating capability.

FUTURE DEVELOPMENTS

Despite the rapid advances in Doppler instrumentation and the established recognition of its clinical value, several avenues of development remain.

FOCUSED-BEAM TRANSDUCERS

Growing recognition of the potential for Doppler measurements to provide more than simple information about flow and directionality and the recent capability to exploit fully all of the detailed information about velocity through real-time spectral analysis has led to a demand for greater sophistication in the Doppler instrument itself. The direct assessment of carotid artery disease and the detection of intracardiac flow abnormalities are two areas of current interest. These applications require refined techniques to sample precise regions for the presence of flow disturbances. The pulsed Doppler provides depth control, but the beam width often covers too large an area. Therefore, efforts are being made to develop narrow-beam transducers that focus on a minimal cross-sectional area at prescribed distances (Figure 26-5).

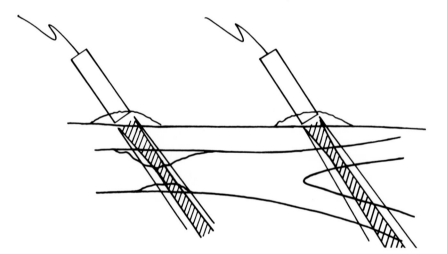

Figure 26-5. Reduced sample volume of focused-beam transducers.

VOLUME FLOWMETERS

Noninvasive determination of total volume flow has long been a goal of researchers interested in monitoring cardiac output and organ perfusion. There are several approaches to this goal, two of which are illustrated in Figure 26-6.

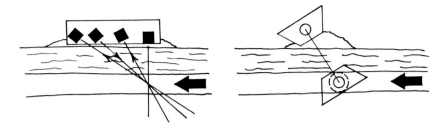

Figure 26-6. Doppler volume flowmeters. *Left:* system based on calculations from vessel diameter and average blood velocity. *Right:* system of concentric pulsed Dopplers.

One method calculates the volume flow from direct, simultaneous measurements of blood velocity and vessel diameter.[2] The transducer consists of a combined Doppler/echo system that measures true velocity (not frequency shift) by three Doppler probes aligned at fixed angles to each other. A fourth crystal operates in the pulse-echo mode and provides vessel diameter measurements from an A-mode signal. The cross-sectional area of the vessel is derived from the diameter and then multiplied by the velocity to produce volume flow. A second method involves a pulsed Doppler using concentric transducer crystals to produce sound beams of different cross-sectional areas.[3] A small central beam (2-mm diameter) is fixed entirely within the vessel of interest, while a large outer beam (12-mm diameter) bathes the entire artery and some adjoining tissue. Normalizing the output from the larger beam by that of the narrow beam causes unknown quantities of probe-to-artery angle and vessel diameter to be factored out, leaving a measurement of true volume flow. This method has the advantage of using only Doppler techniques sampling along the same axis.

SCANNING DOPPLER IMAGER

Doppler imaging has proven to be complementary to static imaging methods because of its sensitivity to fluid motion, not just to structural interfaces. A further advance in this area will be the automatic scanning imager,[4] which will greatly speed the image-formation process. The scanning transducer actually consists of many crystals aligned in a row or matrix pattern, each one being fired in a predetermined sequence (Figure 26-7). As reflected signals return, an image is created without the usual brush-stroke motion of the transducer.

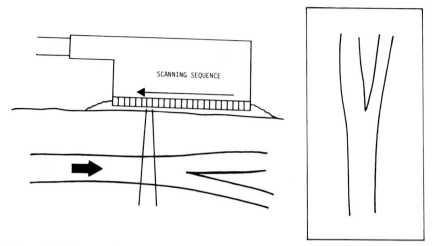

Figure 26-7. Automatic scanning Doppler imager. Reprinted with permission from Hottinger CF, Meindl JD: Blood flow measurement using the attenuation compensated volume flowmeter. Ultrasonic Imaging 1:5, 1979.

FULL DUPLEX IMAGING

The greatest synthesis of diagnostic ultrasonic technologies to date has been the duplex scanner (see Chapter 16). This system incorporates static sector scanning with dynamic Doppler flow sampling to obtain both morphologic and physiologic information. Future advances in this system will lead to a full duplex imager. One major change from the present system will be the extension of the existing single-channel pulsed Doppler to an infinite-gate Doppler capable of sensing flow at multiple depths simultaneously. Also, color coding will be employed to present the variety of information available. With this system, tissue characteristics will be identified by changes in reflectivity, and flow abnormalities will be observed through changes in the entire flow field.

CONCLUSIONS

Much progress has been made during the past two decades in the development and use of Doppler ultrasound in medical diagnosis. Doppler instruments have proven to be sensitive to blood dynamics while remaining simple to use and readily available. Future Doppler devices should provide even more information and improved clinical accuracy.

REFERENCES

1. Rittgers SE, Putney WW, Barnes RW: Real-time spectrum analysis and display of directional Doppler ultrasound blood velocity signals. IEEE Trans Biomed Engr BME 27:723–738, 1980.
2. Uematsu S: Determination of volume of arterial blood flow by an ultrasonic device. J Clin Ultrasound 9:209–216, 1981.
3. Hottinger CF, Meindl JD: Blood flow measurement using the attenuation-compensated volume flowmeter. Ultrasonic Imaging 1:1–15, 1979.
4. Nowicki A, Reid JM: An infinite gate pulse Doppler. Ultrasound Med Biol 7:41–50, 1981.

CHAPTER **27**

MICROCOMPUTER APPLICATIONS IN THE BLOOD FLOW LABORATORY

John T. Collins

With the arrival of small desk-top microcomputers, complete with a range of peripherals and adequate memory, it is time to switch from the central computer and time sharing to the decentralized, individual computer system. With few exceptions, these microcomputers can be classified into three groups: personal, business, and technical. Apple, Radio Shack, Timex, and IBM market personal computers, Xerox, Wang, and Northstar market business computers, and Digital Equipment Corp., Hewlett Packard, and Tektronix specialize in technical computers. These names are only representative; there are hundreds of models on the market. Our computer was acquired in 1979 when there were fewer choices. Since then even some personal computers have all of the capabilities of our system. In light of that fact I have included one of the more popular personal computers in describing a vascular laboratory computer system.

Some vascular laboratories are now using computers principally to maintain patient histories. After a large data base has been entered, it is useful in profiling (e.g., by age, smoking history, and the like) patients who, for example, have undergone a femoral popliteal bypass with a saphenous vein graft. Once the patient data has been entered into computer memory, a program to compile such profiles is straightforward. This capability does require a large amount of computer memory, but computer technology has advanced to the point at which this capability costs less than $25,000, including a computer with 520,000 bytes of memory, a printer, and a 40,000,000-byte disc memory (see Table 27-1 for definitions of these terms).

Table 27-1. A Short Glossary of Computer Terms

Term	Definition
Byte	A measure of computer memory. The computer uses binary words, which are either zero or one in value. These words are called bits. Eight bits equal one byte. One byte is needed for each character stored in memory.
CPU	Central processing unit. This is the microprocessor chip that actually controls the running of the computer.
DOS	Disk operating system. This program allows communication between the disk drive and the CPU.
Modem	Contraction of "modulator demodulator." A device that allows computers to communicate over telephone lines.
RAM	Random access memory. This is memory available to the computer user. It is "volatile" memory, which is lost when the computer is off.
ROM	Read only memory. This is memory that is not erased when the power is off. A computer-game cartridge is a ROM cartridge.

PRACTICAL APPLICATIONS AND LIMITATIONS

A large patient directory file and surgical procedure file can be made with the simplest systems now available. For about $10,000 a Tektronix 4051 computer with 16,000-byte memory and printer can be purchased. Alternatively, an Apple II with 64,000 bytes of memory and a printer now costs about $1,500. Both systems use the simplest large memory device, a magnetic tape cartridge. The Tektronix built-in tape drive uses tapes with a capacity of either 300,000 or 450,00 bytes. The Apple II can use an ordinary audio tape cassette unit containing a 60-minute tape with a capacity of about 200,000 bytes. The primary disadvantage of tape memory is slow data retrieval. At the search speed of 30 inches per second, it takes 12 minutes to read a 300,000-byte tape cartridge. Also, programs and data stored on tape require a bookkeeping system for each filing and retrieval.

Within the limitation of an 8,000- or 16,000-byte memory, several programs can be used in a vascular laboratory for, as examples, the patient directory file and the surgical procedures file. Once computerized, the patient directory file replaces an index card filing system, eliminating the need for new filing cabinets. Formerly, every time a patient visited the laboratory the patient's name, identification number, referring physician, date of test, and whether the test was normal or abnormal was typed on an index card. On subsequent visits, new data were added to the card. Our entire card file from 1972 to 1979 is now stored on magnetic tape cartridges. A separate tape was used for 1980 entries. A list was produced of patients who had tests from 1972 to 1974 so that their reports could be removed from the report file cabinets. Once our card file was transferred to tape, it was possible to obtain a computer count, by year, of the three major vascular tests (Figure 27-1). During budget allocation meetings this tabulation helped us to justify and obtain more space. Also, a monthly census is produced that shows the number of tests done each month with cumulative totals for the current year (Figure 27-2).

TESTS PER YEAR		ARTERIAL	VENOUS	CAROTID
1972	487	283	204	
1973	817	460	357	
1974	1403	697	706	
1975	2224	847	876	501
1976	2983	964	961	1058
1977	3150	1034	972	1144
1978	3953	1259	1241	1453
1979	3811	1356	1329	1126

Figure 27-1. Computer count of tests by year.

NORTHWESTERN MEMORIAL HOSPITAL BLOOD FLOW LAB

	DECEMBER	YEAR	IN	OUT	ABNORMAL	NORMAL
ARTERIAL	125	1391	918	473	1049	345
VENOUS	94	1037	622	415	167	870
CAROTID	125	1367	928	439	476	891
UPPER ARM	19	185	124	61	79	111
PPG	10	151	107	44	110	41
COLD	5	29	10	17	21	8
DIGIT	0	52	26	27	39	13
DRUG	11	96				
SPINAL CORD	2	132				
JOHN DEERE		74				
TOTAL	391	4514				

AVERAGE NUMBER OF TESTS PER DAY = 18.3

Figure 27-2. Monthly and year-to-date census generated by the computer.

COMPONENTS

ANALOG/DIGITAL CONVERTERS

The analog/digital convertor, at a cost of $1,500, is a major advance in the computer. Any instrument in the laboratory with an analog output (Doppler flowmeters, IPG units, pressure monitors, and even the electrocardiograph, for instance, when used during exercise testing) can transfer that information directly into computer memory for processing and storage. There are 16-channel analog/digital converters available for the Apple and Tektronix computers. An arterial report generated by our system is shown in Figure 27-3. Demographic information is initially typed in by the technician performing the test. This arterial report requires about 2,000 bytes of memory to store it on tape. Also shown is the IPG test form that the computer generates (Figure 27-4). Unfortunately, we are not able to operate this system on a daily basis because of computer memory limitations.

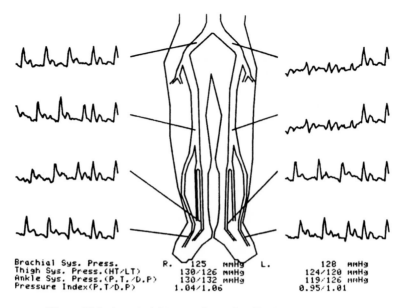

Figure 27-3. An arterial test performed on line by the computer.

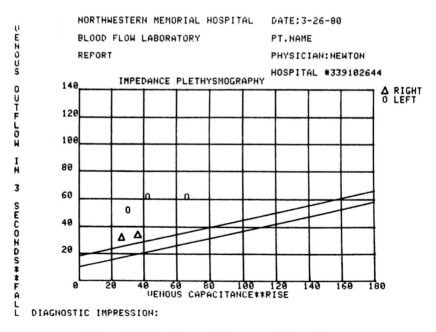

Figure 27-4. Impedance plethysmography by computer.

FLOPPY DISC UNITS

When fully operative, paper files and copies can be eliminated. The larger, faster, and more versatile computers eliminate the disadvantages of a tape memory storage system with the incorporation of a floppy disc unit. These computers have larger memories and fast data retrieval. The Tektronix 4907 File Manager, for instance, costs $4,000, and each removable disc has a capacity of 630,000 bytes. An Apple II disc drive unit costs about $600, and each disc can hold 116,000 bytes on each side. Disc units require controllers that eliminate the bookkeeping requirements of tape storage. Although the 4907 is more expensive, its disc controller programs are built into the unit. The Apple unit disc controller requires 12,000 bytes of computer memory. Disc systems allow access to any file in an average time of 267 milliseconds.

TERMINAL

The next hardware requirement is the peripheral computer terminal, the so-called CRT (for cathode ray tube), used to call up information from disc memory, either displaying it on the video screen or printing it out. Terminals at the receptionist's desk and in the technician's and physician's offices allow a variety of tasks to be performed. The receptionist can call up an appointment program file to schedule patients. Technicians can inquire from the patient directory file if the patients scheduled for testing the next day have been to the laboratory previously. The physician can use the surgical procedure file to obtain a list of patients who have undergone a particular operation. The amount of retrievable material depends on disc and computer memory. The Apple II can handle up to 14 disc drives for total of 1,600,000 bytes, for example, while the Tektronix 4051 can use three File Manager units for a total capacity of 1,890,000 bytes.

It is now possible to purchase fixed-disc systems for the Tektronix 4051 that provide a total capacity of 640,000,000 bytes. In addition to increasing memory, the fixed discs are sealed in the unit, protected from the particles of dust and smoke that can produce major problems with the floppy disc units. A controller is now available that allows Apple II users to have a 5,000,000 byte fixed-disc unit. With this type of memory, the vascular laboratory can function as a real-time report system. Analog data from various tests could easily be entered into computer memory as these data are generated, and reports could be produced before the patient leaves the laboratory. Extensive patient histories can also be stored with this much memory.

Software and Back-Up Procedures

Two problems must be dealt with in even the simplest system. First is the problem of "software," particularly that of developing programs. While none of the programs described here are exceptionally difficult, they do require some familiarity with computer programming. As the system becomes more complex, so do the programs, increasing the need for expert programmers. Software packages for laboratory applications may be offered later at less expense, but such programs may need to be adapted to the needs of the particular laboratory.

The second problem, which is widely ignored, is the need to back up the computer peripheral memory system by making copies of all tapes or floppy discs in use. Data stored on magnetic tape of discs can be erased inadvertently by static electricity, stray magnetic fields, or power-line voltage fluctuations. Therefore, it is mandatory to duplicate all files and programs. The fixed-disc units require a large tape drive with the same capacity as the disc unit. The time lag in backing up any of the modalities is usually based on the amount of retrievable data that is entered. The decision as to how much new information can be added to present computer files before duplicating the data depends on the difficulty of reconstructing data files that have been erased.

Conclusions

The microcomputer revolution allows us to speed computer applications inexpensively in our laboratories. The costs of software and programming are difficult to predict or to budget, but the advantages of relatively inexpensive data storage, analysis, reporting, retrieval, and other aspects of data management argue in favor of the computerized vascular laboratory.

SELF-ASSESSMENT
POSTTEST

Falls B. Hershey

Part I:

NONINVASIVE DIAGNOSIS
OF ARTERIAL OCCLUSIVE DISEASE

CHAPTER 1   **Pathophysiology of Arterial Occlusive Disease**

1. The effects of stenosis on flow through a vessel are (true/false):
   a. Acceleration through the narrow zone
   b. Turbulence at the entrance and exit of the stenosis
   c. Decrease in flow
   d. Drop in pressure
2. Flow and/or pressure are decreased by arterial stenoses that symmetrically (true/false):
   a. Decrease diameter 25%
   b. Decrease diameter 50%
   c. Decrease cross-sectional area 25%
   d. Decrease cross-sectional area 50%
   e. Decrease cross-sectional area 75%
   f. Decrease cross-sectional area 90%

3. A "critical" or "hemodynamically significant" arterial stenosis is defined as (true/false/other):
   a. One that causes intermittent claudication
   b. One that causes TIAs
   c. One that causes pressure or flow decreases distal to the stenosis
   d. One that decreases diameter 50%
4. The effects of vigorous walking on a normal leg include (true/false):
   a. Increased blood flow to the muscles
   b. Decreased ankle pressure
   c. Oxygen and flow debts in the muscles
   d. Reactive hyperemia when exercise stops
5. The effects on a leg of exercise sufficient to cause intermittent claudication include (true/false):
   a. Increased blood flow to the muscles
   b. Insufficient blood flow to the muscles
   c. Increased arterial pressure in the muscles
   d. Decreased ankle pressure
   e. Prolonged reactive hyperemia
   f. Oxygen and flow debts worse than usual
6. Vasodilator drugs (true/false):
   a. Decrease resting peripheral resistance
   b. Increase resting blood flow
   c. Increase blood flow during exercise

CHAPTER 2 Segmental Limb Pressures, Doppler Waveforms, and Stress Testing

1. Segmental pressures taken with cuffs high on the thigh, above the knee, below the knee, and at the ankle are abnormal if (true/false):
   a. Pressure differences between levels ≥ 15 mmHg
   b. Pressure differences between levels ≥ 20 mmHg
   c. Pressure differences between legs at same level ≥ 30 mmHg
2. Ankle/arm index is (true/false/other):
   a. The ratio of the systolic brachial and ankle pressures
   b. Normally over 1
   c. Calculated with the (lowest/highest) arm pressure
   d. Abnormally (low/high) when leg arteries are calcified

3. Resting segmental arterial pressures supply information about (true/false):
   a. The presence of arterial occlusive disease
   b. The etiology of arterial occlusive disease
   c. The pattern of arterial occlusive disease
   d. Arterial aneurysms
   e. The severity of arterial occlusive disease
   f. The presence of intermittent claudication
4. Stress testing with the treadmill at 1½ mph and 10% grade (true/false):
   a. Is unnecessary when resting ankle pressures are less than 40 mmHg
   b. Provides results identical to those of stress testing with reactive hyperemia
   c. Distinguishes between true and pseudoclaudication
   d. Is just as stressful as the cardiac treadmill stress test
   e. Normally shows unchanged or elevated ankle pressures
5. Toe pressures may be taken with the digital cuff and (true/false/other):
   a. Doppler, photoplethysmograph, or strain gauge detection of pulse appearance
   b. Are normally lower than ankle pressures
   c. Are more/less likely to be affected by calcification and poor compressibility of the arteries
   d. Correlate better than ankle pressures with healing of ischemic lesions of the toes and feet

CHAPTER 3   Digital Plethysmography and Pressure Measurements

1. Plethysmographs record changes in:
   a. Volume
   b. Pressure
   c. Flow
   d. Pulses
2. Finger pulse and volume are normally affected by (true/false):
   a. Each heartbeat
   b. Vasoconstriction from cold or excitement
   c. Inspiration and expiration

3. The normal finger pulse wave as recorded by the photoplethysmograph has a (true/false):
   a. Rapid systolic upslope
   b. Rounded peak
   c. Slower, more gradual downslope
   d. "Decrotic" notch
   e. A reversed phase below the zero crossing line
4. Raynaud's phenomenon (true/false):
   a. Is the same as Raynaud's disease
   b. Occurs with occlusions of digital arteries
   c. Usually has some serious underlying cause
5. The normal effect of sympathetic stimuli on the digital photoplethysmograph is (true/false/other):
   a. Increase/decrease/no change in digital volume
   b. Increase/decrease/no change in pulse volume
   c. Not seen with scleroderma
6. Regarding arterial pressures in the toes and at the ankle (true/false/other):
   a. Normal toe pressure is same/greater/less than ankle pressure in the same normal patient
   b. Toe pressures are better/worse predictors of healing of toe or transmetatarsal amputations
   c. Low ankle pressures signify a poor prognosis
   d. High ankle pressures reliably predict healing of ischemic foot lesions

CHAPTER 4   Postoperative Noninvasive Evaluation of Femorotibial Bypass Grafts

1. Causes of vein-graft stenosis include (true/false):
   a. New atherosclerotic plaques in the graft
   b. Technical errors such as improper ligation of tributaries
   c. Intimal and medial fibrosis and hypertrophy
   d. Fibromuscular dysplasia
2. Vein-graft stenosis was detected in these cases (true/false):
   a. Solely by monophasic Doppler velocity tracings over the graft
   b. By decreases in ankle and/or toe pressures
   c. More reliably by toe pressure than by ankle pressure decreases

d. As a result of intermittent claudication
3. Recommended noninvasive follow-up schedules are (true/false):
   a. Frequently in the hospital
   b. Two to four weeks after discharge from the hospital
   c. Monthly for a year
   d. Quarterly for a year
   e. More frequently if pressure indices decrease ≥ 0.15

CHAPTER 5   New Techniques to Assess Aortoiliac Stenosis

1. Signs or symptoms of aortoiliac stenosis include (true/false):
   a. Audible bruits at the groin
   b. Decreased pulses at the groin
   c. Normal nocturnal tumescence and erectile impotence
   d. Intermittent claudication of the calves
   e. Claudication of the hips or thighs
2. Supplementary noninvasive tests to assess aortoiliac stenosis include (true/false):
   a. High-thigh cuffs for proximal thigh pressure measurement
   b. Femoral arterial Doppler waveform tracings
   c. Volume pulse recordings
   d. Femoral arterial pressure measurement
   e. Arteriography

CHAPTER 6   Segmental Volume Pulse Recorder: Improved Anatomic Discrimination by Refinement in Technique

1. The segmental volume pulse recorder (true/false):
   a. Is more useful with two cuffs on the thigh, one below the knee and one at the ankle
   b. Is more accurate when the thigh cuffs are narrow
   c. Is helpful in assessing the combinations of aortoiliac and femoropopliteal occlusions in the same patient
   d. Obtains simultaneous pulse (volume/pressure) recordings from both legs
   e. Is useful to supplement segmental pressure measurements at the same four levels

CHAPTER 7   **Intravenous Digital Angiography in the Assessment of Arterial Disease**

No questions

CHAPTER 8   **Observations on Vasculogenic Impotence**

1. Erection of the penis is a complicated process requiring (true/false):
   a. Normal sympathetic nerve function
   b. Erotic stimuli
   c. Normal parasympathetic nerve function
   d. Normal arterial inflow
   e. Normal venous outflow
2. Resting penile blood pressure is (true/false):
   a. Most easily obtained by listening for arterial signals with the usual Doppler
   b. Obtained by using the 2 cm cuff
   c. Usually equal to the brachial pressure
   d. Less than 60% of brachial pressure in all cases of vasculogenic impotence

Part II:

Noninvasive Diagnosis of Venous Disease

CHAPTER 9   **Venous Anatomy and Pathophysiology**

1. Venous drainage from the normal leg is as follows:
   a. From the foot it runs deep/subcutaneously up into the lower leg
   b. During exercise blood runs from the subcutaneous veins of the lower leg: 1) up the long saphenous vein to the groin or 2) enters the deep veins via the perforating and communicating veins
2. The normal muscle pumping mechanism returns flow from the legs against the force of gravity (true/false):

a. Utilizing leg muscle contraction as the propelling force
b. Ensuring upward flow in the saphenous veins by the one-way valves
c. Confining the pressure inside the thick deep fascia of the leg
d. Reducing the pressure in the superficial veins and foot
e. Directing blood into the deep veins of the calf
3. Postphlebitic venous insufficiency requires (true/false):
a. Varicose veins
b. Incompetence of valves of the deep veins
c. Incompetence of valves of the perforating veins
d. Obstruction of the deep veins

CHAPTER 10 The Diagnosis and Assessment of Venous Disorders in the Office and Laboratory

1. The abnormal physiologic conditions after deep venous thrombosis causing chronic valvular incompetence include (true/false):
a. Poor emptying of the veins of the legs
b. Reflux of blood in the distal (inferior) directions
c. Abnormal ambulatory venous pressures
d. Abnormal resting erect venous pressures
2. Doppler examination of the veins at the groin tests for incompetent valves by (true/false/other):
a. Listening medial/lateral to the femoral pulse
b. Listening for reversed flow with coughing or the Valsalva manuever
c. Recording the reversed flow with the strip-chart recorder
d. Distinguishing between reflux in the common femoral and saphenous veins
e. Compressing the saphenous vein 5–10 cm below the groin
f. Listening while the patient is standing
3. Venous sounds over the pubis are (true/false/other):
a. Abnormal/normal
b. A sign of crossover to bypass an occluded femoral/iliac vein
c. Phasic with respiration
d. Abolished by compressing the affected groin
e. High-pitched or continuous if iliac thrombosis is recent or severe

CHAPTER 11   Doppler Diagnosis of Deep Venous Thrombosis

1. Auditory Doppler diagnosis of deep venous thrombosis (true/false):
   a. Requires the deep Doppler penetration to examine the superior femoral vein in the thigh
   b. Involves an evaluation of the five basic qualities of flow: spontaneity, phasicity, augmentation, competence, and pulsatility
2. The normal venous sounds heard at these sites (true/false):
   a. May be absent over the posterior tibial veins at the ankle
   b. Are normally phasic with respiration and decrease with expiration
   c. Are augmented by compression distally
   d. Are not augmented by compression proximally
   e. Stop with the Valsalva maneuver
   f. Are pulsatile and synchronous with the heartbeat
3. Auditory Doppler examination of the leg veins is highly accurate in detecting (true/false):
   a. Minor calf-vein thrombosis
   b. Obstructions of iliofemoral or popliteal veins
   c. Saphenous phlebitis

CHAPTER 12   Phleborheography in the Diagnosis of Deep Venous Thrombosis

1. The phleborheograph is a multichannel venous recording device that (true/false):
   a. Is highly accurate in the diagnosis of calf-vein thrombosis
   b. Detects thrombi in the legs by accurately measuring segmental volume changes in the legs
   c. Notes decreased respiratory waves resulting from thrombi in the veins
   d. Notes impaired venous outflow, which causes a rise in the baseline of the tracing
2. Experienced clinicians' accuracy in the diagnosis of deep venous thrombosis has been tested and compared with phlebograms and found (true/false):
   a. To be only 50% accurate
   b. To include many false-positive diagnoses
   c. To include many false-negative diagnoses

3. Phleborheography is most helpful in the diagnosis of deep venous thrombosis (or in ruling out the diagnosis) in patients (true/false):
   a. With a massively swollen leg
   b. With tenderness of the calf
   c. With pelvic tumors compressing iliac veins
   d. With chronic deep venous thrombosis

CHAPTER 13   **Venous Plethysmography**

1. Physiologic information yielded by venous plethysmographs include (true/false):
   a. Recording of pulse waveforms
   b. Measurements of pulse waveforms
   c. Recordings of increases of blood volume in the leg
   d. Measurements of arterial inflow to the leg
   e. Measurements of venous outflow from the leg
2. Which of these types of physiologic information (a–e, above) is useful to detect deep venous thrombosis?
3. Venous outflow measurements for the diagnosis of deep venous thrombosis are (true/false):
   a. Made with strain-gauge plethysmographs
   b. Made with impedance plethysmographs
   c. Made with volume pulse recorders
   d. Sensitive to partial obstructions of major deep veins
   e. Insensitive to isolated calf-vein thrombosis
   f. The same or similar with all techniques
4. Conditions that may impair venous outflow and/or mimic deep venous thrombosis include (true/false):
   a. Ruptured Baker's cyst
   b. Ruptured plantaris muscle
   c. Subfascial hematoma from other causes
   d. Acute cellulitis
   e. External compression of the veins by various causes
5. A venous tourniquet is frequently applied to the leg to occlude the superficial subcutaneous veins (true/false):
   a. And to prevent reflux down incompetent superficial veins
   b. To see if reflux occurs below the tourniquet
   c. To localize incompetent perforating veins
   d. To differentiate between primary varicose veins and incompetent perforating veins

CHAPTER 14   **Photoplethysmography in the Evaluation of Chronic Venous Insufficiency**

1. Photoplethysmography in the evaluation of chronic venous insufficiency (true/false/other):
   a. Detects cutaneous blood content at the ankle
   b. Shows decreased cutaneous blood content at the ankle with exercise of the leg in the erect position
   c. Shows that skin refilling time when exercise stops depends on: 1) Doppler ankle pressures and arterial inflow, 2) position of the leg, 3) use of venous tourniquets inflated to 50 mmHg, 4) venous reflux via incompetent valves
2. The venous refilling time noted in the photoplethysmograph (true/false):
   a. Cannot be accurately measured by transducers placed over varices, on areas that move greatly during the exercise phase of the test
   b. Is defined as the number of seconds it takes the PPG curve to reach and maintain a stable level for 5 seconds
   c. Is normally at least 25 seconds
   d. Is shortened by incompetence of venous valves
   e. Is restored to normal by venous tourniquet inflated to 50 mmHg above the knee
   f. Correlates well with walking venous pressures

Part III:

NONINVASIVE DIAGNOSIS
OF CAROTID OCCLUSIVE DISEASE

CHAPTER 15   **The Anatomy and Pathophysiology of Atherosclerotic Extracranial Cerebrovascular Disease**

1. The circle of Willis consists of the (true/false):
   a. Anterior cerebral artery
   b. Middle artery

    c. Posterior cerebral artery

    d. Anterior communicating artery

    e. Posterior communicating artery

2. The circle of Willis (true/false):

    a. Connects all four major inflow arteries to the brain

    b. May serve as outflow from the brain

    c. May receive inflow from the external carotid artery

3. The most frequent pathologic changes in atherosclerotic arterial disease are (answer by ranking in order of frequency):

    a. Narrowing of the artery by plaques

    b. Ulceration of the lining

    c. Dilation and aneurysms

    d. Thrombosis

4. Transient ischemic attacks are focal neurologic deficits that (true/false/other):

    a. Are less than 12 hours/24 hours in duration

    b. Are small strokes

    c. Are caused by microemboli from ulcerated plaques at the carotid bifurcation

    d. Cause positive CT scans of the brain

5. Carotid territory neurologic signs or symptoms include (true/false):

    a. Signs due to the cerebral hemispheres

    b. Signs of vertebrobasilar insufficiency

    c. Weakness of the arm or leg on the same side as the affected carotid

    d. Aphasia

    e. Double vision and other cranial nerve signs or symptoms

CHAPTER 16   Comprehensive Noninvasive Evaluation of Extracranial Cerebrovascular Disease

1. Information desired about atherosclerotic disease at the bifurcation of the carotid artery includes (true/false/other):

    a. Presence or absence of murmurs

    b. Severity of stenosis

    c. Presence of occlusion

    d. Ulceration of any plaques present

2. Ultrasonic techniques of examining the carotid bifurcation for atherosclerosis include (true/false):
   a. Listening for shifts in frequency or turbulence of Doppler signals at the carotid bifurcation
   b. Image formation by B-mode pulse echo from different tissue interfaces, including the arteries
   c. Image formation of the flowing blood stream utilizing a position-sensing arm on the Doppler transducer
   d. Spectral analysis of the Doppler shifts caused by the moving blood
3. Real-time B-mode imaging of the carotid arteries (true/false):
   a. Generates images of the anatomy of the artery wall and its abnormalities
   b. Cannot distinguish between moving and clotted blood
   c. Is blocked by calcific plaques, which shadow and obscure the artery and other structures behind it
4. Characteristics of normal flow in the internal carotid artery include (true/false):
   a. A multiphasic flow pattern
   b. Considerable flow during diastole
   c. High mean flow (average of systolic and diastolic flow)
5. Doppler spectral analysis of the carotid arteries (true/false):
   a. Detects abnormalities not audible to the ear
   b. Reveals only flow-reducing abnormalities
   c. Reveals high peak frequency when stenosis $\geq 50\%$
   d. Is affected by the angle of the Doppler probe
   e. Shows spectral broadening when laminar flow is disturbed by mild stenosis
   f. Shows spectral broadening near the wall of normal arteries
   g. Shows spectral broadening when recording and averaging the flow in the entire width of the artery

CHAPTER 17   K/M Oculoplethysmography and Carotid Phonoangiography

1. Carotid Phonoangiography (true/false):
   a. Records the Doppler murmurs
   b. Records murmurs not audible to the ear
   c. Distinguishes between murmurs radiating up from the heart and those arising at the bifurcation
   d. Reveals diastolic bruits from the external and internal carotid arteries

2. Oculoplethysmography by the Kartchner/McRae method (true/false):
   a. Measures ocular pulses and ocular pulse delays
   b. Measures differences in volumetric filling of the globe of the eye
   c. Notes the reappearance of ocular pulses to measure pressures
   d. Compares ear lobe and ocular pulses
   e. Applies suction cups to the eye and suction of up to 300 mmHg
   f. Detects only hemodynamically significant stenoses

CHAPTER 18   Periorbital Diagnostic Techniques

1. Periorbital cerebrovascular Doppler examinations (true/false/other):
   a. Identify the palpebral, frontal, and supraorbital arteries
   b. Have shown that normal flow in the frontal artery is out of the orbit
   c. Normally show decrease/increase/no change in Doppler flow in the frontal artery with compression of the superficial temporal artery on the same side
   d. Always show reversal of ipsilateral frontal artery flow in the presence of severe internal carotid stenosis
2. Compression of each common carotid artery as performed during the periorbital cerebrovascular Doppler examination (true/false):
   a. Is over the carotid bifurcation
   b. Is only 1 to 3 heartbeats in duration
   c. Normally decreases the Doppler signal in the frontal artery
   d. May decrease the Doppler signal in the opposite frontal artery
3. Supraorbital photoplethysmography records the arterial pulse waves and their response to compression of branches of the external carotid artery including (true/false):
   a. Superficial temporal artery
   b. Middle meningeal artery
   c. Facial artery
   d. Common carotid artery
4. Ocular pneumoplethysmography (OPG-Gee) measures ophthalmic arterial pressures by the reappearance of ocular pulses (true/false).
5. The ophthalmic artery is the first/second/last branch of the internal carotid artery.
6. OPG-Gee is 85%–97% accurate for significant ($\geq 50\%$) stenosis of the internal carotid artery (true/false).

CHAPTER 19   **Direct Doppler Auscultation of the Carotid Arteries**

1. Direct examinations for atherosclerotic lesions of the carotid bifurcation include (true/false):
   a. OPG
   b. CPA
   c. Doppler imaging techniques
   d. Auditory direct Doppler auscultation
   e. Spectral analysis of the Doppler-shifted sounds
2. Direct Doppler auscultation of the carotid bifurcation (true/false):
   a. Requires special Doppler probes
   b. Supplements many imaging methods
   c. Detects stenosis by the sharp increase in velocity through the stenosis
   d. Detects occlusions of the internal carotid artery by absence of the internal carotid artery signal
3. The trained ear of the experienced technician using the continuous-wave Doppler to examine the carotid bifurcation (true/false):
   a. Detects stenosis of the internal carotid artery $\geq$ 50% in 90% of the cases as determined by arteriography
   b. Distinguishes between internal carotid stenosis and internal carotid occlusion in 96%
   c. Compresses the carotid artery with the Doppler probe

CHAPTER 20   **Early Detection of Stroke-Related Lesions by Real-Time Doppler Spectral Analysis**

1. Real-time spectral analysis of the carotid Doppler shifts (true/false):
   a. Provides a continuous display of the Doppler frequency shifts
   b. Uses a bidirectional continuous-wave Doppler to record venous as well as arterial sounds
   c. Distinguishes between flow in the common internal and external carotid arteries
   d. Detects plaques too small to cause stenosis
2. When the spectral waveform from the common carotid artery has low systolic peak velocity, low or no diastolic flow, and increased diastolic flow in the external carotid artery (true/false):
   a. Suspect occlusion of the internal carotid artery
   b. The internal carotid artery is narrowed somewhat

c. The external carotid artery is helping to supply the brain
3. The "window" seen in some internal carotid artery spectral waveforms is (true/false/other):
   a. Normal/abnormal
   b. Systolic/diastolic
   c. Due to the prevalence of high frequencies at the upper part of the frequency envelope, making that part of the waveform grayer
4. Abnormal spectral waveforms show many changes depending on the severity of the stenosis. These include (true/false/other):
   a. Increased/decreased peak frequencies
   b. Loss of the systolic window
   c. Increased diastolic flow
   d. Sharper/blunter systolic peak
   e. Loss of the intensity concentration at the upper part of the waveform

CHAPTER 21 Three-Dimensional Ultrasonic Arteriography

1. The purposes of three-dimensional ultrasonic arteriography include (true/false):
   a. The detection of carotid stenoses that cause minor hemodynamic changes
   b. Making images of the stream in the lumen of the carotid arteries
   c. Making an image of the walls and linings of the carotid arteries
   d. Listening for changes in the Doppler flow sound
   e. Determining cross sections and lumen size at a stenosis

CHAPTER 22 Pulsed-Doppler Ultrasonic Arteriography

1. Pulsed Doppler as used for ultrasonic arteriography:
   a. Visualizes the arterial lumen of carotid arteries when obstructed/unobstructed/both
   b. Is most effective for plaques that narrow the lumen of the internal carotid artery at least $10\%/\geq 40\%/\geq 70\%$
   c. Examines flow in small regions of the lumen/the entire lumen/both
   d. Is used also for spectral analysis in the common carotid artery/internal carotid artery/external carotid artery region of suspected stenosis

2. Spectral analysis with the pulsed Doppler (true/false/other):
   a. Can and should sample the spectra from: 1) the central flow-ing stream, 2) the entire lumen, 3) zones with the highest frequencies, 4) zones of suspected stenosis
   b. Shows more pronounced "windows" than continuous-wave Dopplers
   c. Shows the same spectral pictures as continuous-wave Dopplers
3. Spectral patterns for minor stenoses (true/false/other):
   a. Are more sensitive indicators of stenosis than the image
   b. May even reveal audible changes
   c. Show frequencies that are subnormal/normal/near nor-mal/increased
   d. Show disturbed spectral pattern and spectral broadening during systole/diastole/both
   e. Are not as sensitive or specific for minor stenoses as the ≥ 40% level

CHAPTER 23   Real-Time B-Mode Ultrasonic Carotid Imaging with Gated Doppler

1. Limitations of B-mode imaging of carotid arteries include (true/false/other):
   a. Depth of penetration in fat or muscular necks
   b. Inadequate resolution of 3-MHz imaging units used for ab-dominal or heart studies
   c. Dangers of overheating or damaging the arteries
   d. Artifacts from adjacent vein walls
   e. The need for a supplementary Doppler probe to detect the image/Doppler shift/motion of the blood
   f. The need for high-frequency ultrasound transducers for (true/false) 1) better penetration, 2) better resolution of fine detail
   g. Difficulty in defining residual lumen > 2.5 mm/< 2.5 mm
2. B-mode ultrasonic imaging is more revealing than arteriography in demonstrating (true/false):
   a. Occluded common carotid arteries
   b. Plaques in the carotid bulb
   c. Abnormal motion
   d. Composition of plaque or stenosis
3. The authors propose the combination of B-mode ultrasonic imaging with OPG/CPA because (true/false):

a. B-mode is effective in detecting mild plaques and OPG/CPA is accurate for severe stenosis
b. OPG/CPA gives anatomic information that supplements the functional hemodynamic information from the scan
c. OPG is more effective for patients with TIAs
d. CPA has detected murmurs and plaques that in some cases were missed by ultrasonic imaging

CHAPTER 24 The Predictive Value of Cerebrovascular Studies

1. Predictive value of a positive test is (true/false):
    a. One of the useful calculations of accuracy
    b. The number of true positive tests divided by the sum of all positive tests, expressed as a percentage
    c. The percentage of correct predictions, i.e., the total number of true positives divided by the sum of the true positive and false negative tests
2. The indirect, hemodynamic cerebrovascular tests, including OPG/CPA (K/M), supraorbital directional Doppler, supraorbital PPG, and compression tests of the external carotid collateral circulation (true/false):
    a. Are very accurate for severe stenoses that reduce internal carotid pressure or flow
    b. Are very accurate for the diagnosis of moderate stenoses
    c. Are very accurate for the diagnosis of normal carotids
3. The Bayes theorem permits calculation of (true/false):
    a. Accuracy
    b. Sensitivity
    c. Specificity
    d. Likelihood of disease

CHAPTER 25   Preoperative Screening for Asymptomatic Carotid Obstruction

1. Asymptomatic carotid obstructions are usually discovered by (true/false):
    a. Audible murmurs
    b. Carotid arteriograms
    c. Noninvasive techniques

2. Patients with "hemodynamically significant" carotid stenosis are at increased risk for (true/false):
   a. Symptomatic arteriosclerosis elsewhere
   b. Stroke during or after coronary artery bypass or peripheral vascular reconstructions
   c. Death during or after coronary artery bypass or peripheral vascular reconstructions
   d. TIAs
   e. Hypertension

Part IV:

ASSOCIATED TECHNOLOGICAL CONSIDERATIONS

CHAPTER 26   **Progress in Doppler Instrumentation**

1. The Doppler effect (true/false):
   a. Is caused by a series of waves striking a moving object
   b. Is a shift in: 1) frequency of the waves, 2) intensity, 3) wavelength, 4) pitch
   c. Is proportional to the velocity of the moving objects
   d. Gives: 1) larger shifts with acute angles of the ultrasonic Doppler probe, 2) higher frequencies
   e. Can detect the direction of flow toward or away from the probe
2. Penetration of sound through tissue is (true/false):
   a. Deeper with high-frequency beams
   b. Deeper with low-frequency beams
   c. So important that the best instruments have the deepest penetration
   d. Independent of beam width
   e. Is productive of larger frequency shifts with deeper penetration

CHAPTER 27   **Microcomputer Applications in the Blood Flow Laboratory**

No questions

ANSWERS

PART I:

NONINVASIVE DIAGNOSIS OF
ARTERIAL OCCLUSIVE DISEASE

Chapter 1

Pathophysiology of Arterial
Occlusive Disease

1. a. True
    b. True
    c. True }only for severe stenosis
    d. True
2. a. False
    b. True
    c. False
    d. False
    e. True
    f. True
3. a. True only during exercise
    b. TIAs are critical for the patient
       but are not always accompanied
       by arterial stenosis (see Chapter
       15)
    c. True
    d. True
4. a. True
    b. False
    c. True
    d. True
5. a. True, except for severe multiple
       arterial stenosis or occlusion
    b. True
    c. False
    d. True
    e. True
    f. True
6. a. True
    b. True
    c. False

Chapter 2

Segmental Limb Pressures, Doppler Waveforms, and Stress Testing

1. a. False
    b. True
    c. True
2. a. False
    b. True
    c. Highest
    d. High
3. a. True
    b. False
    c. True
    d. False
    e. True
    f. False, because intermittent
       claudicants may have normal
       resting pressures that are reduc-
       ed only with exercise
4. a. True
    b. False; similar but not identical
    c. True
    d. False
    e. True
5. a. All three are correct
    b. True
    c. Less likely
    d. True

Chapter 3

Digital Plethysmography and
Pressure Measurements

1. a. Volume primarily; the changes
       in volume secondarily reflect
       the arrival of pulses or flow
2. a. True

b. True
c. True
3. a. True
   b. True
   c. True
   d. True
   e. False; this is correct only for Doppler velocity tracings
4. a. False; Raynaud's disease is due solely to digital arterial spasm, not occlusion
   b. True
   c. True
5. a. Decrease
   b. Decrease
   c. True
6. a. Less than
   b. Better
   c. True
   d. False

Chapter 4

Postoperative Noninvasive Evaluation of Femorotibial Bypass Grafts

1. a. True
   b. True
   c. True
   d. False; this disease as observed in the renal or carotid arteries is not yet reported in vein grafts
2. a. True
   b. True
   c. True
   d. False; because some patients' walking was limited by cardiac or pulmonary disease
3. a. True
   b. True
   c. False
   d. True
   e. False; such a decrease signifies the need for arteriography

Chapter 5

New Techniques to Assess Aortoiliac Stenosis

1. a. True
   b. True
   c. False; nocturnal tumescence is absent in vasculogenic impotence
   d. True
   e. True
2. a. True
   b. True
   c. True
   d. False; it is an invasive test
   e. False; it is an invasive test

Chapter 6

Segmental Volume Pulse Recorder: Improved Anatomic Discrimination by Refinement in Technique

1. a. True
   b. True
   c. True
   d. True
   e. True

Chapter 7

Intravenous Digital Angiography in the Assessment of Arterial Disease

No questions

Chapter 8

Observations on Vasculogenic Impotence

1. a. True
   b. True
   c. True
   d. True
   e. False; venous outflow is temporarily blocked

2. a. True
   b. True
   c. True, but may be 60%–70% of brachial pressure, and often equals mean systemic pressure
   d. False; some patients with penile brachial indices ≤ 0.6 have satisfactory erections

PART II:

NONINVASIVE DIAGNOSIS OF VENOUS DISEASE
Chapter 9

Venous Anatomy and Pathophysiology

1. a. Subcutaneously
   b. 2) Enters the deep veins via perforating and communicating veins
2. a. True
   b. False; when the calf muscles relax, a potential space is created in the deep veins and blood is "sucked" from the superficial veins into the deep veins via the perforating veins
   c. True
   d. True
   e. True
3. a. False
   b. True
   c. True
   d. False

Chapter 10

The Diagnosis and Assessment of Venous Disorders in the Office and Laboratory

1. a. True
   b. True

   c. True
   d. False
2. a. Medial
   b. True
   c. Optional and unnecessary
   d. True
   e. True, so as to accomplish (d)
   f. True, so as to increase reflux and make it more audible when present
3. a. Abnormal
   b. Iliac
   c. True, only if venous sounds at the groin are also phasic (signifying recanalization
   d. True
   e. True

Chapter 11

Doppler Diagnosis of Deep Venous Thrombosis

1. a. False; deep penetration is required, but the usual arterial or cerebrovascular Dopplers are 9–10 MHz and better penetration is obtained with the 4–5 MHz instruments
   b. True
2. a. True; especially if the legs are cool
   b. False; normal venous sounds cease during inspiration
   c. True
   d. True; because competent valves present reflux
   e. True
   f. False
3. a. False
   b. True
   c. False; saphenous phlebitis is superficial and usually is easily detectable without Doppler examination, although in the absence of varicosities it may be difficult to distinguish from lymphangitis

Chapter 12

Phleborheography in the Diagnosis of Deep Venous Thrombosis

1. a. True; also true for the ilio-femoral and popliteal veins
   b. True
   c. True
   d. True
2. a. True
   b. True; there are many causes of pain, redness, and swelling of the leg
   c. True; mild cases can be easily missed by physical examination
3. a. True
   b. True
   c. False; because phleborheography cannot distinguish between extrinsic compression and intraluminal clots
   d. False; because persistent venous obstructions cannot be distinguished from new acute obstructions

Chapter 13

Venous Plethysmography

1. a. True
   b. True
   c. True
   d. True
   e. True
2. (c) and (e)
3. a. True
   b. True
   c. True
   d. Usually false, depending on the degree of partial obstructions
   e. True
   f. False
4. a. True
   b. True

   c. True
   d. False
   e. True
5. a. True
   b. True
   c. False; the venous tourniquet both by physical examination and when used as part of the venous plethysmographic examination may signify the level at which reflux occurs, but does not pinpoint the site
   d. True

Chapter 14

Photoplethysmography in the Evaluation of Chronic Venous Insufficiency

1. a. True
   b. True
   c. 1) Irrelevant for the diagnosis of chronic venous insufficiency; 2) same as (1)—the exam is performed with the patient seated, legs dependent and non–weight bearing; 3) true, when the venous tourniquet stops reflux via incompetent superficial veins; 4) true—the main purpose of the examination
2. a. True
   b. True
   c. True
   d. True
   e. True, only if the saphenous or other superficial veins are the sole source of reflux
   f. True

PART III:

NONINVASIVE DIAGNOSIS OF CAROTID OCCLUSIVE DISEASE

Chapter 15

The Anatomy and Pathophysiology of Atherosclerotic Extracranial Cerebrovascular Disease

1. a. True
    b. False
    c. True
    d. True; but there is only one
    e. True
2. a. True
    b. True, for the subclavian steal
    c. True, for severe carotid stenosis, via the orbit of the eye
3. (a), (b), (d), (c)
4. a. Less than 24 hours
    b. False; but they are precursors of strokes
    c. Usually; but not always from the carotid bifurcation
    d. False
5. a. True
    b. False
    c. False
    d. True
    e. False

Chapter 16

Comprehensive Noninvasive Evaluation of Extracranial Cerebrovascular Disease

1. a. True; murmurs do not affect treatment, but signify the need to investigate their cause
    b. True
    c. True
    d. True

2. a. True; see Chapter 19
    b. True
    c. True
    d. True
3. a. True
    b. True
    c. True
4. a. False; this is true for the external carotid or peripheral arteries
    b. True
    c. True
5. a. True
    b. False
    c. True
    d. True
    e. True
    f. True
    g. True

Chapter 17

K/M Oculoplethysmography and Carotid Phonoangiography

1. a. False; no Doppler is needed
    b. True
    c. True
    d. False; only from the internal
2. a. True
    b. True
    c. False; correct for the OPG-Gee
    d. True
    e. False; cups are held in place with mild suction of 40–60 mmHg
    f. True

Chapter 18

Periorbital Diagnostic Techniques

1. a. False; only the frontal and supraorbital arteries
    b. True
    c. Increase; augmentation
    d. False; frequently but not always

2. a. False (never); only low in the neck
    b. True
    c. True, but only on the same side as the carotid compression
    d. True, when it is a collateral source
3. a. True
    b. False; middle meningeal is not accessible for compression
    c. True
    d. True
4. True
5. First
6. False for $\geq$ 50% stenosis; True for $\geq$ 70% stenosis

Chapter 19

Direct Doppler Auscultation of the Carotid Arteries

1. a. False
    b. True
    c. True; see Chapter 16
    d. True
    e. True; see Chapter 16
2. a. False; it requires only the usual directional continuous-wave Doppler detectors
    b. True; for some B-mode scanners
    c. True; for imaging devices that print images of the flowing streams
    d. True; plus some compensatory changes in the common and external carotid artery
3. a. True
    b. True
    c. False; or you may extinguish the flow and cause false-positive signals

Chapter 20

Early Detection of Stroke-Related Lesions by Real-Time Doppler Spectral Analysis

1. a. True
    b. False; excludes the venous sounds as they flow toward the probe
    c. True
    d. True
2. a. True
    b. False; it would have to be narrowed very much
    c. True
3. a. Normal
    b. Systolic
    c. True
4. a. Increased
    b. True
    c. True; occurs only in the external carotid artery and only with severe stenosis of the internal carotid artery
    d. Blunter
    e. True

Chapter 21

Three-Dimensional Ultrasonic Arteriography

1. a. True
    b. True
    c. False; true for the B-mode scanners
    d. True
    e. True

Chapter 22

Pulsed-Doppler Ultrasonic Arteriography

1. a. Unobstructed
    b. $\geq$ 40%
    c. Both; small regions are sampled and "dots" stored on the oscilloscope to build the flow map image of the entire lumen
    d. Internal carotid artery and any regions of suspected stenosis
2. a. 1), 3), 4); suspect severe stenosis when peak frequencies

are unusually high
  b. True
  c. False
3. a. True
  b. True
  c. Normal or near normal
  d. Systole
  e. True; sensitivity for $\geq 90\%$
    stenosis is 97%.

Chapter 23

Real-Time B-Mode Ultrasonic Carotid Imaging with Gated Doppler

1. a. True
  b. True
  c. False; but avoid prolonged use around the eye
  d. True
  e. True
  f. 1) False, 2) true
  g. <2.5 mm; however, these are readily diagnosed by the OPG, which is also performed
2. a. True; for severe cases with patent internal carotid artery not visualized by arteriography
  b. True; ultrasonic carotid imaging shows plaques which thicken the wall but which do not necessarily narrow the lumen
  c. True; motion of the wall of the artery or of flaps or plaque within the carotid lumen
  d. True; reveals calcium in plaque, hemorrhage beneath plaque
3. a. True
  b. False; the opposite is correct
  c. False; ultrasonic imaging is more effective in revealing the ulcerations that are a common cause of TIAs
  d. True

Chapter 24

The Predictive Value of Cerebrovascular Studies

1. a. True
  b. True
  c. True
2. a. True
  b. False   (see Figure 24-1)
  c. True
3. a. False
  b. False
  c. False
  d. True

Chapter 25

Preoperative Screening for Asymptomatic Carotid Obstruction

1. a. True
  b. True; discover asymptomatic obstructions on the side opposite from the sypmptomatic or suspected side
  c. True (same answer as [b])
2. a. True
  b. False; not according to this study
  c. True
  d. True
  e. False; not proven

PART IV:

ASSOCIATED TECHNOLOGICAL CONSIDERATIONS

Chapter 26

Progress in Doppler Instrumentation

1. a. True
  b. 1) True, 2) false, 3) false 4) true
  c. True
  d. 1) True, 2) false
  e. True

2. **a.** False
   b. True
   c. False; one must compromise for the best frequency resolution compatible with sufficient penetration for the intended use
   d. False
   e. False

Chapter 27

Microcomputer Applications in the Blood Flow Laboratory

No questions

INDEX

Index

pulsed Doppler, 262–263
pulse–echo (B-mode) imaging, 184, 187, 190–194
Ultrasound, Doppler (*see* Doppler ultrasound)

Vagus nerve, 161
Valsalva maneuver, 105, 122
Valve incompetence, 97–101, 103–115, 143–147, 153–154
Valves, venous, 89–90, 97–101
Varicosities (*see* Veins, varicose)
Vascular resistance (*see* Resistance)
Vasodilating drugs, 14–15
Vein grafts (*see* Grafts)
Vein stripping, superficial, 155
Veins (*see also* Venous system; specific names)
  communicating, 89–90
  deep, 88–90, 97–101
  perforating, 89–90, 97–101
  superficial, 88–90, 97–101
  tree–barking (defined), 135
  varicose, 97–101, 104, 106–107, 146, 149, 155
Velocity: of blood, 3–5
Vena cava: and Doppler examination, 124
Venography (*see also* Phlebography), 103, 114–115
Venous capacitance
  defined, 110
  in venous thrombosis, 111–112
Venous disorders (*see also* specific disorders and techniques)
  Doppler diagnosis, 117–124
  insufficiency, 105–109
  and phleborheography, 126–137
  techniques of diagnosis, 103–115
  thrombosis, 110–115, 117–124
Venous Doppler examination (*see* Doppler examination, venous)
Venous insufficiency, 99–100
  defined, 105
  diagnosis, 103–115
  differentiating between deep and superficial, 103–115
  limitations of Doppler examination, 149
  and photoplethysmography, 104, 107
  sites of clinical importance, 105
Venous insufficiency, chronic, 149–155
  and photoplethysmography, 149–155
  scope of the problem, 149
  and venous reflux plethysmography, 143–147

and venous volume plethysmography (*see also* Phleborheography), 142-143
Venous outflow
  and compression maneuvers, 128
  defined, 111
  plethysmographic examination, 139–141
  and rhythmic compression, 128
  in venous thrombosis, 111–112
Venous system
  anatomy, 88–102
  causes of extrinsic compression, 124
  collateral circulation, 103, 110
  diagnosis, 103–115
  dynamics, 95–101
  edema formation, 94–95
  effect of exercise, 97–101
  hydrostatics, 91–92
  incompetence, 97–101
  muscle pump mechanism, 89, 92, 94, 97–101
  pathophysiology, 88–102
  physiology, 90–101
  pressure–volume relationships, 92–94
  resistance, 90–91
  valves, 89–90, 97–101
  volume measurements, 141–143
Vertebral arteries, 158–162, 164–165, 167–168, 173–174
Vertebral "steal," 158
Vertebrobasilar system
  anatomy, 164
  insufficiency, 160, 170–173
Vertigo, 173
Viscosity: of blood, 2–5
Volume pulse recorder, 68
Volume pulse recordings
  in aortoiliac disease, 63–65
  compared to arteriography, 63
  predictive values, 63
  results, 63
  sensitivity, 63
  specificity, 63
  technique, 61

Waveform
  in digital plethysmography, 26–41
  Doppler, 17–19, 21–22
Wavelength (defined), 282

Xenon (^{133}Xe) clearance method of measuring blood flow, 10, 23

Zero–crossing detectors, 185–186

371